T0259089

Ambulatory Anesthesiology

Editors

JEFFREY L. APFELBAUM
THOMAS W. CUTTER

ANESTHESIOLOGY CLINICS

www.anesthesiology.theclinics.com

Consulting Editor
LEE A. FLEISHER

June 2014 • Volume 32 • Number 2

ELSEVIER

1600 John F. Kennedy Boulevard • Suite 1800 • Philadelphia, Pennsylvania, 19103-2899

http://www.theclinics.com

ANESTHESIOLOGY CLINICS Volume 32, Number 2
June 2014 ISSN 1932-2275, ISBN-13: 978-0-323-29916-9

Editor: Jennifer Flynn-Briggs
Developmental Editor: Susan Showalter

Anesthesiology Clinics (ISSN 1932-2275) is published quarterly by Elsevier Inc., 360 Park Avenue South, New York, NY 10010-1710. Months of issue are March, June, September, and December. Periodicals postage paid at New York, NY and at additional mailing offices. Subscription prices are $160.00 per year (US student/resident), $330.00 per year (US individuals), $400.00 per year (Canadian individuals), $533.00 per year (US institutions), $674.00 per year (Canadian institutions), $225.00 per year (Canadian and foreign student/resident), $455.00 per year (foreign individuals), and $674.00 per year (foreign institutions). To receive student and resident rate, orders must be accompanied by name of affiliated institution, date of term, and the *signature* of program/residency coordinator on institutions letterhead. Orders will be billed at individual rate until proof of status is received. Foreign air speed delivery is included in all *Clinics'* subscription prices. All prices are subject to change without notice. POSTMASTER: Send address changes to *Anesthesiology Clinics,* Elsevier Health Sciences Division, Subscription Customer Service, 3251 Riverport Lane, Maryland Heights, MO 63043. Customer Service (orders, claims, online, change of address): Elsevier Health Sciences Division, Subscription Customer Service, 3251 Riverport Lane, Maryland Heights, MO 63043. Tel: 1-800-654-2452 (U.S. and Canada); 314-447-8871 (outside U.S. and Canada). Fax: 314-447-8029. E-mail: journalscustomerservice-usa@elsevier.com (for print support); journalsonlinesupport-usa@elsevier.com (for online support).

Reprints. For copies of 100 or more of articles in this publication, please contact the Commercial Reprints Department, Elsevier Inc., 360 Park Avenue South, New York, NY 10010-1710. Tel.: 212-633-3874; Fax: 212-633-3820; E-mail: reprints@elsevier.com.

Anesthesiology Clinics, is also published in Spanish by McGraw-Hill Inter-americana Editores S. A., P.O. Box 5-237, 06500 Mexico D. F., Mexico.

Anesthesiology Clinics, is covered in *MEDLINE/PubMed (Index Medicus), Current Contents/Clinical Medicine, Excerpta Medica, ISI/BIOMED*, and *Chemical Abstracts*.

Contributors

CONSULTING EDITOR

LEE A. FLEISHER, MD, FACC, FAHA
Robert D. Dripps Professor and Chair of Anesthesiology and Critical Care; Professor of Medicine; Perelman School of Medicine, University of Pennsylvania, Philadelphia, Pennsylvania

EDITORS

JEFFREY L. APFELBAUM, MD
Professor and Chairman, Department of Anesthesia and Critical Care, Pritzker School of Medicine, University of Chicago, Chicago, Illinois

THOMAS W. CUTTER, MD, MAEd
Professor, Associate Chairman, Department of Anesthesia and Critical Care, Pritzker School of Medicine, University of Chicago, Chicago, Illinois

AUTHORS

HAIRIL RIZAL ABDULLAH, MBBS, MMed
Associate Consultant, Department of Anesthesiology, Singapore General Hospital, Singapore

ELIZABETH A. ALLEY, MD
Department of Anesthesia, Virginia Mason Medical Center, Seattle, Washington

JENNIFER ANDERSON, MD
Assistant Professor, Department of Anesthesia and Critical Care, University of Chicago, Chicago, Illinois

MAGDALENA ANITESCU, MD, PhD
Associate Professor; Director, Pain Management Fellowship Program, Department of Anesthesia and Critical Care, University of Chicago Medical Center, Chicago, Illinois

DAVID A. AUGUST, MD, PhD
Instructor, Harvard Medical School, Boston, Massachusetts

SUHABE BUGRARA, BSc
Computer Science Department, Stanford University, Stanford, California

FRANCES CHUNG, MBBS, FRCPC
Professor, Department of Anesthesiology, Toronto Western Hospital, University Health Network, University of Toronto, Toronto, Ontario, Canada

DAVID M. DICKERSON, MD
Assistant Professor, Department of Anesthesia and Critical Care, University of Chicago Medicine, Chicago, Illinois

RICHARD P. DUTTON, MD, MBA
Executive Director, Anesthesia Quality Institute, Park Ridge; Chief Quality Officer, American Society of Anesthesiologists; Clinical Associate, Department of Anesthesia and Critical Care, University of Chicago, Chicago, Illinois

LUCINDA L. EVERETT, MD
Associate Professor, Harvard Medical School, Boston, Massachusetts

TONG J. GAN, MD, MHS, FRCA, MB, FFARCSI
Professor, Department of Anesthesiology, Duke University Medical Center, Durham, North Carolina

ORI GOTTLIEB, MD
Assistant Professor, Department of Anesthesia and Critical Care, University of Chicago, Chicago, Illinois

SAMIR R. JANI, MD, MPH
Resident in Anesthesia, Beth Israel Deaconess Medical Center, Boston, Massachusetts

RAYMOND S. JOSEPH, MD
Staff Anesthesiologist, Department of Anesthesiology, Virginia Mason Medical Center, Seattle, Washington

BASSAM KADRY, MD
Clinical Instructor, Department of Anesthesiology, Perioperative and Pain Medicine, Stanford University School of Medicine, Stanford, California

STEPHEN M. KLEIN, MD
Associate Professor, Department of Anesthesiology, Duke University Medical Center, Durham, North Carolina

P. ALLAN KLOCK Jr, MD
Professor; Vice-Chairman for Clinical Affairs, Department of Anesthesia and Critical Care, University of Chicago, Chicago, Illinois

XIAOXIA LIU, MS
Statistician, Brigham and Women's Hospital, Boston, Massachusetts

ALEX MACARIO, MD, MBA
Professor, Department of Anesthesiology, Perioperative and Pain Medicine, Stanford University School of Medicine, Stanford, California

WALTER MAURER, MD
Head, Department of General Anesthesia, Anesthesiology Institute, Cleveland Clinic, Cleveland, Ohio

M. STEPHEN MELTON, MD
Assistant Professor, Department of Anesthesiology, Duke University Medical Center, Durham, North Carolina

DOUGLAS G. MERRILL, MD, MBA
Professor of Anesthesiology; Geisel School of Medicine; Director, Center for Perioperative Services, Dartmouth-Hitchcock Medical Center, Dartmouth, Grantham, New Hampshire

MICHAEL F. MULORY, MD
Department of Anesthesia, Virginia Mason Medical Center, Seattle, Washington

KAREN C. NIELSEN, MD
Associate Professor, Department of Anesthesiology, Duke University Medical Center, Durham, North Carolina

JOEL PASH, DO, BCom, FRCPC
Clinical Instructor, Department of Anesthesiology, Perioperative and Pain Medicine, Stanford University School of Medicine, Stanford, California; Clinical Assistant Professor, Department of Anesthesia, University of Calgary, Calgary, Alberta, Canada

BEVERLY K. PHILIP, MD
Professor of Anaesthesia; Departments of Anesthesiology, Perioperative and Pain Medicine, Brigham and Women's Hospital, Harvard Medical School, Boston, Massachusetts

RAVIRAJ RAVEENDRAN, MBBS, MD
Clinical Fellow, Department of Anesthesiology, Toronto Western Hospital, University Health Network, University of Toronto, Toronto, Ontario, Canada

J. DEVIN ROBERTS, MD
Assistant Professor, Department of Anesthesia and Critical Care, University of Chicago, Chicago, Illinois

DANIEL RUBIN, MD
Assistant Professor, Department of Anesthesia and Critical Care, University of Chicago, Chicago, Illinois

FRANCIS V. SALINAS, MD
Staff Anesthesiologist, Department of Anesthesiology, Virginia Mason Medical Center, Seattle, Washington

JUDITH JURIN SEMO, JD
PLLC, Washington, DC

FRED E. SHAPIRO, DO
Assistant Professor of Anesthesia, Beth Israel Deaconess Medical Center, Boston, Massachusetts

BOBBIEJEAN SWEITZER, MD
Professor, Anesthesia and Critical Care; Director, Anesthesia Perioperative Medicine Clinic; Professor of Medicine, University of Chicago, Chicago, Illinois

JOHN E. TETZLAFF, MD
Professor of Anesthesiology, Cleveland Clinic Lerner College of Medicine of Case Western Reserve University, Cleveland, Ohio

MARCY TUCKER, MD, PhD
Assistant Professor, Department of Anesthesiology, Duke University Medical Center, Durham, North Carolina

RICHARD D. URMAN, MD, MBA
Assistant Professor of Anaesthesia; Departments of Anesthesiology, Perioperative and Pain Medicine, Brigham and Women's Hospital, Harvard Medical School, Boston, Massachusetts

MARY ANN VANN, MD
Assistant Professor of Anesthesia, Harvard Medical School; Department of Anesthesia, Critical Care and Pain Medicine, Beth Israel Deaconess Medical Center, Boston, Massachusetts

JOHN J. VARGO, MD, MPH
Professor of Medicine, Cleveland Clinic Lerner College of Medicine of Case Western Reserve University, Cleveland, Ohio

Contents

Foreword: Ambulatory Anesthesia   xv

Lee A. Fleisher

Preface: The Four Ps: Place, Procedure, Personnel, and Patient   xvii

Jeffrey L. Apfelbaum and Thomas W. Cutter

Perioperative Management of Co-Morbidities

Perioperative Evaluation and Management of Cardiac Disease in the Ambulatory
Surgery Setting   309

J. Devin Roberts and BobbieJean Sweitzer

> Preoperative cardiac evaluation focuses on risk assessment and reduc-
> tion. Diagnostic testing and interventions are used only when the risk of
> adverse outcomes is high and intervention will lower the risk. The evalua-
> tion is performed in a stepwise fashion according to guidelines in the
> literature.

Perioperative Consideration of Obstructive Sleep Apnea in Ambulatory Surgery   321

Raviraj Raveendran and Frances Chung

> The prevalence of obstructive sleep apnea (OSA) is increasing and a signif-
> icant number of patients with OSA are undiagnosed. The suitability of
> ambulatory surgery in patients with OSA remains controversial, and the
> evidence regarding the safety of ambulatory surgery for patients with
> OSA is limited. Preoperative screening and careful selection of patients
> for ambulatory surgery is the most important step. Patients diagnosed
> and suspected of having OSA should be managed with a systematic algo-
> rithm to improve outcomes.

Management of Diabetes Medications for Patients Undergoing Ambulatory Surgery   329

Mary Ann Vann

> A stress-free actively managed perioperative experience is crucial to suc-
> cessful ambulatory surgery for diabetes patients. Practitioners who inte-
> grate diabetes treatment regimens into their perioperative management
> can facilitate a good outcome, smooth recovery, and rapid return to nor-
> mal life. Hypoglycemia, hyperglycemia, and glucose variability must be
> avoided and patients should be maintained near their usual blood glucose.

Regional Anesthesia

Peripheral Nerve Blocks for Ambulatory Surgery   341

Francis V. Salinas and Raymond S. Joseph

> Peripheral nerve blocks (PNBs) provide significant improvement in postop-
> erative analgesia and quality of recovery for ambulatory surgery. Use of

continuous PNB techniques extend these benefits beyond the limited duration of single-injection PNBs. The use of ultrasound guidance has significantly improved the overall success, efficiency, and has contributed to the
increased use of PNBs in the ambulatory setting. More recently, the use of
ultrasound guidance has been demonstrated to decrease the risk of local
anesthetic systemic toxicity. This article provides a broad overview of the
indications and clinically useful aspects of the most commonly used upper
and lower extremity PNBs in the ambulatory setting. Emphasis is placed
on approaches that can be used for single-injection PNBs and continuous
PNB techniques.

Neuraxial Anesthesia for Outpatients   357

Elizabeth A. Alley and Michael F. Mulory

Neuraxial anesthesia for outpatient surgery can provide excellent anesthesia for certain patients. The short-acting local anesthetic 2-chloroprocaine
has an appropriate length of action for short outpatient procedures with
a very low risk of transient neurologic symptoms. Epidural anesthesia
with short-acting agents can provide good outpatient anesthesia for
procedures lasting 90 minutes or longer.

Anesthesia for Procedures

Anesthesia for Ambulatory Diagnostic and Therapeutic Radiology Procedures   371

Daniel Rubin

The radiology suite presents the anesthesia provider with a unique set of
challenges such as ionizing radiation, intravascular contrast, magnetic
fields, physical separation and barriers from the patient, so-called borrowed space, and the large range of procedures performed. Most of these
procedures will continue to be performed without the presence of an
anesthesia team but, because of the ever-increasing complexity of the
procedures being performed and the increasing comorbidities of patients,
the anesthesia provider will likely be called more often to provide care. A
thorough understanding of these challenges is essential to providing
a safe anesthetic in a difficult environment.

**Ambulatory Anesthesia for the Cardiac Catheterization and Electrophysiology
Laboratories**   381

J. Devin Roberts

The cardiac catheterization laboratory (CCL) and electrophysiology laboratory (EPL) environments present unique clinical challenges. These challenges include unfamiliar work areas and staff, limited space with physical
barriers separating the patient from the care provider, remote locations,
and procedures with rare but potentially catastrophic clinical complications. Ambulatory anesthesiologists must familiarize themselves with
these new surroundings and practice vigilant preoperative planning and
continual communication with the proceduralist and team. In the future,
the need for anesthesiologists in the CCL and EPL will continue to grow
as procedures increase in complexity and duration.

Nonoperating Room Anesthesia for the Gastrointestinal Endoscopy Suite   387

John E. Tetzlaff, John J. Vargo, and Walter Maurer

Anesthesia services are increasingly being requested for gastrointestinal (GI) endoscopy procedures. The preparation of the patients is different from the traditional operating room practice. The responsibility to optimize comorbid conditions is also unclear. The anesthetic techniques are unique to the procedures, as are the likely events that require intervention by the anesthesia team. The postprocedure care is also unique. The future needs for anesthesia services in GI endoscopy suite are likely to expand with further developments of the technology.

Chronic Pain: Anesthesia for Procedures   395

Magdalena Anitescu

Chronic pain is a symptom that patients fear significantly. To treat and alleviate pain, physicians perform various interventions for which patients often need to be immobile for long periods of time. To improve patient satisfaction and relief anxiety of those complex procedures, pain physicians use various anesthetic techniques for their pain-relieving procedures that range from local skin infiltration to general anesthesia with endotracheal intubation. This article describes the anesthetic techniques used in interventional pain procedures and their indications, side effects, and complications.

Pediatric Ambulatory Anesthesia   411

David A. August and Lucinda L. Everett

Pediatric patients often undergo anesthesia for ambulatory procedures. This article discusses several common preoperative dilemmas, including whether to postpone anesthesia when a child has an upper respiratory infection, whether to test young women for pregnancy, which children require overnight admission for apnea monitoring, and the effectiveness of nonpharmacological techniques for reducing anxiety. Medication issues covered include the risks of anesthetic agents in children with undiagnosed weakness, the use of remifentanil for tracheal intubation, and perioperative dosing of rectal acetaminophen. The relative merits of caudal and dorsal penile nerve block for pain after circumcision are also discussed.

Initial Results from the National Anesthesia Clinical Outcomes Registry and Overview of Office-Based Anesthesia   431

Fred E. Shapiro, Samir R. Jani, Xiaoxia Liu, Richard P. Dutton, and Richard D. Urman

Safe office-based anesthesia practices dictate proper patient and procedure selection, appropriate provider qualifications, adequately equipped facilities, and effective administrative infrastructure. Analysis of patient outcomes can help reduce mortality and morbidity by identifying high-risk patients and procedures. We analyzed data from the Anesthesia Quality Institute National Anesthesia Clinical Outcomes Registry. Analysis included patient demographics and outcomes, procedure and anesthesia type and duration, and case coverage by provider. Increased regulation and standardization of care, such as the use of checklists and professional guidelines, can advance safe practices. There is increasing emphasis on continuous quality improvement, electronic health records, and outcomes data reporting.

Airway Management   445

Jennifer Anderson and P. Allan Klock Jr

In this article, recent literature related to airway management in the ambulatory surgery setting is reviewed. Practical pointers to improve clinical success and avoid complications of newer airway management techniques are provided.

New Medications and Techniques in Ambulatory Anesthesia   463

M. Stephen Melton, Karen C. Nielsen, Marcy Tucker, Stephen M. Klein, and Tong J. Gan

Novel anesthetic and analgesic agents are currently under development or investigation to improve anesthetic delivery and patient care. The pharmacokinetic and analgesic profiles of these agents are especially tailored to meet the challenges of rapid recovery and opioid minimization associated with ambulatory anesthesia practice.

Postop Issues/Care/Discharge

Postoperative Issues: Discharge Criteria   487

Hairil Rizal Abdullah and Frances Chung

With the continuous increase in the numbers and complexity of cases being done as ambulatory procedures, striking a balance between operational efficiency, patient safety, and patient satisfaction has become increasingly difficult. This article summarizes the latest evidence and consensus with regard to discharging an ambulatory patient home, the use of patient recovery scoring systems for protocol-based decision making, the concept of fast-track recovery, and requirements for patient escort. Fast-tracking (ie, bypassing the postanesthesia care unit) is an acceptable and safe pathway, provided careful patient selection and assessment are performed.

Acute Pain Management   495

David M. Dickerson

This article updates acute pain management in ambulatory surgery and proposes a practical three-step approach for reducing the impact and incidence of uncontrolled surgical pain. By identifying at-risk patients, implementing multimodal analgesia, and intervening promptly with rescue therapies, the anesthesiologist may improve outcomes, reduce cost, and optimize the patient's experience and quality of recovery.

Long-Acting Serotonin Antagonist (Palonosetron) and the NK-1 Receptor Antagonists: Does Extended Duration of Action Improve Efficacy?   505

M. Stephen Melton, Karen C. Nielsen, Marcy Tucker, Stephen M. Klein, and Tong J. Gan

In a growing outpatient surgical population, postdischarge nausea and vomiting (PDNV) is unfortunately a common and costly anesthetic complication. Identification of risk factors for both postoperative nausea and vomiting and PDNV is the hallmark of prevention and management. New pharmacologic interventions with extended duration of action, including palonosetron and aprepritant, may prove to be more efficacious.

Administrative Issues

Scheduling of Procedures and Staff in an Ambulatory Surgery Center   517

Joel Pash, Bassam Kadry, Suhabe Bugrara, and Alex Macario

For ambulatory surgical centers (ASC) to succeed financially, it is critical for ASC managers to schedule surgical procedures in a manner that optimizes operating room (OR) efficiency. OR efficiency is maximized by using historical data to accurately predict future OR workload, thereby enabling OR time to be properly allocated to surgeons. Other strategies to maintain a well-functioning ASC include recruiting and retaining the right staff and ensuring patients and surgeons are satisfied with their experience. This article reviews different types of procedure scheduling systems. Characteristics of well-functioning ASCs are also discussed.

Practice Management/Role of the Medical Director   529

Douglas G. Merrill

Although the nature of ambulatory surgery has changed over the years, the ideal role of the medical director mirrors its earliest iterations, focusing on excellent customer service and high quality of care. These efforts are supported by 3 modern methods of quality management borrowed from industry: intentional process improvement, standard care pathways, and monitoring outcomes to determine the efficacy of each. These methods are critical to master in order to lead the facility and providers to the highest quality of care and service.

Legal Aspects of Ambulatory Anesthesia   541

Judith Jurin Semo

This article informs anesthesiologists of some of the legal issues they may encounter in connection with ambulatory surgical center-based or office-based practice. The primary legal issues that anesthesiologists face in connection with practice in such settings can be broken down into practice-related issues and ownership-related issues. Given the complexity of legal issues relating to ambulatory anesthesia, anesthesiologists are advised to consult counsel at an early stage so as to understand the issues that may apply to their practices.

Accreditation of Ambulatory Facilities   551

Richard D. Urman and Beverly K. Philip

With the continued growth of ambulatory surgical centers (ASC), the regulation of facilities has evolved to include new standards and requirements on both state and federal levels. Accreditation allows for the assessment of clinical practice, improves accountability, and better ensures quality of care. In some states, ASC may choose to voluntarily apply for accreditation from a recognized organization, but in others it is mandated. Accreditation provides external validation of safe practices, benchmarking performance against other accredited facilities, and demonstrates to patients and payers the facility's commitment to continuous quality improvement.

Anesthesia Information Management Systems in the Ambulatory Setting: Benefits and Challenges   559

Ori Gottlieb

Adopting an anesthesia information management system (AIMS) is a challenge for anesthesia departments. The transition requires a physician champion and the support of members in every section. This change can be facilitated by visiting similar institutions that are already using AIMS, shadow charting for a sufficient period of time, and understanding that optimization continues after the go-live date. Once implemented, the benefits outweigh the challenges, but understanding where the potential obstacles lie is critical to removing them efficiently and effectively. As different AIMS continue to spread throughout the medical world, so will their benefits.

Quality Management and Registries   577

Richard P. Dutton

This article provides a review of key concepts in quality management (QM) for ambulatory anesthesia. The importance of collecting data from every case is emphasized, and important outcome measures are recommended. The use of specific data collection tools and methodologies is discussed, including the national registry projects of the Society for Ambulatory Anesthesia and the Anesthesia Quality Institute. A brief overview is provided of how to use QM data to improve patient outcomes within an anesthesia practice.

Index   587

ANESTHESIOLOGY CLINICS

FORTHCOMING ISSUES

September 2014
Vascular Anesthesia
Charles Hill, *Editor*

December 2014
Orthopedic Anesthesia
Nabil Elkassabany and Edward Mariano,
Editors

RECENT ISSUES

March 2014
Pediatric Anesthesiology
Alan Jay Schwartz, Dean B. Andropoulos,
and Andrew Davidson, *Editors*

December 2013
Abdominal Transplantation
Claus U. Niemann, *Editor*

September 2013
Obstetric Anesthesia
Robert Gaiser, *Editor*

June 2013
Cardiac Anesthesia
Colleen G. Koch, *Editor*

RELATED INTEREST

Clinics in Plastic Surgery, July 2013 (Volume 40, Issue 3, Pages 447–452)
Management of Postoperative Nausea and Vomiting in Ambulatory Surgery:
The Big Little Problem, 20 May 2013
Mary Keyes, *Editor*

NOW AVAILABLE FOR YOUR iPhone and iPad

Foreword

Ambulatory Anesthesia

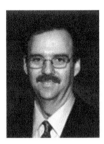

Lee A. Fleisher, MD, FACC, FAHA
Consulting Editor

Ambulatory anesthesia has grown tremendously and is now the predominant type of surgical and anesthesia care provided. The remarkable trend to move patients to the outpatient arena was driven by advances in ambulatory anesthesia. Importantly, these advances have occurred in multiple domains, including patient comorbidity management, drug development, regulatory issues, and most recently, assessing outcomes. In this issue of *Anesthesiology Clinics*, a remarkable group of experts in the field have written outstanding reviews to provide state-of-the-art information in all of these realms. In addition, the editors have chosen to include important reviews on both office-based care and the ever-increasing important area of anesthesia for procedural specialists.

In choosing editors for an ambulatory anesthesia issue, it was easy to approach Drs Thomas Cutter and Jeffrey Apfelbaum. Dr Cutter is the section chief of Ambulatory Anesthesia and a Professor in the Departments of Anesthesia/Critical Care and Surgery at the University of Chicago, where he also holds the administrative position of Medical Director of Perioperative Services. He was a past president of the Society for Ambulatory Anesthesia and the current president of the Illinois Society of Anesthesiologists. Dr Apfelbaum is Professor and Chair of Anesthesia and Critical Care at the University of Chicago Medical Center and the Pritzker School of Medicine in Chicago. He was President of ASA in 2008 and currently serves as Chair of its Committee on Standards and Practice Parameters. He also was President of the Illinois Society of Anesthesiologists, the Society for Ambulatory Anesthesia, the Society of Academic Anesthesiology Associations, and the Association of Academic Anesthesiology Chairs. Together, they have solicited an outstanding compendium of authors to update us on this critical field of care.

Lee A. Fleisher, MD, FACC, FAHA
Perelman School of Medicine
University of Pennsylvania
Philadelphia, PA 19104, USA

E-mail address:
lee.fleisher@uphs.upenn.edu

Anesthesiology Clin 32 (2014) xv
http://dx.doi.org/10.1016/j.anclin.2014.03.002   **anesthesiology.theclinics.com**
1932-2275/14/$ – see front matter © 2014 Published by Elsevier Inc.

Preface

The Four Ps: Place, Procedure, Personnel, and Patient

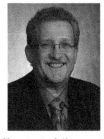 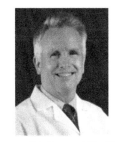

Jeffrey L. Apfelbaum, MD   Thomas W. Cutter, MD, MAEd
Editors

PATIENT INGRESS

As with all anesthetics, perioperative management may be divided into preoperative, intraoperative, and postoperative management. Preoperatively, one of the things that makes the practice of ambulatory anesthesia unique is the appropriate selection of patients. Most ambulatory anesthesiologists have encountered the patient who is deemed an inappropriate candidate because of his or her comorbidities. A question often asked of experienced ambulatory practitioners is whether there is a checklist or the like that can be applied to determine appropriate patients for the outpatient setting. This checklist might include answers to questions such as, "what is the maximum body mass index; should I care for a patient with a difficult airway; is a spinal anesthetic appropriate; are patients with an implantable cardiac defibrillator (ICD) acceptable?" There is potential value in creating such a checklist for the anesthesia provider and the proceduralist, but there are potential problems as well. To uniformly refuse service to all individuals with a given condition likely unduly limits access and does not allow the facility to take full advantage of its potential. Rather than a checklist that limits itself to just one aspect, it is best to recognize that it is not just the *patient* selection process that is important, but one must also consider the *providers*, the *procedure*, and the facility (*place*), taking into account the comorbidities of the patient, the skillsets of and access to providers, the procedure itself, and the availability of equipment in, and the location of, the facility.

Facilities (*place*) where ambulatory anesthesia is practiced include hospitals, where there can be a designated suite of operating rooms for these cases or where they can be interspersed throughout the larger operating room suite. Alternatively, there can be a separate dedicated building where ambulatory procedures are performed, referred to as an "on-campus" setting. Outpatient procedures can also be performed in a free-standing surgicenter located some distance away from a major hospital. The final

Anesthesiology Clin 32 (2014) xvii–xxi
http://dx.doi.org/10.1016/j.anclin.2014.03.001
1932-2275/14/$ – see front matter © 2014 Published by Elsevier Inc.

anesthesiology.theclinics.com

location is that of the office, which is probably the ne plus ultra of ambulatory anesthesia. Obviously, each of these settings has its advantages and limitations in terms of its ability to care for the more complex patient because of the available personnel and equipment and the proximity to other facilities for support or even transfer.

The number of *providers* and their level of training also impact the selection process. The skillset of the ancillary staff is important, especially when it comes to postanesthesia care. Having a receptionist with no medical training who also serves as the individual who monitors the patient after the procedure limits the complexity of both the procedure and the anesthetic technique. Having two trained and capable postanesthesia care unit nurses may mean that more complex procedures and anesthetics may be performed. Having an anesthesia technician may provide more equipment support so more sophisticated techniques (eg, fiberoptic bronchoscopy) may be available. Thus, the caliber and quantity of primary and support personnel influence the selection process.

The *procedure* is clearly an important part of the equation. In the 1990s, criteria for an acceptable procedure included minimal blood loss/fluid shift, duration of less than 90 minutes with simple equipment, minimal postoperative care, and minimal pain able to be treated with oral medications.[1] In the twenty-first century, the requirement is merely that the patient be able to go home the same day or, in some settings, within 23 hours. There really are no hard and fast rules that can be applied to distinguish an ambulatory procedure from an inpatient procedure other than the ability to safely go

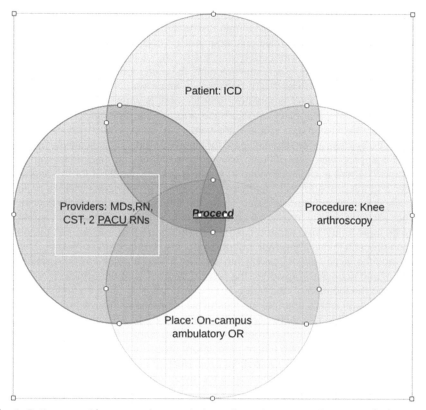

Patient: ICD

Providers: MDs,RN, CST, 2 PACU RNs

Proceed

Procedure: Knee arthroscopy

Place: On-campus ambulatory OR

Fig. 1. Patient, providers, procedure, and place all overlap: proceed. CST, certified surgical technician; MD, medical doctor; OR operating room; PACU, postanesthesia care unit; RN, registered nurse.

home the same day. When an anesthesiologist can provide an anesthetic from which the patient should be able to recover within a few hours, the limiting feature becomes the postoperative care associated with the procedure.

The final factor in the equation is the *patient*. Some may believe that only American Society of Anesthesiologists physical status class 1 or 2 patients should be cared for in an ambulatory setting, but this fails to take into account the impact of the place, the procedure, and the personnel. For example, a patient with obstructive sleep apnea can safely receive a lower extremity regional anesthetic with intravenous sedation and analgesia in many ambulatory facilities. There is little if any evidence that an otherwise healthy patient with a body mass index above a certain level is at increased risk for an ambulatory procedure, but there is the caveat that the operative table must be able to support the weight. While some may be loathe to care for a patient with an ICD in an office-based practice or a surgicenter, performing a procedure for this patient in an on-campus or integrated facility may be entirely appropriate. Thus, one must look at a variety of factors and integrate them into a meaningful whole to determine the appropriateness of admission to an ambulatory setting. **Figs. 1** and **2** illustrate this principle, where a patient with an ICD is acceptable in an on-campus setting but not in an office setting.

PATIENT EGRESS

The defining aspect of an ambulatory anesthetic is the patient's ability to safely and comfortably leave the facility the same day. There are at least four sequelae to

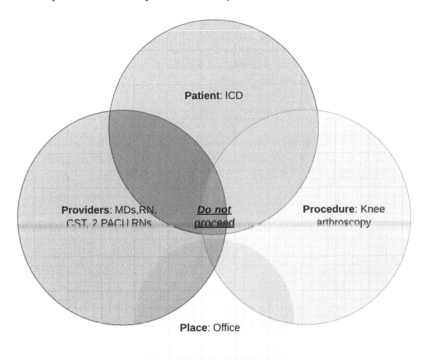

Fig. 2. Patient, providers, procedure, and place do not all overlap: do not proceed.

consider that are dependent on the anesthesiologist's preoperative, intraoperative, and postoperative management. While these will be dealt with in greater detail in other articles, they can be summarized to provide an overall recommendation for perioperative management. These "barriers" to discharge include pain, postoperative nausea and vomiting, excessive sedation, and significant pathophysiologic derangements.

Pain is regarded as the most common and most important adverse postoperative outcome.[2–4] Multimodal therapy using low-dose opioids, nonsteroidal anti-inflammatory drugs, and regional anesthesia serves to mitigate this. Postoperative nausea and vomiting can likely be regarded as the second most significant impediment and is also amenable to a multimodal approach, both to avoid the problem and to treat it. Excessive sedation also results in delayed discharge,[5] so preoperative and intraoperative sedative-hypnotics and intraoperative and postoperative opioids should be used judiciously. Morbid events, such as cardiac ischemia, hyperglycemia, cerebral vascular accident, or persistent hypotension, may also delay discharge, but the preoperative selection process and overall perioperative management should minimize this. Managing to avoid the sequelae of these comorbidities and other "complications" is of paramount importance to ensure a safe and timely discharge to home.

For this issue of *Anesthesiology Clinics*, our authors have detailed many of the clinical and logistical perioperative ambulatory anesthesia concerns that may lead to suboptimal outcomes and offer ways to manage them. We have also included articles on the administrative aspect of the practice of ambulatory anesthesia, since quite often it is the anesthesiologist who serves as the medical director and administrative go-to person in the facility. We finish with a glimpse of the future, including articles on the electronic medical record and the application of quality assurance registries in the ambulatory domain. We hope to provide a relatively broad overview of the practice of ambulatory anesthesia while also yielding a deeper understanding of some of the more common or pressing issues.

SUMMARY

The bottom line is that proper preoperative selection and preparation and the application of certain intraoperative techniques will best ensure that those who walk in to an ambulatory surgery facility will be able to walk out the same day.

Jeffrey L. Apfelbaum, MD
Department of Anesthesia and Critical Care
Pritzker School of Medicine
University of Chicago
5841 South Maryland Avenue, MC 4028
Chicago, IL 60637, USA

Thomas W. Cutter, MD, MAEd
Department of Anesthesia and Critical Care
Pritzker School of Medicine
University of Chicago
5841 South Maryland Avenue, MC 4028
Chicago, IL 60637, USA

E-mail addresses:
japfelbaum@dacc.uchicago.edu (J.L. Apfelbaum)
tcutter@dacc.uchicago.edu (T.W. Cutter)

REFERENCES

1. White PF, Song D. New criteria for fast-tracking after outpatient anesthesia: a comparison with the modified Aldrete's scoring system. Anesth Analg 1999;88: 1069–72.
2. Macario A, Weinger M, Truong P, et al. Which clinical anesthesia outcomes are both common and important to avoid? The perspective of a panel of expert anesthesiologists. Anesth Analg 1999;88:1085–91.
3. Swan BA, Maislin G, Traber K. Symptom distress and functional status changes during the first seven days after ambulatory surgery. Anesth Analg 1998;86: 739–45.
4. Chung F, Un V, Su J. Postoperative symptoms 24 hours after ambulatory anaesthesia. Can J Anaesth 1996;43:1121.
5. Atiyeh L, Philip B. Adverse outcomes after ambulatory anesthesia: surprising results. Anesthesiology 2002;96:A30.

Perioperative Management
of Co-Morbidities

Perioperative Evaluation and Management of Cardiac Disease in the Ambulatory Surgery Setting

J. Devin Roberts, MD[a],*, BobbieJean Sweitzer, MD[b]

KEYWORDS

- Ambulatory surgery • Aortic stenosis • Implantable electronic devices
- Coronary artery disease • Endocarditis prophylaxis • Heart failure • Hypertension

KEY POINTS

- The busy ambulatory surgery anesthesiologist needs a concise and practical approach to cardiac evaluation.
- Despite the prolific publication of guidelines in the literature, thorough perioperative cardiac risk stratification can be difficult, especially in a busy ambulatory surgery setting.
- The emphasis of preoperative cardiac evaluation should focus on identification and stratification of patient risk while attempting to avoid routine testing and prophylactic revascularization.
- Diagnostic testing and interventions are used only when the risk of adverse outcomes is high and intervention will lower risk.

INTRODUCTION

Within the last decade the emphasis during preoperative cardiac evaluation has been on identifying and stratifying patient risk and less on routine testing and prophylactic revascularization. Therapeutic interventions have focused on medications and other strategies to modify cardiovascular morbidity and mortality.[1,2] Anesthesia for ambulatory surgery is infrequently associated with adverse cardiac outcomes, but details of specific patient conditions are often limited. Few preoperative trials are available to guide patient management decisions. The busy ambulatory surgery anesthesiologist needs a concise and practical approach to cardiac evaluation.

[a] Department of Anesthesia and Critical Care, University of Chicago, 5841 South Maryland Ave MC4028, Chicago, IL 60637, USA; [b] Departments of Anesthesia and Critical Care, Anesthesia Perioperative Medicine Clinic, University of Chicago, 5841 South Maryland Ave MC4028, Chicago, IL 60637, USA
* Corresponding author.
E-mail address: JRoberts@dacc.uchicago.edu

Anesthesiology Clin 32 (2014) 309–320
http://dx.doi.org/10.1016/j.anclin.2014.02.012

HYPERTENSION

Hypertension, defined as 2 or more blood pressure (BP) measurements greater than 140/90, affects one billion individuals worldwide. Ischemic heart disease is the most common form of organ damage associated with hypertension. Hypertension is associated with risk of myocardial infarction (MI)[3] or even death and it increases perioperative cardiac risk 1.3-fold.[4]

A general recommendation is that elective surgery be delayed if hypertension is severe: diastolic BP greater than 115 mm Hg or systolic BP greater than 200 mm Hg. The American College of Cardiology Foundation (ACCF) and American Heart Association (AHA) guidelines suggest that the risk of delaying a procedure be considered before deciding to improve the patient's medical status. It is unclear whether delay improves outcomes.[4,5]

FUNCTIONAL CAPACITY

The inability to exercise indicates cardiac risk. Patients able to perform at least 4 metabolic equivalents, such as climbing 2 flights of stairs, have low cardiac risk despite other preexisting cardiac risk factors.[6]

CORONARY ARTERY DISEASE

Coronary artery disease (CAD) is often undiagnosed before a patient's first ischemic event. Although smoking, hypertension, older age, male sex, hypercholesterolemia, and family history of CAD are useful to assess symptoms or abnormal diagnostic tests, they do not predict greater risk for perioperative cardiac events. The Revised Cardiac Risk Index is a simple validated risk index for predicting perioperative cardiac risk in noncardiac surgery (**Table 1**).[7,8] According to the 2009 ACCF/AHA guidelines, asymptomatic patients undergoing low-risk procedures in ambulatory facilities do not usually

Table 1 Revised cardiac risk index components and expected cardiac risk	
Components of Revised Cardiac Risk Index	**Points Assigned**
High-risk surgery (intraperitoneal, intrathoracic, or suprainguinal vascular procedure)	1
Ischemic heart disease (by any diagnostic criteria)	1
History of congestive heart failure	1
History of cerebrovascular disease	1
Diabetes mellitus requiring insulin	1
Creatinine >2.0 mg/dL (176 μmol/L)	1
Revised Cardiac Risk Index Score	**Risk of Major Cardiac Events[a]**
0	0.4%
1	1.0%
2	2.4%
≥3	5.4%

[a] Defined as cardiac death, nonfatal MI, or nonfatal cardiac arrest.
Data from Lee TH, Marcantonio ER, Mangione CM, et al. Derivation and prospective validation of a simple index for prediction of cardiac risk of major noncardiac surgery. Circulation 1999;100:1043–9; and Devereaux OJ, Goldman L, Cook DJ, et al. Perioperative cardiac events in patients undergoing noncardiac surgery: a review of the magnitude of the problem, the pathophysiology of the events and methods to estimate and communicate risk. CMAJ 2005;173:627–34.

require preoperative assessment of functional status or cardiac risk factors. Certain high-risk conditions (**Fig. 1**), however, may prompt postponement of low-risk procedures pending further evaluation.

HEART FAILURE

If not an emergency, surgery is postponed in patients with decompensated, new onset, or untreated heart failure.[9,10] The goal of the anesthesiologist is to detect

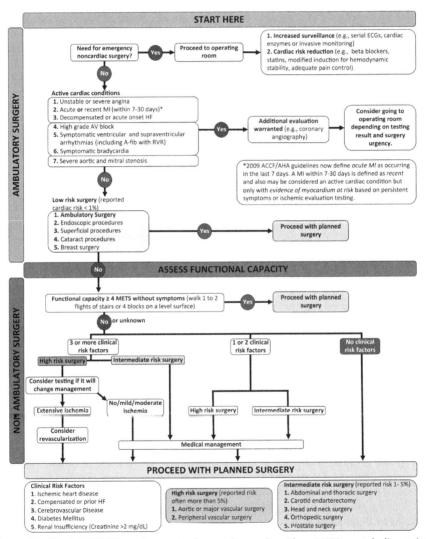

Fig. 1. Modified ACC/AHA cardiac evaluation and care algorithm. METS, metabolic equivalents. (*Adapted from* Fleisher LA, Beckman JA, Brown KA, et al. 2009 ACCF/AHA focused update on perioperative beta blockade incorporated into the ACC/AHA 2007 guidelines on perioperative cardiovascular evaluation and care for noncardiac surgery: a report of the American College of Cardiology Foundation/American Heart Association Task Force on Practice Guidelines. Circulation 2009;120:e169–276.)

patients with heart failure through a focused history and physical examination. Current ACCF/AHA guidelines recommend preoperative echocardiography (or another noninvasive measure of ventricular function) for patients with dyspnea of unknown origin or recently altered clinical status with known heart failure.[1]

CORONARY STENTS

Percutaneous coronary intervention (PCI) to reduce perioperative cardiac risk is reserved for patients experiencing active unstable CAD. PCI in other situations subjects patients to the risks of stent thrombosis with stenosis and prolonged or lifelong antiplatelet therapy.[1] Patients who have undergone PCI require a careful evaluation of stent type and time of placement. Management decisions are made in collaboration with the patient's cardiologist and surgeon. Patients with a bare metal stent placed within 30 days should absolutely *not* undergo elective surgery. Elective surgery is delayed for 1 year after placement of a drug-eluting stent.[11] It may be safe to proceed with surgery only after 6 months; however, these decisions are made with the patient's cardiologist.[12–14] With unavoidable surgery, dual antiplatelet therapy (ie, thienopyridine and aspirin) is continued unless the bleeding risk outweighs a high risk of thrombosis.[1,15] Patients are monitored for postoperative myocardial injury (eg, serial troponin measurements), which poses an additional challenge in the ambulatory setting. They may require urgent postoperative interventions, making them less than ideal candidates for free-standing ambulatory centers.

The concerns in patients with previous PCI are stent thrombosis, MI, or death. Perioperative stent thrombosis is best treated with immediate PCI.[16] Although opinions differ,[17] complex or high-risk patients may not be best suited for centers lacking immediate access to interventional cardiology. Bridging strategies with unfractionated or low-molecular-weight heparin as substitutes for antiplatelet therapy are inappropriate for patients with coronary stents. Heparin administration can paradoxically *increase* platelet aggregation and the risk of stent thrombosis.[18]

CARDIOVASCULAR IMPLANTABLE ELECTRONIC DEVICES: PACEMAKERS AND IMPLANTABLE CARDIOVERTER DEFIBRILLATORS

More than 100,000 cardiovascular implantable electronic devices (CIEDs) are implanted yearly in the United States.[1] During the preoperative evaluation, the anesthesiologist determines the type of device and the features (eg, device inhibition, antitachyarrhythmia functions, or rate-modulation) that may be affected during surgery. A preoperative electrocardiogram (ECG) reveals the presence of active pacing; a chest radiograph shows the type of device and possibly the manufacturer's code.

Pacemakers are designated with a 5-letter code (**Table 2**). Ideally, these devices are interrogated preoperatively during consultation with the cardiologist or electrophysiology nurse (**Box 1**). Electrocautery (especially above the umbilicus), radiofrequency ablation, magnetic resonance imaging, or radiation therapy can produce electromagnetic interference. Electromagnetic interference can inhibit pacing. An implantable cardioverter defibrillator (ICD) can misinterpret interference as an arrhythmia, inappropriately shocking the patient.[19]

As CIEDs become more complex, it is best to apply a magnet only when its specific effect is known or in emergency situations. Although not always the case, magnet application usually causes pacemakers to switch to an asynchronous mode. ICD antitachyarrhythmia functions will be disabled but any underlying pacemaker functions will remain intact (**Box 2**).

Table 2
Pacemaker nomenclature

Position I	Position II	Position III	Position IV	Position V
Chamber(s) paced	Chamber(s) sensed	Response to sensing	Rate modulation	Multisite pacing
O = None	O = None	O = None	O = None	O = None
A = Atrium	A = Atrium	I = Inhibited	R = Rate Modulation	A = Atrium
V = Ventricle	V = Ventricle	T = Triggered	—	V = Ventricle
D = Dual (A + V)	D = Dual (A + V)	D = Dual (T + I)	—	D = Dual (A + V)

From Bernstein AD, Daubert JC, Fletcher RD, et al. The revised NASPE/BPEG generic code for anti-bradycardia, adaptive-rate, and multisite pacing. North American Society of Pacing and Electro-physiology/British Pacing and Electrophysiology Group. Pacing Clin Electrophysiol 2002;25:260–4; with permission.

AORTIC STENOSIS

Severe aortic stenosis is associated with a high perioperative risk.[20] Undiagnosed stenosis can be particularly hazardous in the ambulatory surgery setting if neuraxial anesthesia is anticipated. A reduction in preload and cardiac output, especially with coexisting CAD, can initiate a potentially irreversible cycle of cardiac malperfusion and arrest. Classic symptoms of severe stenosis are angina, exertional dyspnea, and syncope. A systolic ejection murmur, best heard in the right upper sternal border and often radiating to the neck, is often present and may warrant preoperative echo-cardiography (**Box 3**).

Box 1
Proposed principles for CIED management

The perioperative management of CIEDs must be individualized to the patient, type of CIED, and procedure being performed. A single recommendation for all CIED patients is not appropriate.

The CIED team is defined as the physicians and physician extenders who monitor the CIED function of the patient.

The surgical or procedural team should communicate with the CIED team to identify the type of procedure and likely risk of EMI.

The CIED team should communicate with the procedure team to deliver a prescription for the perioperative management of patients with CIEDs.

For most patients, the prescription can be made from a review of the records of the CIED clinic. A small percentage of patients may require consultation from CIED specialists if the information is not available.

It is inappropriate to have industry-employed allied health professionals independently develop this prescription.

Abbreviation: EMI, electromagnetic interference.
From Crossley GH, Poole JE, Rozner MA, et al. The Heart Rhythm Society (HRS)/American Society of Anesthesiologists (ASA) expert consensus statement on the perioperative management of patients with implantable defibrillators, pacemakers and implantable monitors: facilities and patient management: executive summary. Heart Rhythm 2011;8:e1–8; with permission.

Box 2
Preoperative recommendations for CIEDs

- Inactivation of ICDs is not absolutely necessary for all procedures
- Not all pacemakers need to be altered to pace asynchronously in all patients or for all procedures
- Pacemakers can be reprogrammed or magnets can be used to force pacemakers to pace asynchronously to prevent inhibition
- ICDs can be reprogrammed or magnets can be used to inhibit ICD arrhythmia detection and tachyarrhythmia functions
- Magnets can NOT/will NOT force pacemakers in ICDs to pace asynchronously
- Inactivation of ICDs is recommended for all procedures above the umbilicus involving electrocautery or radiofrequency ablation
- It is preferable to change to asynchronous pacing in pacemaker-dependent patients for procedures involving electrocautery or radiofrequency ablation above the umbilicus

The procedure team provides the following information to the CIED team:

- Type of procedure
- Anatomic site of procedure
- Patient position during procedure
- Will electrocautery (and type of cautery) be used?
- Are there other sources of EMI
- Other issues, such as likelihood of damage to leads (eg, chest procedures), anticipated large blood loss, surgery in close proximity to CIED

The CIED team provides the following information to the procedure team:

- Type of device (eg, pacemaker, ICD)
- Indication for device (eg, sick sinus syndrome, primary or secondary prevention of lethal arrhythmias)
- Programing (eg, pacing mode, rate, rate responsive, heart rates for shock delivery)
- Is the patient pacemaker dependent and what is the underlying heart rate/rhythm
- Magnet response
  - Pacing rate
  - Is the device responsive to a magnet?
  - Will ICD functions resume automatically with magnet removal?
  - Does magnet need to be placed off-center?

Abbreviation: EMI, electromagnetic interference.
From Crossley GH, Poole JE, Rozner MA, et al. The Heart Rhythm Society (HRS)/American Society of Anesthesiologists (ASA) expert consensus statement on the perioperative management of patients with implantable defibrillators, pacemakers and implantable monitors: facilities and patient management: executive summary. Heart Rhythm 2011;8:e1–8; with permission.

PROSTHETIC HEART VALVES

The type and position of prosthetic valves determine the need for continual perioperative anticoagulation. Generally, mechanical valves require continual anticoagulation; bioprosthetic valves do not. A multidisciplinary team that includes the patient's cardiologist and surgeon decides anticoagulation and bridging strategies.

Box 3
Indications for echocardiographic evaluation of murmurs

Class I

Echocardiography is recommended for asymptomatic patients with diastolic murmurs, continuous murmurs, holosystolic murmurs, late systolic murmurs, murmurs associated with ejection clicks, or murmurs that radiate to the neck or back (level of evidence: C)

Echocardiography is recommended for patients with heart murmurs and symptoms or signs of heart failure, myocardial ischemia/infarction, syncope, thromboembolism, infective endocarditis, or other clinical evidence of structural heart disease (level of evidence: C)

Echocardiography is recommended for asymptomatic patients who have grade 3 or louder mid-peaking systolic murmurs (Level of Evidence: C)

Class IIa

Echocardiography can be useful for the evaluation of asymptomatic patients with murmurs associated with other abnormal cardiac physical findings or murmurs associated with an abnormal ECG or chest radiograph (level of evidence: C)

Echocardiography can be useful for patients whose symptoms and/or signs are likely noncardiac in origin but in whom a cardiac basis cannot be excluded by standard evaluation (level of evidence: C)

Class III

Echocardiography is not recommended for patients who have a grade 2 or softer midsystolic murmur identified as innocent or functional by an experienced observer (level of evidence: C)

From Bonow RO, Carabello BA, Chatterjee K, et al. 2008 Focused update incorporated into the ACC/AHA 2006 guidelines for the management of patients with valvular heart disease: a report of the American College of Cardiology/American Heart Association Task Force on Practice Guidelines (Writing Committee to Revise the 1998 Guidelines for the Management of Patients with Valvular Heart Disease). Circulation 2008;118:e523–661.

PREOPERATIVE TESTING

In the ambulatory surgery setting when little is known regarding a patient's cardiac status, a practitioner may be tempted to acquire a preoperative ECG. Routine preoperative ECGs, however, are not indicated, especially for patients without cardiac symptoms (**Box 4**).[21] Echocardiography may be indicated for the evaluation of valvular or ventricular dysfunction.

PERIOPERATIVE MEDICAL MANAGEMENT

Patients already taking β-blockers continue these medications throughout the perioperative period (**Box 5**). The initiation of β-blockers in low-risk patients seems to be associated with harm.[2,22,23] Because statins reduce perioperative cardiac risk,[24,25] they are continued perioperatively.

Aspirin is continued perioperatively except for patients undergoing intraspinal or intracranial procedures. The risk of bleeding complications from continuing aspirin for most procedures is low.[26] If aspirin is discontinued preoperatively, it is restarted as soon as possible following surgery.

PROPHYLAXIS FOR INFECTIVE ENDOCARDITIS

Recent guidelines have dramatically reduced the number of conditions and procedures warranting prophylaxis. Prophylaxis is now recommended only for patients

---

Box 4
Recommendations for preoperative resting 12-lead ECG

Class 1

Preoperative resting 12-lead ECG is recommended for patients with at least 1 clinical risk factor who are undergoing vascular surgical procedures (level of evidence: B)

Preoperative resting 12-lead ECG is recommended for patients with known coronary heart disease, peripheral arterial disease, or cerebrovascular disease who are undergoing intermediate-risk surgical procedures (level of evidence: C)

Class IIa

Preoperative resting 12-lead ECG is reasonable in persons with no clinical risk factors who are undergoing vascular surgical procedures (level of evidence: B)

Class IIb

Preoperative resting 12-lead ECG may be reasonable in patients with at least 1 clinical risk factor who are undergoing intermediate-risk operative procedures (level of evidence: B)

Class III

Preoperative and postoperative resting 12-lead ECGs are not indicated in asymptomatic persons undergoing low-risk surgical procedures (level of evidence: B)[a]

Class I indication: Evidence and/or general agreement that a given procedure or treatment is beneficial, useful, and effective.
Class IIa indication: There is conflicting evidence and/or a divergence of opinion about the usefulness/efficacy of a procedure or treatment, but the weight of evidence/opinion is in favor of usefulness/efficacy.
Class IIb indication: There is conflicting evidence and/or a divergence of opinion about the usefulness/efficacy of a procedure or treatment, and usefulness/efficacy is not well established.
Class III indication: Procedure or treatment is not recommended/indicated because risks are greater than potential therapeutic benefits.
  [a] According to ACCF/AHA guidelines, all ambulatory procedures are considered low risk.
  From Fleisher LA, Beckman JA, Brown KA, et al. 2009 ACCF/AHA focused update on perioperative beta blockade incorporated into the ACC/AHA 2007 guidelines on perioperative cardiovascular evaluation and care for noncardiac surgery: a report of the American College of Cardiology Foundation/American Heart Association Task Force on Practice Guidelines. Circulation 2009;120:e169–276; with permission.

---

with cardiac conditions that produce the highest risk of possible infection (**Box 6**).[27] As always, prophylaxis is recommended only for "dirty" procedures (eg, oral, gastrointestinal, infected tissue).

PUTTING IT ALL TOGETHER: A STEPWISE PRACTICAL APPROACH FOR AMBULATORY SURGERY

Most practitioners have adopted the 2009 ACCF/AHA guidelines for cardiac evaluation before noncardiac surgery, which are to be updated in 2014.[1] The goal is to identify perioperative cardiac risk to determine if the risk can be modified before surgery. The guidelines are designed to be followed in a stepwise fashion and are based on literature and expert consensus (see **Fig. 1**).

First the urgency and risk of surgery and active cardiac conditions are identified. For unavoidable emergency surgery, additional monitoring and medical management are warranted. If patients are at high risk, care in an ambulatory center may not be ideal. If

---

Box 5
Recommendations for use of perioperative β-blockers from the ACCF and AHA

Class I Indications

β-blockers should be continued in patients undergoing surgery who are already receiving β-blockers for treatment of conditions with ACCF/AHA class I guideline indications for the drugs.

Class IIa Indications

β-blockers titrated to heart rate and BP are probably recommended for patients undergoing vascular surgery who are at high cardiac risk owing to CAD or the finding of cardiac ischemia on preoperative stress testing.

β-blockers titrated to heart rate and BP are reasonable for patients in whom preoperative assessment for vascular surgery identifies high cardiac risk, as defined by the presence of more than 1 clinical risk factor.

β-blockers titrated to heart rate and BP are reasonable for patients in whom preoperative assessment identifies CAD or high cardiac risk, as defined by the presence of 2 or more clinical risk factors, who are undergoing intermediate-risk surgery.

From Fleisher LA, Beckman JA, Brown KA, et al. 2009 ACCF/AHA focused update on perioperative beta blockade incorporated into the ACC/AHA 2007 guidelines on perioperative cardiovascular evaluation and care for noncardiac surgery: a report of the American College of Cardiology Foundation/American Heart Association Task Force on Practice Guidelines. Circulation 2009;120:e169–276; with permission.

---

active cardiac conditions exist and surgery is nonemergent, the procedure is delayed to allow further evaluation (**Table 3**). Because ambulatory surgery is considered low risk if the patient is without active cardiac conditions, further evaluation is unnecessary (see **Fig. 1**).

Box 6
Cardiac conditions requiring endocarditis prophylaxis

Prosthetic heart valves or prosthetic material used for cardiac valve repair

Previous infective endocarditis

Congenital heart disease (CHD)[a]

Unrepaired cyanotic CHD, including palliative shunts and conduits

Completely repaired congenital heart defect with prosthetic material or device, whether placed by surgery or by catheter intervention, during the first 6 months after the procedure[b]

Repaired CHD with residual defects at the site or adjacent to the site of a prosthetic patch or prosthetic device (which inhibited endothelialization)

Cardiac transplantation recipients who develop cardiac valvulopathy

[a] Antibiotic prophylaxis is no longer recommended for forms of CHD not listed in this table.
[b] Prophylaxis is recommended because prosthetic material is usually endothelialized after 6 months of the procedure.
From Wilson W, Taubert K, Gewitz M, et al. Prevention of infective endocarditis. Guidelines from the American Heart Association. A Guideline from the American Heart Association Rheumatic Fever, Endocarditis, and Kawasaki Disease Committee, Council on Cardiovascular Disease in the Young, and the Council on Clinical Cardiology, Council on Cardiovascular Surgery and Anesthesia, and the Quality of Care and Outcomes Research Interdisciplinary Working Group. Circulation 2007;16:1736–54.

Table 3
Active cardiac conditions for which the patient should undergo evaluation and treatment before noncardiac surgery (class I, level of evidence: B)

Condition	Examples
• Unstable coronary syndromes • Decompensated heart failure (NYHA functional class IV; worsening or new-onset heart failure)	• Unstable or severe angina (CCS class III or IV)[a] • Acute MI[b] or recent MI with ischemic risk[c]
Significant arrhythmias	• High-grade atrioventricular block • Mobitz II atrioventricular block • Third-degree atrioventricular heart block • Symptomatic ventricular arrhythmias • Supraventricular arrhythmias (including atrial fibrillation) with uncontrolled ventricular rate (HR >100 bpm at rest) • Symptomatic bradycardia • Newly recognized ventricular tachycardia
Severe valvular disease	• Severe aortic stenosis (mean pressure gradient >40 mm Hg, aortic valve area <1.0 cm², or symptomatic) • Symptomatic mitral stenosis (progressive dyspnea on exertion, exertional presyncope, or heart failure)

Abbreviations: bpm, beats per minute; CCS, Canadian Cardiovascular Society; HF, heart failure; HR, heart rate; NYHA, New York Heart Association.
[a] May include "stable" angina in patients who are unusually sedentary.
[b] Acute MI is within 7 d.
[c] The American College of Cardiology National Database Library defines recent MI as greater than 7 d but less than or equal to 1 month (within 30 d).
From Fleisher LA, Beckman JA, Brown KA, et al. 2009 ACCF/AHA Focused update on perioperative beta blockade incorporated into the ACC/AHA 2007 Guidelines on Perioperative Cardiovascular Evaluation and Care for Noncardiac Surgery: A Report of the American College of Cardiology Foundation/American Heart Association Task Force on Practice Guidelines. Circulation 2009;120:e169–276; with permission.

PREOPERATIVE CARDIAC EVALUATION ON THE HORIZON

Despite the prolific publication of guidelines in the literature, thorough perioperative cardiac risk stratification can be difficult especially in a busy ambulatory surgery setting. Focused transthoracic perioperative echocardiography by anesthesiologists represents a valuable additional diagnostic modality. The examination can be performed with relative ease after training and can stratify cardiac risk and identify pathologic abnormality that predicts adverse perioperative cardiac events.[28]

REFERENCES

1. Fleisher LA, Beckman JA, Brown KA, et al. 2009 ACCF/AHA focused update on perioperative beta blockade incorporated into the ACC/AHA 2007 guidelines on perioperative cardiovascular evaluation and care for noncardiac surgery: a report of the American College of Cardiology Foundation/American Heart Association Task Force on Practice Guidelines. Circulation 2009;120:e169–276.
2. POISE Study Group. Effects of extended-release metoprolol succinate in patients undergoing non-cardiac surgery (POISE trial): a randomised controlled trial. Lancet 2008;371:1839–47.

3. Wax DB, Porter SB, Lin HM, et al. Association of preanesthesia hypertension with adverse outcomes. J Cardiothorac Vasc Anesth 2010;24:927–30.

4. Howell SJ, Sear JW, Foex P. Hypertension, hypertensive heart disease and perioperative cardiac risk. Br J Anaesth 2004;92:570–83.

5. Weksler N, Klein M, Szendro G, et al. The dilemma of immediate preoperative hypertension: to treat and operate, or to postpone surgery? J Clin Anesth 2003;15:179–83.

6. Morris CK, Ueshima K, Kawaguchi T, et al. The prognostic value of exercise capacity: a review of the literature. Am Heart J 1991;122:1423–31.

7. Ford MK, Beattie WS, Wijeysundera DN. Prediction of perioperative cardiac complications and mortality by the Revised Cardiac Risk Index: A systematic review. Ann Intern Med 2010;152:26–35.

8. Lee TH, Marcantonio ER, Mangione CM, et al. Derivation and prospective validation of a simple index for prediction of cardiac risk of major noncardiac surgery. Circulation 1999;100:1043–9.

9. Hernandez AF, Whellan DJ, Stroud S, et al. Outcomes in heart failure patients after major noncardiac surgery. J Am Coll Cardiol 2004;44:1446–53.

10. Balion C, Santaguida P, Hill S, et al. Testing for BNP and NT-proBNP in the diagnosis and prognosis of heart failure. Evidence Report/Technology Assessment No. 142. (Prepared by the McMaster University Evidence-based Practice Center under Contract No. 290-02-0020). Rockville (MD): Agency for Healthcare Research and Quality; 2006. AHRQ Publication No. 06-E014.

11. Assali A, Vaknin-Assa H, Lev E, et al. The risk of cardiac complications following noncardiac surgery in patients with drug-eluting stents implanted at least six months before surgery. Catheter Cardiovasc Interv 2009;74:837–43.

12. Brotman DJ, Bakhru M, Saber W, et al. Discontinuation of antiplatelet therapy prior to low-risk noncardiac surgery in patients with drug-eluting stents: a retrospective cohort study. J Hosp Med 2007;2:378–84.

13. Rabbitts JA, Nuttall GA, Brown MJ, et al. Cardiac risk of noncardiac surgery after percutaneous coronary intervention with drug-eluting stents. Anesthesiology 2008;109:596–604.

14. Wijeysundera DN, Wijeysundera HC, Yun L, et al. Risk of elective major noncardiac surgery after coronary stent insertion: a population-based study. Circulation 2012;126:1355–62.

15. Grines CL, Bonow RO, Casey DE, et al. Prevention of premature discontinuation of dual antiplatelet therapy in patients with coronary artery stents: a science advisory from the American Heart Association, American College of Cardiology, Society for Cardiovascular Angiography and Interventions, American College of Surgeons, and American Dental Association, with representation from the American College of Physicians. Circulation 2007;115:813–8.

16. Berger PB, Bellot V, Bell MR, et al. An immediate invasive strategy for the treatment of acute myocardial infarction early after noncardiac surgery. Am J Cardiol 2001;87:1100–2.

17. Thomas VR, Boudreaux AM, Papapietro SE, et al. The perioperative management of patients with coronary artery stents: surveying the clinical stakeholders and arriving at a consensus regarding optimal care. Am J Surg 2012;204:453–61.

18. Webster SE, Payne DA, Jones CI, et al. Anti-platelet effect of aspirin is substantially reduced after administration of heparin during carotid endarterectomy. J Vasc Surg 2004;40:463–8.

19. Crossley GH, Poole JE, Rozner MA, et al. The Heart Rhythm Society (HRS)/American Society of Anesthesiologists (ASA) expert consensus statement on the

perioperative management of patients with implantable defibrillators, pacemakers and arrhythmia monitors: facilities and patient management: Executive summary. Heart Rhythm 2011;8:e1–18.

20. Kertai MD, Bountioukos M, Boersma E, et al. Aortic stenosis: an underestimated risk factor for perioperative complications in patients undergoing noncardiac surgery. Am J Med 2004;116:8–13.

21. Tait AR, Parr HG, Tremper KK. Evaluation of the efficacy of routine preoperative electrocardiograms. J Cardiothorac Vasc Anesth 1997;11:752–5.

22. Lindenauer PK, Pekow P, Wang K, et al. Perioperative beta-blocker therapy and mortality after major noncardiac surgery. N Engl J Med 2005;353:349–61.

23. Bouri S, Shun-Shin MJ, Cole G, et al: Meta-analysis of secure randomised controlled trials of β-blockade to prevent perioperative death in non-cardiac surgery. Available at: http://heart.bmj.com/content/early/2013/07/30/heartjnl-2013-304262.full. Accessed September 17, 2013.

24. Dunkelgrun M, Boersma E, Schouten O, et al. Bisoprolol and fluvastatin for the reduction of perioperative cardiac mortality and myocardial infarction in intermediate-risk patients undergoing noncardiovascular surgery: a randomized controlled trial (DECREASE-IV). Ann Surg 2009;249:921–6.

25. Schouten O, Boersma E, Hoeks SE, et al. Fluvastatin and perioperative events in patients undergoing vascular surgery. N Engl J Med 2009;361:980–9.

26. Burger W, Chemnitius JM, Kneissl GD, et al. Low-dose aspirin for secondary cardiovascular prevention - cardiovascular risks after its perioperative withdrawal versus bleeding risks with its continuation - review and meta-analysis. J Intern Med 2005;257:399–414.

27. Wilson W, Taubert KA, Gewitz M, et al. Prevention of infective endocarditis: guidelines from the American Heart Association: A guideline from the American Heart Association Rheumatic Fever, Endocarditis, and Kawasaki Disease Committee, Council on Cardiovascular Disease in the Young, and the Council on Clinical Cardiology, Council on Cardiovascular Surgery and Anesthesia, and the Quality of Care and Outcomes Research Interdisciplinary Working Group. Circulation 2007;116:1736–54.

28. Cowie B. Focused transthoracic echocardiography predicts perioperative cardiovascular morbidity. J Cardiothorac Vasc Anesth 2012;26:989–93.

Perioperative Consideration of Obstructive Sleep Apnea in Ambulatory Surgery

Raviraj Raveendran, MBBS, MD, Frances Chung, MBBS, FRCPC*

KEYWORDS

- Obstructive sleep apnea • Ambulatory surgery • Anesthetic management
- Perioperative outcome

KEY POINTS

- The prevalence of obstructive sleep apnea (OSA) is increasing and a significant number of patients with OSA are undiagnosed.
- The suitability of ambulatory surgery in patients with OSA remains controversial, and the evidence regarding the safety of ambulatory surgery for patients with OSA is limited.
- Preoperative screening and careful selection of patients for ambulatory surgery is the most important step.
- Patients diagnosed and suspected of having OSA should be managed with a systematic algorithm to improve outcomes.

INTRODUCTION

Obstructive sleep apnea (OSA) syndrome is the most common type of sleep disorder and is characterized by repetitive episodes of upper airway obstruction that occur during sleep, usually associated with a reduction in blood oxygen saturation. A significant number of patients with OSA are undiagnosed when they present for elective surgery.[1] Approximately 10% to 20% of surgical patients, of whom 81% had not been previously diagnosed with OSA,[2,3] were found to be at high risk based on screening. Increases in the prevalence of OSA and surgical procedures performed on an outpatient basis pose a challenge to anesthesiologists. The suitability of ambulatory surgery in patients with OSA remains controversial because of the concerns of increased perioperative complications, including postdischarge death. Currently, evidence regarding

Department of Anesthesiology, Toronto Western Hospital, University Health Network, University of Toronto, 399 Bathurst Street, Toronto, Ontario M5T2S8, Canada
* Corresponding author. Department of Anesthesia, Room 405, 2McL, 399 Bathurst Street, Toronto, Ontario M5T2S8, Canada.
E-mail address: Frances.chung@uhn.ca

Anesthesiology Clin 32 (2014) 321–328
http://dx.doi.org/10.1016/j.anclin.2014.02.011
1932-2275/14/$ – see front matter © 2014 Elsevier Inc. All rights reserved.

the safety of ambulatory surgery for patients with OSA is limited. To emphasize the importance of proper patient selection for ambulatory surgery, both the American Society of Anesthesiologists (ASA)[4] and the Society for Ambulatory Anesthesia (SAMBA)[5] have published guidelines in this area.

RISK FACTORS AND PATHOPHYSIOLOGY

The prevalence of OSA among the general population aged 30 to 70 years is 5% in women and 14% in men,[6] and is 78% in morbidly obese patients scheduled for bariatric surgery.[7] Various pathophysiologic, demographic, and lifestyle factors predispose individuals to OSA, including anatomic abnormalities that may cause a mechanical reduction in airway lumen (eg, craniofacial deformities, macroglossia, retrognathia), endocrine diseases (eg, Cushing disease, hypothyroidism), connective tissue diseases (eg, Marfan syndrome), male sex, age older than 50 years, neck circumference greater than 40 cm, and lifestyle factors, including smoking and alcohol consumption.[8] OSA is associated with multiple comorbidities, such as myocardial ischemia, heart failure, hypertension, arrhythmias, cerebrovascular disease, metabolic syndrome, insulin resistance, gastroesophageal reflux, and obesity.

DIAGNOSTIC CRITERIA OF OSA

The gold standard for the definitive diagnosis of OSA is an overnight polysomnography or sleep study. The apnea hypopnea index (AHI), defined as the average number of abnormal breathing events per hour of sleep, is used to determine the presence and severity of OSA. An apneic event refers to cessation of airflow for 10 seconds, whereas hypopnea occurs with reduced airflow with desaturation of 4% or greater. The American Academy of Sleep Medicine (AASM) diagnostic criteria for OSA require either an AHI of 15 or greater or an AHI of 5 or greater with symptoms such as daytime sleepiness, loud snoring, or observed obstruction during sleep.[9] OSA is considered to be mild for an AHI of 5 to 14, moderate for an AHI of 15 to 30, and severe for an AHI greater than 30.

METHODS FOR PERIOPERATIVE SCREENING FOR OSA

Because routine screening with polysomnography is costly and resource-intensive, several screening tools have been developed.[10] The SAMBA guidelines recommend using the STOP-Bang questionnaire as a first step because of its simplicity. The questionnaire was originally developed in the surgical population but has been validated in various patient populations (**Table 1**).[11–13] Patients with STOP-Bang scores of 0 to 2 may be considered at low risk of OSA; 3 to 4 as intermediate risk; and 5 to 8 as high risk.[12] The specificity of STOP-Bang can be improved by using a number greater than 3. The addition of a serum bicarbonate level can also help improve specificity. In those deemed at high risk of OSA via the STOP-Bang questionnaire, the oxygen desaturation index, which is derived from nocturnal oximetry, can then be used to further indicate OSA.[12,14,15] These screening tests do not differentiate OSA from other sleep disorders, such as obesity hypoventilation syndrome and central sleep apnea, and therefore a blood gas and polysomnography are indicated to diagnose hypercarbia and effortless apnea, respectively.

PREOPERATIVE EVALUATION OF THE PATIENT WITH SUSPECTED OR DIAGNOSED OSA FOR AMBULATORY SURGERY

In 2006, the ASA developed guidelines on the perioperative management of patients with OSA[4] based on the severity of OSA, the invasiveness of surgery, the type of

Table 1			
STOP-Bang screening questionnaire			
S	Snoring: Do you snore loudly (louder than talking or loud enough to be heard through closed doors)?	Yes	No
T	Tired: Do you often feel tired, fatigued, or sleepy during the daytime?	Yes	No
O	Observed: Has anyone observed you stop breathing during your sleep?	Yes	No
P	Blood Pressure: Do you have or are you being treated for high blood pressure?	Yes	No
B	BMI: BMI >35 kg/m^2?	Yes	No
A	Age: Age >50 y?	Yes	No
N	Neck circumference: Neck circumference >40 cm?	Yes	No
G	Gender: Male?	Yes	No

Low risk of OSA: 0–2; intermediate risk: 3–4; high risk: 5–8.
Abbreviation: BMI, body mass index.
Adapted from Chung F, Yegneswaran B, Liao P, et al. STOP questionnaire: a tool to screen patients for obstructive sleep apnea. Anesthesiology 2008;108:812–21, with permission; and Chung F, Subramanyam R, Liao P, et al. High STOP-Bang score indicates a high probability of obstructive sleep apnoea. Br J Anaesth 2012;108:768–75, with permission.

anesthesia, and the need for postoperative opioids. The scores range from 0 to 9, and patients with a score of 3 or less may safely undergo ambulatory surgery. In 2012, SAMBA recommended guidelines based on more recent evidence.[5] The STOP-Bang questionnaire should be used as a screening tool, and patients with a known diagnosis of OSA who are compliant with continuous positive airway pressure (CPAP) and have optimized comorbid conditions may be considered for ambulatory surgery (**Fig. 1**). Patients who are noncompliant with CPAP may not be appropriate for ambulatory surgery. Patients with a presumed diagnosis of OSA based on the screening tool and optimized comorbid conditions can be considered for most types of ambulatory surgery if postoperative pain relief can be provided predominantly with

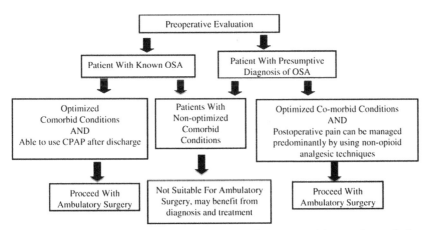

Fig. 1. Decision making in preoperative selection of patients with OSA for ambulatory surgery. (*From* Joshi GP, Ankichetty SP, Gan TJ, et al. Society for Ambulatory Anesthesia consensus statement on preoperative selection of adult patients with obstructive sleep apnea scheduled for ambulatory surgery. Anesth Analg 2012;115(5):1060–8; with permission.)

nonopioid analgesic techniques. In contrast to the ASA OSA guidelines, laparoscopic upper abdominal procedures (eg, gastric banding) may be safely performed on an outpatient basis provided the perioperative precautions are followed. No guidance was provided for patients with OSA undergoing upper airway surgery.

OUTCOME OF PATIENTS WITH OSA UNDERGOING AMBULATORY SURGERY

Studies on inpatient surgeries have shown serious cardiac and pulmonary complication in patients with OSA,[16] but only a few studies have examined postoperative complications in patients with OSA undergoing ambulatory surgery. The recent systematic review by SAMBA analyzed 5 prospective and 2 retrospective trials studying various ambulatory procedures, including general surgery,[3] orthopedic surgery,[17] laparoscopic bariatric surgery,[18,19] and upper airway surgery.[20,21] It compared the postoperative outcome in 1491 patients with OSA, 2036 patients at low risk for OSA, and 2095 patients without OSAs. None of the studies reported clinically significant adverse outcomes, such as the need for a surgical airway, incidence of anoxic brain injury, delayed discharge, unanticipated hospital admission, or death. Patients with OSA had a higher incidence of postoperative hypoxemia, but no differences were seen in the need for ventilatory assistance or reintubation. In a prospective cohort study, those patients with greater propensity for OSA had an increase in laryngoscopy attempts, a more difficult laryngoscopic view grade, and increased use of fiberoptic intubation.[3] Furthermore, the use of intraoperative ephedrine, metoprolol, and labetolol was greater in patients with OSA, but no difference was seen in unanticipated hospital admission.[3] A recent study on 404 ambulatory head and neck procedures in patients with OSA revealed a 0% complication and readmission rate.[22] All of these studies indicate that patients with OSA may safely undergo ambulatory surgery if they are carefully selected and receive appropriate perioperative care.

PERIOPERATIVE CARE OF PATIENTS WITH OSA FOR AMBULATORY SURGERY

General anesthesia in patients with OSA is often challenging, because the administration of sedatives, anesthetics, and analgesics could further worsen pharyngeal obstruction in a preexisting dysfunctional airway (**Table 2**). For general anesthesia, the anticipation of difficult intubation and the use of short-acting opioids, such as propofol, desflurane, or sevoflurane, may minimize airway-related complications.[23] Intraoperative use of opioid-sparing agents (eg, nonsteroidal anti-inflammatory drugs [NSAIDs], cyclooxygenase-2 [COX-2] inhibitors, paracetamol, tramadol, and adjuvants such as the anticonvulsants pregabalin and gabapentin) may reduce postoperative opioid requirements. During emergence, extubating the patient while awake with adequate reversal of neuromuscular blockade in a semiupright posture decreases the incidence of oxygen desaturation in the immediate postoperative period. Local and regional anesthesia techniques may be preferable to general anesthesia, because they avoid manipulation of the airway and reduce the postoperative requirement for analgesia.[23] One should consider a secured airway over an unprotected one for procedures requiring deep sedation.[23] For shoulder surgery, interscalene block in patients with OSA indicates careful evaluation. Phrenic nerve blockade may be minimized through using ultrasound, a small volume of local anesthetic, and a catheter technique for titrating the dose.[24] Patients with OSA undergoing painful ambulatory surgery, such as shoulder repair, anterior cruciate ligament repair, foot arthrodesis, and reconstructive plastic surgeries, may be at higher risk of adverse events because they require a larger amount of postoperative analgesic, which may include opioids.

Table 2
Perioperative precautions and risk mitigation for patients with OSA

Anesthetic Concern	Principles of Management
Premedication	Avoid sedating premedication Consider α_2-adrenergic agonists (clonidine, dexmedetomidine)
Potential difficult airway (difficult mask ventilation and tracheal intubation)	Optimal positioning (head-elevated laryngoscopy position) if patient obese Adequate preoxygenation Consider CPAP preoxygenation Two-handed triple airway maneuvers Anticipate difficult airway; personnel must be familiar with a specific difficult airway algorithm
Gastroesophageal reflux disease	Consider proton pump inhibitors, antacids, rapid sequence induction with cricoid pressure
Opioid-related respiratory depression	Minimize opioid use Use of short-acting agents (remifentanil) Multimodal approach to analgesia (nonsteroidal anti-inflammatory drugs, acetaminophen, tramadol, ketamine, gabapentin, pregabalin, dexmedetomidine, clonidine, dexamethasone, melatonin) Consider local and regional anesthesia when appropriate
Carry-over sedation effects from longer-acting intravenous and volatile anesthetic agents	Use of propofol/remifentanil for maintenance of anesthesia Use of insoluble potent anesthetic agents (desflurane) Use of regional blocks as a sole anesthetic technique
Excessive sedation in monitored anesthetic care	Use of intraoperative capnography for monitoring of ventilation
Postextubation airway obstruction	Verify full reversal of neuromuscular blockade Extubate only when fully conscious and cooperative Nonsupine posture for extubation and recovery Resume use of positive airway pressure device after surgery

Adapted from Seet E, Chung F. Management of sleep apnea in adults - functional algorithms for the perioperative period: continuing professional development. Can J Anaesth 2010;57:849–64; with permission.

POSTOPERATIVE DISPOSITION AND UNPLANNED ADMISSION AFTER AMBULATORY SURGERY

Patients with known or suspected OSA receiving general anesthesia should have extended monitoring for an additional 60 minutes after they have met the modified Aldrete criteria for discharge (**Fig. 2**). Recurring adverse respiratory events, such as oxygen saturation less than 90% on nasal cannula, bradypnea at less than 8 breaths per minute, apnea lasting more than 10 seconds, or pain-sedation mismatch, are indications for extended monitoring and admission.[25] Ideally, ambulatory surgical centers that manage patients with OSA should have the resources to handle postoperative problems associated with OSA and a transfer agreement with an appropriate inpatient facility. The anesthesiologist and surgeon should agree on postoperative analgesic prescription, and patients should be educated to use mostly acetaminophen, NSAIDs, and COX2 inhibitors and to limit or avoid opioids. Postoperatively, patients should be advised to sleep in a semiupright position, such as in a recliner, and to apply their positive airway pressure devices when sleeping, even during the daytime.

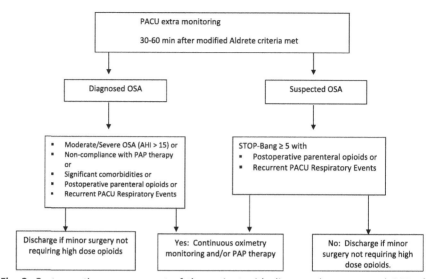

Fig. 2. Postoperative management of the patient with diagnosed or suspected OSA after general anesthesia. (*Adapted from* Seet E, Chung F. Management of sleep apnea in adults - functional algorithms for the perioperative period: continuing professional development. Can J Anesth 2010;57:849–64; with permission.)

SUMMARY

Anesthesiologists play an important role in identifying, evaluating, and optimizing patients with OSA.[26] Careful selection and preparation of patients with either diagnosed or suspected OSA is critical for patient safety. Understanding the perioperative risk and practicing perioperative risk mitigation can minimize cancellations and complications. Educating patients and the surgical team will improve the perioperative outcome. With proper screening and algorithm-based management, most patients with OSA may be safely anesthetized in the ambulatory surgery setting.

REFERENCES

1. Singh M, Liao P, Kobah S, et al. Proportion of surgical patients with undiagnosed obstructive sleep apnoea. Br J Anaesth 2013;110:629–36.
2. Finkel KJ, Searleman AC, Tymkew H, et al. Prevalence of undiagnosed obstructive sleep apnea among adult surgical patients in an academic medical center. Sleep Med 2009;10:753–8.
3. Stierer TL, Wright C, George A, et al. Risk assessment of obstructive sleep apnea in a population of patients undergoing ambulatory surgery. J Clin Sleep Med 2010;6:467–72.
4. Gross JB, Bachenberg KL, Benumof JL, et al. Practice guidelines for the perioperative management of patients with obstructive sleep apnea: a report by the ASA Task Force on perioperative management of patients with obstructive sleep apnea. Anesthesiology 2006;104:1081–93.
5. Joshi GP, Ankichetty SP, Gan TJ, et al. Society for Ambulatory Anesthesia Consensus statement on preoperative selection of adult patients with obstructive sleep apnea scheduled for ambulatory surgery. Anesth Analg 2012;115:1060–8.

6. Peppard PE, Young T, Barnet JH, et al. Increased prevalence of sleep-disordered breathing in adults. Am J Epidemiol 2013. http://dx.doi.org/10.1093/aje/kws342.

7. Lopez PP, Stefan B, Schulman CI, et al. Prevalence of sleep apnea in morbidly obese patients who presented for weight loss surgery evaluation: more evidence for routine screening for obstructive sleep apnea before weight loss surgery. Am Surg 2008;74:834–8.

8. Chung F, Elsaid H. Screening for obstructive sleep apnea before surgery: why is it important? Curr Opin Anaesthesiol 2009;22:405–11.

9. Iber C, Ancoli-Israel S, Cheeson A, et al. The AASM manual for the scoring of sleep and associated events, rules, terminology and technical specifications. Westchester (IL): American Academy of Sleep Medicine; 2007.

10. Abrishami A, Khajehdehi A, Chung F. A systematic review of screening questionnaires for obstructive sleep apnea. Can J Anaesth 2010;57:423–38.

11. Chung F, Yegneswaran B, Liao P, et al. STOP questionnaire: a tool to screen patients for obstructive sleep apnea. Anesthesiology 2008;108:812–21.

12. Farney RJ, Walker BS, Farney RM, et al. The STOP-Bang equivalent model and prediction of severity of obstructive sleep apnea: relation to polysomnographic measurements of the apnea/hypopnea index. J Clin Sleep Med 2011;7:459–65.

13. Chung F, Subramanyam R, Liao P, et al. High STOP-Bang score indicates a high probability of obstructive sleep apnoea. Br J Anaesth 2012;108:768–75.

14. Chung F, Chau E, Yang Y, et al. Serum bicarbonate level improves specificity of STOP-Bang screening for obstructive sleep apnea. Chest 2013;143: 1284–93.

15. Chung F, Liao P, Elsaid H, et al. Oxygen desaturation index from nocturnal oximetry: a sensitive and specific tool to detect sleep-disordered breathing in surgical patients. Anesth Analg 2012;114:993–1000.

16. Kaw R, Chung F, Pasupuleti V, et al. Meta-analysis of the association between obstructive sleep apnoea and postoperative outcome. Br J Anaesth 2012;109: 897–906.

17. Liu SS, Chisholm MF, John RS, et al. Risk of postoperative hypoxemia in ambulatory orthopedic surgery patients with diagnosis of obstructive sleep apnea: a retrospective observational study. Patient Saf Surg 2010;4:9. http://dx.doi.org/ 10.1186/1754-9493-4-9.

18. Kurrek MM, Cobourn C, Wojtasik Z, et al. Morbidity in patients with or at high risk for obstructive sleep apnea after ambulatory laparoscopic gastric banding. Obes Surg 2011;21:1494–8.

19. Watkins BM, Montgomery KF, Ahroni JH, et al. Adjustable gastric banding in an ambulatory surgery center. Obes Surg 2005;15:1045–9.

20. Hathaway B, Johnson JT. Safety of uvulopalatopharyngoplasty as outpatient surgery. Otolaryngol Head Neck Surg 2006;134:542–4.

21. Kieff DA, Busaba NY. Same-day discharge for selected patients undergoing combined nasal and palatal surgery for obstructive sleep apnea. Ann Otol Rhinol Laryngol 2004;113:128–31.

22. Baugh R, Burke B, Fink B, et al. Safety of outpatient surgery for obstructive sleep apnea. Otolaryngol Head Neck Surg 2013;148:867–72.

23. Seet E, Chung F. Management of sleep apnea in adults - Functional algorithms for the perioperative period: continuing professional development. Can J Anaesth 2010;57:849–64.

24. Al-Nasser B. Review of interscalene block for postoperative analgesia after shoulder surgery in obese patients. Acta Anaesthesiol Taiwan 2012;50:29–34.

25. Gali B, Whalen FX, Schroeder D, et al. Identification of patients at risk for postoperative respiratory complications using a preoperative obstructive sleep apnea screening tool and postanesthesia care assessment. Anesthesiology 2009;110: 869–77.
26. Ankichetty S, Chung F. Consideration for patients with obstructive sleep apnea undergoing ambulatory surgery. Curr Opin Anaesthesiol 2011;24:605–11.

Management of Diabetes Medications for Patients Undergoing Ambulatory Surgery

Mary Ann Vann, MD

KEYWORDS

- Ambulatory anesthesia • Ambulatory surgery • Diabetes mellitus
- Perioperative hyperglycemia • Perioperative insulin

KEY POINTS

- Perioperative hyperglycemia is typically due to the neuroendocrine stress response and the discontinuation of insulin and other antihyperglycemic medications.
- Blood glucose (BG) should be maintained in a patient's usual range because acute variations may be harmful.
- Hypoglycemia treatments should be readily available for fasting patients.
- For type 1 diabetic patients, basal insulins should be administered at or near customary doses.
- For type 2 diabetic patients, oral medications may be withheld on the day of surgery until meals resume; intermediate-acting or sole peakless insulin regimens usually require modification.

PREOPERATIVE INQUIRIES

Patients should be questioned about duration and type of diabetes, compliance with medications, level of glycemic control, and frequency of self-monitoring of BG (SMBG). Their understanding of and skill in managing their treatment regimen must be evaluated prior to altering medications preoperatively. Practitioners should ascertain the incidence and frequency of hypoglycemia, the BG at which symptoms occur, and the presence of hypoglycemia unawareness.

Medications for Type 2 Diabetes Mellitus

Among diabetics, 72% take oral hypoglycemic drugs,[1] with metformin the first-line oral hypoglycemic. Patients with renal insufficiency may develop lactic acidosis, and metformin is often held prior to radiologic procedures requiring contrast. Insulin secretagogue

The author has no interests to disclose.
Department of Anesthesia, Critical Care and Pain Medicine, Beth Israel Deaconess Medical Center, Harvard Medical School, 330 Brookline Avenue, Boston, MA 02215, USA
E-mail address: mvann@bidmc.harvard.edu

Anesthesiology Clin 32 (2014) 329–339
http://dx.doi.org/10.1016/j.anclin.2014.02.008
1932-2275/14/$ – see front matter © 2014 Elsevier Inc. All rights reserved.

drugs, such as sulfonylureas (eg, glinides) and meglitinides may cause perioperative hypoglycemia. **Table 1** provides additional information on hypoglycemic drugs.

Insulin

Although only 5% to 10% of all diabetics have type 1 diabetes mellitus, 26% take insulin (**Table 2**).[1] The preferred regimen of physiologic insulin dosing (also called basal bolus) mimics endogenous insulin production by providing basal, prandial or nutritional, and correction doses.[2] Continuous subcutaneous insulin infusions via an insulin pump or long-acting peakless insulin analogs are used for basal dosing. Basal insulin comprises approximately 50% of a patient's total daily dose (TDD) of insulin, which covers basal metabolic needs and should not cause hypoglycemia.[3] Patients administer variable boluses of rapid-acting nutritional insulin to match the carbohydrate content of meals. The final element of a physiologic insulin regimen is correction of elevated BG.

Peakless insulin alone or intermediate-acting or premixed insulins are alternative regimens used mostly by type 2 diabetes mellitus patients. For these patients, insulin supplements oral medications and endogenous insulin production but may cause hypoglycemia while fasting. Type 2 diabetes mellitus patients are insulin resistant and usually require higher insulin doses for the same level of BG control.[4] Administration of premixed or fixed combinations of intermediate- and short- or rapid-acting insulins poses a challenge perioperatively, because each should be dosed independently. Components of premixed NPH insulin and regular insulin are available, but for Humalog (Lilly, Indianapolis, IN, USA) Mix, intermediate-acting lispro protamine is not offered alone and NPH insulin must be substituted. Split dosing for most patients should occur at an ambulatory facility.

Insulin Pumps

More than 20% of type 1 diabetes mellitus patients in the United States use insulin pumps.[5,6] The pump delivers multiple basal infusion rates of a rapid-acting insulin analog (RAIA), lispro, aspart, or glulisine, which matches diurnal rhythms and activity and also provides adjustable nutritional and correction insulin boluses. The lowest basal rate should be used perioperatively, although some authors advocate reducing this rate by 10% to 20% to prevent hypoglycemia.[6] Basal insulin is vital for metabolic functions, and replacement insulin must be administered if the pump is discontinued. An insulin-deficient patient's BG rises 45 mg/dL per hour if basal insulin is withheld.[7]

HYPOGLYCEMIA

Hypoglycemia is a common occurrence in type 1 and advanced type 2 diabetic patients. Elderly patients are at increased risk due to fewer symptoms and diminished counter-regulatory responses.[8,9] The alert value for hypoglycemia, BG less than 70, allows for a response prior to symptoms in well-controlled patients.[10] Severe hypoglycemia, BG less than 40 or cognitive impairment, typically requires assistance to correct. Thresholds for hypoglycemic symptoms are dynamic and are reduced by frequent low BG and elevated by poor glycemic control.

There are 2 levels of symptoms during hypoglycemia. Sympathoadrenal activation with mild hypoglycemia produces neurogenic symptoms, such as sweating, palpitations, hunger, and tremor. At lower BG, neuroglycopenic symptoms of fatigue, confusion, visual changes, and seizures occur.[3,11] Hypoglycemia unawareness or hypoglycemia-associated autonomic failure minimizes or eliminates a patient's neurogenic symptoms, so neuroglycopenic symptoms are the only response to low BG. This unawareness can be diminished by elevating BG targets.

Table 1
Oral and injectable antihyperglycemics/hypoglycemics

Drug Class Examples	Action	Risk of Hypoglycemia[a]	Adverse Effects
Oral medications			
Biguanide Metformin	*Sensitizer* Antihyperglycemic, decreases glucose production, increases insulin action	Low	Lactic acidosis in susceptible patients (renal failure), certain cases (radiologic)
Meglitinides Repaglidine, nateglinide	*Secretagogue* Stimulates insulin release from beta cells	Yes—moderate risk	Hypoglycemia
Sulfonylureas First generation: chlopropamide, tolbutamide Second-generation glinides: glyburide, glipizide, glimepiride, gliquidone	*Secretagogue* Stimulates insulin release from beta cells	Yes—highest-risk first generation, hypoglycemic effects up to 12–24 h Glimepiride (long-acting glyburide) more likely	Weight gain
Thiazolidindiones Pioglitazone, rosiglitazone	*Sensitizer* Decreases insulin resistance, glucose production	Low	Hepatotoxicity, fluid retention, CHF, cardiac events, bone fractures, bladder cancer
α-Glucosidase inhibitors Acarbose, miglitol	Reduce intestinal absorption of starch, disaccharides	Low	Gastrointestinal symptoms
Dipeptidyl peptidase 4 inhibitors Sitagliptin, saxagliptin, linagliptin, vildagliptin	*Incretin* drugs: increase insulin production, decrease glucose production	Low	Respiratory tract infection
Injectable medications			
Glucagon-like peptide 1 receptor agonists Exenatide Bydureon (once-weekly dose of exenatide)	*Incretin* drugs: increase insulin production, decrease glucose production	Low	Gastrointestinal symptoms, caution in renal insufficient patients
Pramlintide	An *incretin* drug, analog of amylin: increases insulin production, decreases glucose production	Low Increases risk of hypoglycemia with insulin	Gastrointestinal symptoms

Abbreviation: CHF, congestive heart failure.
[a] Drugs that do not cause hypoglycemia solely may do so in combination.
Data from Refs.[24–27]

Table 2
Insulin types[a] and times to effect

Rapid-acting insulin analogs			
Lispro (Humalog)	10–20 min	30–90 min	3–4 h
Aspart (NovoLog)	10–20 min	30–90 min	3–4 h
Glulisine (Apidra)	10–20 min	30–90 min	3–4 h
Regular insulin			
Humulin R, Novolin R	30–60 min	2–4 h	6–8 h
Intermediate-acting insulins			
NPH	1.5–4 h	4–10 h	10–20 h
70% NPH/30% regular (70/30)	30–60 min	3–12 h	10–20 h
50% NPL/50% lispro (Humalog mix)	10–20 min	1–4 h	10–20 h
Long-acting peakless insulins			
Glargine	1–3 h	No peak	20–24 h
Detemir	1–3 h	No peak	20–24 h

[a] Selected common insulins for comparison.
Data from Refs.[12,22,28]

Ambulatory surgery patients should travel with appropriate hypoglycemic treatments. The usual treatment of hypoglycemia is 15 to 20 g of glucose or other simple sugar. For fasting patients, this is best accomplished with 4 to 8 oz of clear juice or a sugary drink. Glucose gels or tablets are not recommended because they may be particulate. For patients with an intravenous line, 250 mL D5W or 25 mL D50 provides 12.5 g dextrose. BG should be measured 15 minutes after treatment and additional glucose administration may be required.

SIGNIFICANCE OF DIABETES IN SURGICAL OUTPATIENTS
Glycemic Disturbances

Common reasons for hyperglycemia in the perioperative period include the neuroendocrine stress response, withholding insulin and antihyperglycemic medications, and certain drugs.[2,12] Major negative effects of hyperglycemia for surgical patients include decreased immune function, prothrombotic state, and poor wound healing.[13,14]

Evidence for Glucose Control in Critical Care and Surgical Patients

A meta-analysis of intensive insulin therapy (IIT) for critically ill patients showed no decrease in mortality but a greatly increased risk of hypoglycemia in these aggressively treated patients.[15] Frequent bouts of severe hypoglycemia during IIT increased the risk of death.[16,17] For surgical patients, a meta-analysis found no benefit on mortality from perioperative insulin infusions despite the required substantial investment of resources, polices, and manpower.[13,14] BG values less than 180 mg/dL are recommended for hospitalized and surgical patients.[2,13]

PERIOPERATIVE MANAGEMENT OF DIABETES MEDICATIONS
Insulin Dosing

Day prior to surgery
Patients may take their usual insulin doses on the day prior to surgery unless they experience nocturnal hypoglycemia (**Table 3**); if so, they may reduce bedtime or evening insulin by 20% to 30%. Basal insulin dosing should be maintained provided it is

Table 3
Day-of-surgery insulin dosing

Regimen	Dosing for Early Case	Dose Adjustment for Later Case	During Case in OR	Dosing in PACU
Basal insulins (in physiologic regimens)				
Insulin pump	Maintain basal rate or decrease by 20%–30% if patient reports hypoglycemia	Maintain basal rate or decrease by 20%–30%	Maintain basal or decreased rate in OR if possible	Maintain basal rate if possible Bolus with food
Peakless single or bid dosing (eg, glargine, detemir)	Give usual morning dose or decrease by 20%–30% if patient reports hypoglycemia	Give usual morning dose or decrease by 20%–30%	Not appropriate	Not appropriate
Intermediate insulins or peakless nonbasal dosing[a]				
Peakless single or bid dosing (sole insulin[a]) (eg, glargine, detemir)	Options: give full dose prior to minor case; hold full dose until after case; give % of dose	Give % of dose based on expected time to first meal	Not appropriate	Give if held: full dose or calculated % of insulin
Intermediate-acting insulin: single or bid dosing (eg, NPH insulin)	Options: same as above	Give same as above	Not appropriate	Give if held: full-dose or calculated % of insulin
Premixed or fixed combination of long- and short-acting insulins (eg, 70/30)	Options: hold morning dose; give full or calculated amount of long-acting insulin (70%) only	Give calculated amount of long-acting insulin (70%) only	Not appropriate	Give if held: full-dose or calculated amount of insulin (long acting or combination)
Nutritional or correction dose insulin (RAISs recommended)	Give: as needed for hyperglycemia: use rule of 1800/1500 or patient's usual correction factor	Give: as needed for hyperglycemia: use rule of 1800/1500 or patient's usual correction factor	Give: as needed for hyperglycemia: use rule of 1800/1500 or patient's usual correction factor	Give: as needed for hyperglycemia or when food intake resumes: use rule of 1800/1500 or patient's usual correction factor

Abbreviations: OR, operating room; PACU, postanesthesia care unit.
[a] Peakless insulin as a sole insulin is not considered basal dosing.

only 50% of TDD. Insulin pumps should deliver usual sleep basal rates. For type 2 diabetes mellitus patients on peakless insulin only, bedtime doses may be reduced or omitted. NPH insulin given at dinnertime can be continued because the peak occurs prior to sleep. Doses of NPH insulin at bedtime may be reduced if a patient reports hypoglycemia when breakfast is delayed.

Day of surgery
Patients should bring their insulin with them on the day of surgery. This confirms the medication and allows them to receive doses of their own insulin. Patients on a physiologic insulin regimen may take their usual peakless basal insulin on the morning of surgery.[18] Peakless insulin given solely should be held or reduced as calculated from the dosing interval and predicted or actual time of fasting (**Box 1**).[3] Early arrival and management at the facility is recommended for patients taking intermediate-acting insulin preparations. For brief early morning cases, NPH or sole peakless insulin can be held until after the procedure. For longer procedures or later in the day, the sole basal or intermediate insulin can be reduced (see **Box 1**). This formula applies to

---

Box 1

Day-of-surgery adjustment of single peakless or intermediate-acting insulins (eg, glargine as sole agent, NPH insulin, or premixed insulins)

This formula uses the predicted or actual time of fasting and the usual time interval between doses of insulin:

$$\frac{[\text{Dosing interval (h)} - \text{Hours of fast during interval}]}{\text{Dosing interval (h)}} = \text{fraction of insulin to give}$$

Examples

Case: adult patient undergoing carpal tunnel release under block with sedation. He is estimated to be eating normally by 10:00 AM due to this minimally disruptive anesthesia technique.

A. If this patient usually takes 1 dose of 32 U of glargine at 7:00 AM daily (dosing interval is 24 hours, time of fast *predicted* as 3 hours), $(24 - 3)/24 = 21/24$, he would receive seven-eighths of his morning dose or 28 U (give before or after case).

B. If patient in scenario A is in the PACU, his morning insulin was held and his case is done in 1 hour, so he *actually* only misses 2 hours of food intake: $(24 - 2)/24 = 11/12$, he would essentially receive his usual dose, or 30–32 U of glargine, in the PACU.

C. If this patient usually takes 24 U of glargine twice daily at 7:00 AM and 7:00 PM (dosing interval is 12 hours) and he is *predicted* to eat at 10 AM, $(12 - 3)/12 = 9/12$, he would receive three-quarters of his usual morning dose or 18 U (give before or after case).

D. Patient (same scenario as C) usually takes 50 U of premixed NPH insulin/regular insulin 70/30 twice a day. His NPH insulin dose is only 35 U twice daily and this is the amount of insulin that should be used in calculation. He would receive three-quarters of the 35 U or 27 U of NPH insulin only (*not the mix*).

E. Patient (same scenario as C) is scheduled later in the day and is expected to eat at 1:00 PM. He is expected to miss 6 hours of food intake. He has not taken morning insulin: $(12 - 6)/12 = 6/12$, he would receive one-half his usual morning dose or 12 U, which should be given prior to surgery to supplement endogenous insulin. His BG, however, should be checked frequently until he is eating normally.

From Vann MA. Perioperative management of ambulatory surgical patients with diabetes mellitus. Curr Opin Anaesthesiol 2009;22(6):718–24; with permission.

premixed or fixed-combination insulins but pertains only to the intermediate-acting component.

Correction doses of insulin

The same insulin used for nutritional doses is used to treat hyperglycemia. Perioperatively, it is recommended to administer RAIA subcutaneously for correction dosing.[3,12,19] This allows a fairly quick reduction of BG with short duration of action so patients can be observed until peak effect has passed. Subcutaneous insulin is easy to administer, avoids large swings in BG, and duplicates a patient's normal routine. Hypoglycemia may occur from overlapping, or stacking, repeat doses. Subcutaneous insulin absorption occurs fastest from the abdomen, followed by arms, thighs, and buttocks,[20] but is affected by perfusion, heat, and cold. Regular insulin infusions require protocols and resources[14] beyond the scope of most ambulatory centers and intravenous boluses of regular insulin may cause potentially harmful swings in BG, because action commences in 5 to 6 minutes but lasts only 30 to 40 minutes.[3,21]

Methods for determining the appropriate correction dose include following a nonindividualized protocol or sliding scale, using a patient's usual correction factor, or calculating the dose based on a patient's TDD of insulin (**Box 2**). It is unclear whether insulin-naïve patients should receive their first insulin in an ambulatory surgical setting or be controlled prior to surgery.

Insulin pumps

An insulin pump may be continued during general anesthesia with certain safeguards, including limiting pump use to cases lasting less than 1 to 2 hours,[6,22] securing the infusion site and tubing away from the surgical field, isolating the pump from patient contact, shielding from radiographs to minimize potential interference,[5] and checking BG every hour to ensure proper pump function. Subcutaneous doses of RAIA should be given by syringe, not the pump, to correct elevated BG. A standardized perioperative insulin pump checklist is advisable (**Box 3**).[5]

Oral Medications

Both oral medications and noninsulin injectables should be held on the day of surgery. They may be restarted when regular meals are expected.[2]

Box 2
Calculation for correction dose insulin using rule of 1800/1500

1800 ÷ TDD = the mg/dL decrease in BG with each unit of rapid-acting insulin given (or 1500 for patients *less* sensitive to insulin)

TDD of insulin = basal + *nutritional doses*

    For example: 30 U glargine (once a day) + *30 U lispro* (6 U at breakfast, 10 U at lunch, and 14 U at dinner) = 60 U

Correction dose: How much will this patient's BG decrease with 1 U of lispro?

1800 ÷ 60 = 30 mg/dL predicted decrease in BG with each unit of insulin

    To decrease this patient's BG by 150 mg/dL, administer 5 U of lispro.

1500 ÷ 60 = 25 mg/dL predicted decrease in BG with each unit of insulin (lower, patient is *less* sensitive to insulin)

    To decrease this patient's BG by 150 mg/dL, administer 6 U of lispro.

Box 3
Recommended elements for insulin pump checklist

1. Pump information

   Manufacturer

   Functioning? (Y/N)

   On/off switch

   Battery life checked? (Y/N)

   Insulin type

2. Programmed settings information

   Basal rate settings

   Current setting

   Insulin-to-CHO ratio

   Correction factor OR TDD of insulin

3. Supplies

   Fresh tubing, not kinked? (Y/N)

   Adequate insulin in reservoir? (Y/N)

4. Insertion site

   Fresh site (Y/N) (How long?)

   Location of site

   Need for isolation from electrical hazards? (Y/N)

   Need for shielding from radiograph? (Y/N)

5. Blood sugar measurements

   Admission

   Q1–2 hours during stay

6. Plan for correction dosing

   RAIA vials/syringes for dosing available

   Formula for dosing:

   Patient's correction factor (see Box 2 above)

   Rule of 1800/1500 calculation (see Box 2 above for TDD)

7. Pump failure plan

8. Treatment of hypoglycemia plan

9. Diabetes provider (endocrinologist) contact information

Abbreviation: CHO, carbohydrate.

ANESTHESIA CARE
Scheduling

A minimally stressful anesthetic and surgery performed early in the day least disrupts a diabetic patient's medications and meals.[12,19] Intermediate and premixed insulin regimens usually require dosing alterations that necessitate early arrival at the facility.

| **Box 4** |
| **Factors that may affect perioperative POC capillary BG measurements** |
| Hypoglycemia |
| Oxygen administration |
| Acetaminophen |
| Hypotension, use of vasopressors |
| Anemia |
| pH changes |
| Active warming or cooling |
| Vitamin C excess |

Glucose Measurement

Point-of-care (POC) capillary BG meters are commonly used in hospitals and ambulatory centers and testing should take place every 1 to 2 hours. The U.S. Food and Drug Administration allows a 20% variance in BG readings from actual values[8] and, when a patient is hypoglycemic, meters typically overestimate BG levels.[23] For hemodynamically stable patients, POC testing is likely to agree with laboratory values.[13] **Box 4** lists factors that can affect BG readings.

Abnormal Blood Glucose Values

No particular BG value necessarily warrants treatment or cancellation of surgery. During ambulatory surgery, patients' BG should be maintained near their normal level unless they display evidence of ketoacidosis, hyperosmolar coma, or dehydration.[6,12,13] Acute and temporary corrections of BG are not always beneficial.[13] If surgery proceeds for a hyperglycemic patient, there are risks of further elevations of BG postoperatively.

Postoperative Care

The metabolic effects of ambulatory surgery may not appear until patients are home and well into the postoperative period.[13] SMBG should be encouraged to avoid unexpected consequences of hyper- or hypoglycemia. Providing patients with clear written instructions on postoperative management of medications and a contact person for their diabetes care can ensure their safety.[19]

REFERENCES

1. National Diabetes Fact Sheet: national estimates and general information on diabetes and prediabetes in the United States 2011. Available at: http://www.cdc.gov/diabetes/pubs/pdf/ndfs_2011.pdf. Accessed August 22, 2013.
2. American Diabetes Association. Standards of Medical Care in Diabetes – 2013. Diabetes Care 2013;36(Suppl 1):s4–66.
3. Vann MA. Perioperative management of ambulatory surgical patients with diabetes mellitus. Curr Opin Anaesthesiol 2009;22(6):718–24.
4. Lipshutz AK, Gropper MA. Perioperative glycemic control. Anesthesiology 2009; 110:408–21.
5. Boyle ME, Seifert KM, Beer KA, et al. Guidelines for application of continuous subcutaneous insulin infusion (insulin pump) therapy in the perioperative period. J Diabetes Sci Technol 2012;6(1):184–90.

6. Abdelmalak B, Ibrahim M, Yared JP, et al. Perioperative glycemic management in insulin pump patients undergoing noncardiac surgery. Curr Pharm Des 2012; 18(38):6204–14.

7. Clement S, Braithwaite SS, Magee MF, et al. Management of diabetes and hyperglycemia in hospitals. Diabetes Care 2004;27:553–91.

8. Seaquist ER, Anderson J, Childs B, et al. Hypoglycemia and diabetes: a report of a workgroup of the American Diabetes Association and The Endocrine Society. J Clin Endocrinol Metab 2013;98:1845–59.

9. Maynard G, O'Malley CW, Kirsh SR. Perioperative Care of the Geriatric Patient with Diabetes or Hyperglycemia. Clin Geriatr Med 2008;24:649–65.

10. Cryer PE. Preventing hypoglycaemia: what is the appropriate glucose alert value? Diabetologia 2009;52:35–7.

11. Cryer PE. The barrier of hypoglycemia in diabetes. Diabetes 2008;57:3169–76.

12. Joshi GP, Chung F, Vann MA, et al, Society for Ambulatory Anesthesia. Society for Ambulatory Anesthesia consensus statement on perioperative blood glucose management in diabetic patients undergoing ambulatory surgery. Anesth Analg 2010;111(6):1378–87.

13. Akhtar S, Barash PG, Inzucchi SE. Scientific principles and clinical implications of perioperative glucose regulation and control. Anesth Analg 2010;110:478–97.

14. Gandhi GY, Murad MH, Flynn DN, et al. Effect of perioperative insulin infusion on surgical morbidity and mortality: systemic review and meta-analysis of randomized trials. Mayo Clin Proc 2008;83:418–30.

15. Griesdale DE, de Souza RJ, van Dam RM, et al. Intensive insulin therapy and mortality among critically ill patients: a meta-analysis including NICE-SUGAR study data. CMAJ 2009;180(8):821–7.

16. Egi M, Bellomo R, Stachowski E, et al. The interaction of chronic and acute glycemia with mortality in critically ill patients with diabetes. Crit Care Med 2011;39:105–11.

17. The NICE-SUGAR Study Investigators. Hypoglycemia and risk of death in critically ill patients. N Engl J Med 2012;367:1108–18.

18. Umpierrez GE, Smiley D, Jacobs S, et al. Randomized study of basal-bolus insulin therapy in the inpatient management of patients with type 2 diabetes undergoing general surgery (RABBIT 2 surgery). Diabetes Care 2011;34(2):256–61.

19. Dhatariya K, Levy N, Kilvert A, et al, Joint British Diabetes Societies. NHS Diabetes guideline for the perioperative management of the adult patient with diabetes. Diabet Med 2012;29(4):420–33.

20. Heinemann L, Krinelke L. Insulin infusion set: the Achilles heel of continuous subcutaneous insulin infusion. J Diabetes Sci Technol 2012;6(4):954–64.

21. Inzucchi SE. Management of hyperglycemia in the hospital setting. N Engl J Med 2006;355:1903–11.

22. Ferrari LR. New insulin analogues and insulin delivery devices for the perioperative management of diabetic patients. Curr Opin Anaesthesiol 2008;21:401–5.

23. Rebel A, Rice MA, Fahy BG. Accuracy of point-of-care glucose measurements. J Diabetes Sci Technol 2012;6(2):396–411.

24. Ha WC, Oh SJ, Kim JH, et al. Severe hypoglycemia is a serious complication and becoming an economic burden in diabetes. Diabetes Metab J 2012;36:L280–4.

25. Chen D, Lee SL, Peterfreund RA. New therapeutic agents for diabetes mellitus: implications for anesthetic management. Anesth Analg 2009;108:1803–10.

26. Bailey CJ, Day C. Fixed-dose single tablet antidiabetic combinations. Diabetes Obes Metab 2009;11:527–33.

27. Garber AJ, Abrahamson MJ, Barzilay JI, et al. American association of clinical endocrinologists' comprehensive diabetes management algorithm 2013 consensus statement - executive summary. Endocr Pract 2013;19(3):536–57.
28. Borgoño CA, Zinman B. Insulin therapy insulins: past, present, and future. Endocrinol Metab Clin North Am 2012;41:1–24.

Regional Anesthesia

Peripheral Nerve Blocks for Ambulatory Surgery

Francis V. Salinas, MD*, Raymond S. Joseph, MD

KEYWORDS

- Peripheral nerve blocks • Continuous peripheral nerve blocks • Ultrasound guidance
- Ambulatory surgery

KEY POINTS

- Peripheral nerve blocks (PNBs) provide significant improvement in postoperative analgesia and quality of recovery for ambulatory surgery.
- Use of continuous PNB techniques extend these benefits beyond the limited duration of single-injection PNBs.
- The use of ultrasound guidance has significantly improved the overall success, efficiency, and has contributed to the increased use of PNBs in the ambulatory setting. More recently, the use of ultrasound guidance has been demonstrated to decrease the risk of local anesthetic systemic toxicity.

INTRODUCTION

Peripheral nerve blocks (PNBs) for ambulatory surgery, and in particular for orthopedic surgery, may be used as either the primary anesthetic or more commonly as an analgesic adjunct to general anesthesia. The benefits of PNBs for ambulatory surgery include reductions in postoperative pain, opioid requirements, and postoperative nausea and vomiting, and possibly decreased time to functional recovery.[1,2] Poorly controlled pain after ambulatory surgery may lengthen stay in the postanesthesia care unit, and possibly even require hospitalization.[3–5] Thus, PNBs have also been shown to facilitate postanesthesia care unit bypass and decrease time to achieve discharge criteria after ambulatory upper and lower extremity orthopedic surgery.[6–9] Recent data indicate that for patients undergoing arthroscopic shoulder surgery in the beach chair position, regional anesthesia with sedation compared with general anesthesia significantly decreases the incidence of critical cerebral deoxygenation events.[10]

The benefits of single-injection PNB techniques are primarily determined by the physical properties of the local anesthetic agent (and analgesic adjuncts) chosen for

Disclosure: None.
Department of Anesthesiology, Virginia Mason Medical Center, 1100 Ninth Avenue, B2-AN, Seattle, WA 98101–2756, USA
* Corresponding author.
E-mail address: Francis.Salinas@vmmc.org

Anesthesiology Clin 32 (2014) 341–355
http://dx.doi.org/10.1016/j.anclin.2014.02.005   anesthesiology.theclinics.com

a particular procedure. Even with concentrated long-acting local anesthetic agents (eg, bupivacaine 0.5% and ropivacaine 0.5%–7.5%), the duration of postoperative analgesia typically last only for 12 to 24 hours. There are several potential disadvantages when injecting a large volume of concentrated local anesthetic agents, including an increased potential for local anesthetic systemic toxicity and residual dense sensory and motor block (**Box 1**), which is bothersome for some patients. In contrast, although continuous PNBs (CPNBs) do require additional time for placement, they have been shown to consistently provide superior analgesia compared with opioid-based analgesia and single-injection PNB techniques (**Box 2**).[11–13] It has been demonstrated that CPNBs may be successfully managed in the ambulatory setting if patient selection, patient expectations, and patient education are thoroughly addressed in the perioperative setting (**Box 3**, **Figs. 1** and **2**).[13–16]

For PNBs to gain more widespread use in the ambulatory setting, they must not only have predictably high success rates, but also be performed in an efficient manner, with few complications. The use of ultrasound guidance (USG) for PNBs provides improvements in overall block success (defined as surgical anesthesia), block onset, block quality, and decreases in local anesthetic requirements when compared with peripheral nerve stimulation (PNS).[17–21] More recent evidence provides further support that USG not only increases the success rate of CPNB placement, but also consistently decreases the block procedure time for peripheral nerve catheter placement, even in patients who are obese.[22,23] Although USG has not been shown to completely eliminate the most feared complications of local anesthetic systemic toxicity and peripheral nerve injury, recent evidence from large databases indicates that its use (compared with PNS techniques) significantly decreases the incidence of local anesthetic systemic toxicity.[24–26] Accompanying editorials largely support the view that

---

Box 1
Advantages and disadvantages of single-injection peripheral nerve block techniques

Advantages

- Provides effective analgesia for surgical procedures not expected to have moderate-to-severe postoperative pain for greater than 12–24 hours

- Decreased cost for equipment and supplies: does not require continuous peripheral nerve catheter kits (specialized needles, catheters), infusion pumps, and additional local-anesthetic infusion

- Decreased time for placement

- Single-injection techniques within training of most anesthesiologists

- Does not require dedicated 24-hour availability (acute pain service and/or 24-hour pager availability for outpatient management)

Disadvantages

- Risk of severe rebound pain ("midnight syndrome") in the ambulatory setting on resolution of single-injection analgesia

- Limited flexibility

  o Short-acting agents provide rapid onset of surgical anesthesia but a limited duration of analgesia (<6–8 hours)

  o Long-acting agents have slower onset of surgical anesthesia

  o Prolonged dense sensory analgesia and motor block may not be desirable in postoperative setting

Box 2
Advantages and disadvantages of continuous peripheral nerve block techniques

Advantages

- Provides effective analgesia for surgical procedures that are expected to result in moderate-to-severe pain lasting greater than 24 hours not expected to be well controlled with moderately potent oral analgesic (opioids) agents

- May allow more painful procedures traditionally requiring hospitalization to be converted to an outpatient or overnight admission procedure

- Increased flexibility in the perioperative setting

   ○ May use more concentrated short-acting (lidocaine 1.5% or mepivacaine 1.5%) local anesthetic agent resulting in rapid onset of surgical anesthesia (when desired) by needle or catheter

   ○ May redose shorter-acting local anesthetic agents tailored to expected duration of surgical procedure

   ○ May use more dilute (ropivacaine, 0.1%–0.2%, or bupivacaine, 0.1%–0.125%) local anesthetic agents to facilitate sensory-motor dissociation

Disadvantages

- Requires specialized equipment (catheter kits, infusion pumps, and infusate)

- Requires added skill set to place catheters

- Requires 24-hour 7-day-a-week management by a dedicated call-person and/or acute pain service

USG has become the dominant technique for placement of single-injection PNBs and CPNBs (**Box 4**).[27,28] A recent survey also indicates ultrasound-guided PNBs are universally taught across anesthesia training programs, and the primary barriers to ultrasound use were lack of teaching faculty training and timely availability of ultrasound equipment.[29]

The following sections provide a broad overview of the indications and clinically useful aspects of the most commonly used upper and lower extremity PNBs in the ambulatory setting. Emphasis is placed on approaches that can be used for single-injection PNBs and CPNBs techniques.

Box 3
Advantages of ultrasound guidance for peripheral nerve blocks

- Increased block success (surgical anesthesia) for specific blocks: brachial plexus blocks and popliteal sciatic nerve blocks for foot surgery

- Increased block quality

- Increased success rate for continuous peripheral nerve catheter placement

- Decreased procedural time for block placement

- Decreased number of needle passes

- Decrease in unintended vascular punctures

- Decreased local anesthetic requirements

- Decreased incidence of local anesthetic systemic toxicity

Adapted from Refs.[17–23]

To remove the catheter:

1. Remove the clear tape covering the catheter on your skin.

2. Grip the catheter about 2 inches from the point where it enters the skin.

3. Pull the catheter gently. It should come out with minimal resistance.

4. If it does not come out easily, DO NOT TRY TO REMOVE IT WITH FORCE, call the anesthesiologist to obtain further instructions.

5. Make sure all of the catheter came out (tip of the catheter is black - see arrow).

6. Cover the site with a bandaid.

Pump Instructions: How It works-
A small plastic tube (catheter) has been placed close to the nerves that control the feeling and movement of your arm. A numbing medication is pumped through the catheter, decreasing your pain.

A normal pump will purr like a cat, about every 30 seconds.

After pressing the 'boost' button, the motor will run every 3 seconds and return to normal function after the 'boost' dose is delivered.

Follow up:

● We will call you every day until the catheter is removed.
● If you are not at home, we will attempt to leave a message.

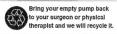 Bring your empty pump back to your surgeon or physical therapist and we will recycle it.

Feedback:
We are always working to improve our patient's experience and value your opinion. Please share your insights with us when we call.

Fig. 1. Standardized patient instructions on pump functions and perineural catheter removal.

UPPER EXTREMITY PNBS

The choice of brachial plexus block approaches is largely determined by the type of surgery (anatomic location of surgical stimulus) and individual patient anatomy.

Interscalene Block

An interscalene block refers to the injection of local anesthetic within the interscalene groove between the anterior and middle scalene muscles (**Fig. 3**). It is the most

General Considerations:

● Protect your arm. The blocked extremity is numb and often very weak.
● Be careful with hot, cold, hard, or sharp surfaces as you can get injured as your body will not feel pain or pressure.
● Avoid pulling or tugging on the catheter.
● Keep the catheter insertion site dry.
● Follow your surgeon's instructions regarding positioning, activity, and surgical dressing.
● Use caution with activity. While your arm is numb, your balance may be affected.

Normal reversible side-effects:
Slight redness and drooping of the eyelid on the same side as the pain catheter, hoarse voice and mild shortness of breath.
Shortness of breath may be worse while lying flat, so you may have to sit yourself up with several pillows.

General Considerations:

● Protect your leg and foot. The blocked extremity is numb and often very weak.
● Be careful with hot, cold, hard, or sharp surfaces as you can get injured as your body will not feel pain or pressure.
● Avoid pulling or tugging on the catheter.
● Keep the catheter insertion site dry.
● Follow your surgeon's instructions regarding positioning and surgical dressing.

RISK FOR FALLING!!!
Your nerve block can create a very weak leg and foot. This makes it potentially dangerous to stand or walk. Follow your surgeon's instructions regarding activity and use of crutches or walkers. Make sure you have plenty of help any time you get up.

Fig. 2. Standardized patient instructions and precautions for brachial plexus and lower extremity (femoral or sciatic) perineural catheters.

Box 4
Checklist for selection criteria for ambulatory continuous peripheral nerve blocks

Procedure with anticipated moderate-to-severe postoperative pain

Procedure with anticipated mild-to-moderate postoperative pain, but patient with clinically significant intolerance (eg, severe nausea or vomiting, obstructive sleep apnea) to postoperative opioid analgesia

Assess for chronic preoperative pain and/or chronic opioid consumption

Has a working telephone and can be reliably contacted

Patient (or designated caregiver) speaks English well enough to facilitate telephone follow-up

Mental status intact, no psychosocial issues that would cloud assessment of block

Lives within reasonable distance (and has reliable transportation) of a medical facility (could be primary care office, local emergency room, or urgent care)

No contraindications to regional anesthesia

Address concerns regarding clinical consequences of associated phrenic nerve block (interscalene or supraclavicular approaches)

Address concerns regarding baseline risk (preblock) of falling

---

commonly used approach to provide anesthesia-analgesia after shoulder procedures in the outpatient setting because it reliably blocks the upper roots (C5-C6 roots forming the upper trunk and the C7 root forming the middle trunk) of the brachial plexus.[30] Injection of local anesthetics at this level often spares the lower roots (C8, T1) making this block less suitable for procedures at or below the elbow.[31] The intense analgesia that is achieved with this block provides a dramatic reduction in opioid consumption after shoulder surgery; however, the duration of these blocks with conventional local anesthetics lasts less than 24 hours.[32] To provide extended analgesia of the shoulder, a catheter may be placed in the interscalene groove followed by continuous administration of a dilute local anesthetic solution (**Fig. 4**). This may extend the length of analgesia (from hours to days) and reduce the frequency of opioid-related side effects from

A   **B**

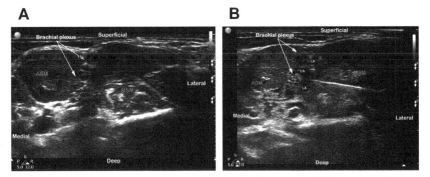

Fig. 3. (A) Sonographic image of the interscalene brachial plexus (ISBP). The brachial plexus elements appear as hypoechoic structures surrounded by hyperechoic connective tissue and are located between the anterior scalene muscle (ASM) and middle scalene muscle (MSM). (B) An example of USG short-axis in-plane technique (SAX-IP) for a single-injection ISBP. The block needle is advanced from lateral-to-medial through the MSM and approaches the posterior aspect of the roots-trunks of ISBP. Local anesthetic (LA) is seen surrounding the ISBP.

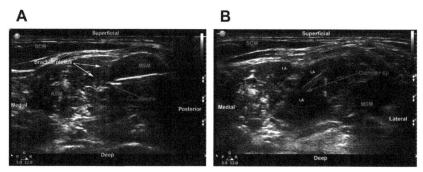

Fig. 4. (*A*) Sonographic image of USG continuous interscalene block using the SAX-IP technique. Note the larger 17-gauge needle to facilitate the passage of a 19-gauge perineural catheter. (*B*) The sonographic image confirms placement of the interscalene catheter and LA within the interscalene groove, immediately posterior to the ISBP. Note LA is also seen anterior to the ISBP. SCM, sternocleidomastoid muscle.

oral analgesics.[33–35] For procedures where brachial plexus analgesia provides complete coverage of the operative site, nonsteroidal anti-inflammatory drugs and acetaminophen alone may be adequate for analgesia in addition to an interscalene infusion of local anesthetics, thus completely eliminating the requirement for oral opioids. The most common side effects of interscalene blockade are ipsilateral phrenic nerve block and Horner syndrome. If a particular patient may not tolerate temporary paralysis of the hemidiaphragm, a catheter may be inserted with a shorter-acting local anesthetic and the patient may be observed in the postanesthesia care unit for complaints of subjective shortness of breath or respiratory compromise before being discharged home. Alternatively, USG has facilitated the use of significant reduction in local anesthetic volumes and/or concentrations to decrease (although not completely eliminate) phrenic nerve block when interscalene block is primarily for postoperative analgesia.[36–39] Large prospective case series have demonstrated a very low incidence of severe complications with either USG or PNS with the interscalene approach to brachial plexus block.[40–42]

Supraclavicular Block

Before the more widespread use of USG, many anesthesiologists had avoided the supraclavicular approach to brachial plexus block because of the concern of pneumothorax. Single-injection blocks at this site may provide similar analgesia to interscalene blocks but often miss the cape of the shoulder supplied by the cervical plexus (C2-C4).[30] The ability to visualize and differentiate the first rib from the pleura and important vascular structures (**Fig. 5**) with ultrasound has caused more widespread use of this block in clinical practice.[41,43–45] Contrary to popular belief, if the supraclavicular approach is to be used for surgical anesthesia, even with USG, it still requires the use of relatively large volumes of local anesthetic (approximately 30 mL). The addition of a catheter and infusion of local anesthetic at this site extends analgesia as with other techniques.[46,47]

Infraclavicular Block

This block is ideally suited for surgeries of the elbow, forearm, wrist, and hand where a single injection of local anesthetic may spread to the posterior, medial, and lateral cords and their corresponding terminal branches (**Fig. 6**). This is the last site where a single injection of local anesthetic may be deposited before the musculocutaneous

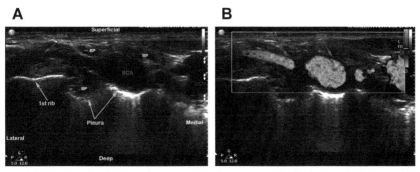

Fig. 5. (*A*) Sonographic image of USG approach to a supraclavicular brachial plexus block. The first rib (with typical posterior acoustic dropout) and the pleura (located deep to the inferior trunk-divisions of brachial plexus [BP], and with a typical "shimmering" appearance) both appear hyperechoic. The dorsal scapular artery (DSA) is seen coming directly off the subclavian artery (SCA) and appears to pass through the inferior and middle trunks of the BP. The subclavian vein (SCV) is seen medial to the anterior scalene muscle. (*B*) Color flow Doppler representation of **Fig. 3**A, confirming and clearly demonstrating the DSA branching directly off the SCA.

and axillary nerves branch from the brachial plexus.[30] Because this block is below the clavicle, concerns for phrenic nerve block are also diminished at this injection site making it an ideal technique for patients with pulmonary compromise. The steep trajectory of this block may also make USG needle visualization difficult. Frequent small injections of local anesthetic or saline may be required as a surrogate indicator of needle tip location until proper spread of local anesthetic deposited posterior to the axillary artery creates the "double bubble" sign. As with PNS, local anesthetic should be targeted at the posterior cord, which facilitates subsequent spread to the medial and lateral cords. In fact, a single injection posterior to the axillary artery has been shown to be as effective (and more efficient) as an injection near each of the three separate cords.[48–52] The addition of a catheter at this site may indefinitely extend analgesia. In addition, these catheters are well tolerated by patients (much

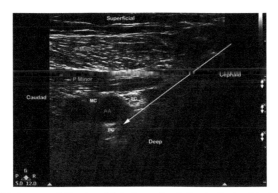

Fig. 6. Sonographic image of the brachial plexus for infraclavicular block. Note the neuro-vascular bundle is located deep to the pectoralis major and minor muscles. The axillary artery (AA) is located cephalad to the axillary vein (AV), and is surrounded by the cords of the brachial plexus. The *arrow* depicts a typical needle approach with the optimal target for needle placement (or catheter insertion) deep to the axillary artery. The posterior cord (PC) is typically located deep to the AA. LC, lateral cord; MC, medial cord.

like subclavian central lines) and an occlusive dressing keeps them securely in place. When compared with the supraclavicular approach, infraclavicular catheters provide superior analgesia requiring patients to take fewer supplemental opioids for break-through pain for procedures at or distal to the elbow.[53] When USG is used, blocks may be facilitated by abduction of the arm, which allows for the posterior movement of the clavicle and reduction of skin to nerve distance to enhance needle visualization.[54,55]

Axillary Block

The blockade of the terminal branches of the brachial plexus to the forearm, wrist, and hand is known as the axillary block. It is performed in the axillary fossa by a wide variety of techniques (landmark, periarterial, transarterial, PNS, and USG).[30] It is a widely used block for ambulatory surgery given its long history, relative safety profile, and ease of compressibility in the event of a vascular puncture. Although the orientation of the median, ulnar, and radial nerves around the axillary artery are variable,[56–58] an injection of anesthetics anterior and posterior to it under direct visual guidance (ultrasound) is as effective as an injection around each of the terminal branches around the artery (**Fig. 7**).[59]

The placement of catheters in the axilla has been reported,[60,61] but the inherent instability of this location makes fixation of these catheters more difficult than those placed at more proximal sites. We recommend the use of interscalene catheters for shoulder procedures and infraclavicular catheters for elbow, forearm, and hand procedures. Growing concerns about the use of intra-articular injections and/or continuous infusions of local anesthetic into the shoulder joint and the devastating complication of postarthroscopic glenohumeral chrondrolysis will likely further increase the need for continuous interscalene blocks.[62,63] A supraclavicular might be used based on practitioner experience; surgical procedure; and patient factors, such as body mass index or mobility.

LOWER EXTREMITY PNBS

The benefits of lower extremity PNBs are increasingly recognized in the surgical literature.[64]

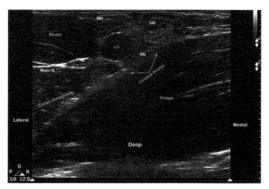

Fig. 7. Sonographic image of the brachial plexus for the axillary approach. The median nerve (MN), ulnar nerve (UN), and radial nerve (RN) are located around the axillary artery (AA). The musculocutaneous nerve (Musc N) is most often located within the body of the coracobrachialis muscle. The brachial plexus lies directly superficial to the conjoint tendon.

Femoral Nerve Block

The femoral nerve contributes sensory innervation to the hip joint, knee joint, and the medial aspect of the ankle joint.[65] The femoral nerve is located just lateral to the femoral artery and deep to the fascia iliaca (**Fig. 8**). USG has been shown to increase the quality of sensory block and to facilitate the efficient placement of continuous femoral nerve block (FNB).[20,66] It also provides sensory motor innervation to the anterior thigh, quadriceps muscles, and the skin of the medial lower leg. Although FNB is most commonly used to provide postoperative analgesia after minor (knee arthroscopy) and major knee surgery (arthroscopic anterior cruciate ligament [ACL] reconstruction), it has also been reported to provide effective rescue analgesia after ambulatory hip arthroscopy.[67] Although the anesthesia literature strongly supports the analgesic benefits of single-injection[68] and continuous FNB[69,70] for arthroscopic ACL reconstruction, the surgical literature has recently called these benefits into question,[71] especially with the increasing use of autologous hamstring grafts.[72] A recent systematic review and meta-analysis demonstrated an increased risk of falls associated with continuous FNBs in orthopedic surgery patients undergoing major lower extremity knee surgery.[73] Given the concerns about the risk of falls associated with FNB, the use of USG has facilitated the development of selective blockade of the saphenous nerve within the adductor canal[74] (with associated block of the nerve to the vastus medialis and sensory contribution of the obturator nerve to the knee joint) or deep to the distal aspect of the sartorius muscle. These selective approaches have been shown to improve analgesia after minor[75,76] and major knee surgery[77] with a clinically significant decrease in quadriceps motor block.[78,79] Further research is needed to evaluate the risk-benefit ratio of continuous FNB for arthroscopic ACL repair, and the indications and possible benefits of the recently developed adductor canal block for ambulatory knee surgery. Recent data indicate that blockade of the femoral nerve[80] or proximal saphenous nerve[81,82] has been shown to provide significant benefit in ambulatory ankle surgery.

Sciatic Nerve Block

Popliteal sciatic nerve blocks have consistently been shown to improve analgesia and quality of recovery after major ambulatory foot and ankle surgery.[2,83–85] The sciatic

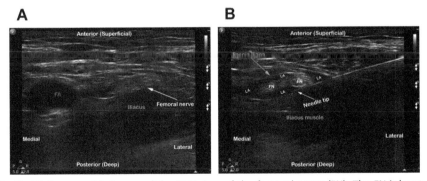

A   **B**

Fig. 8. (A) Sonographic image of the SAX view of the femoral nerve (FN). The FN is located just lateral to the femoral artery (FA) and immediately superficial to the iliacus muscle. (B) Sonographic image of the USG SAX-IP technique for single-injection FNB. The needle approach is from lateral-to-medial. The needle tip is manipulated to facilitate circumferential local anesthetic (LA) distribution if desired. Note the enhanced appearance of the hyperechoic fascia iliaca just superficial to the FN after the LA has been injected.

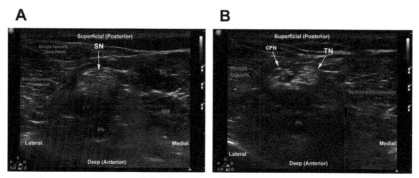

Fig. 9. (*A*) Sonographic image of the SAX view of the sciatic nerve (SN) in the popliteal fossa. The SN is easily identified as a hyperechoic polyfasicular (honeycomb appearance) structure located deep to the popliteal vein (PV) and artery (PA). The distal aspects of the semimembranosus (SM) and semitendinosis (ST) muscles are medial to the SN and the biceps femoris forms the lateral border of the popliteal fossa. (*B*) SAX view just distal to the bifurcation of the SN with the common peroneal nerve (CPN) and tibial nerve (TN) beginning to diverge.

nerve is most commonly blocked within the popliteal fossa.[30] USG facilitates identification of the common sciatic nerve and bifurcation into the tibial nerve and common peroneal nerve trunks (**Fig. 9**), and has been shown to increase block success for single-injection and continuous sciatic nerve blocks compared with PNS.[20,22] USG further improves the efficacy of popliteal sciatic nerve block by facilitating separate blockade of the individual tibial nerve and common peroneal nerve trunks just distal to the sciatic nerve bifurcation.[86,87] More recent data indicate that USG-facilitated injection just deep to the paraneural sheath of the popliteal sciatic nerve block provides even further improvements in block onset and block success.[88,89]

SUMMARY

PNBs provide significant improvements in postoperative analgesia and quality of recovery for ambulatory surgery. Use of CPNB techniques further improves these benefits beyond the duration of single-injection PNBs. The use of USG has significantly improved the success, safety, and efficiency of PNBs, and as a result has contributed to the increased use of PNBs in the ambulatory setting.

REFERENCES

1. Liu SS, Strodtbeck WM, Richman JM, et al. A comparison of regional versus general anesthesia for ambulatory anesthesia: a meta-analysis of randomized controlled trials. Anesth Analg 2005;101(6):1634–42.
2. Capdevila X, Dadure C, Bringuier S, et al. Effect of patient-controlled perineural analgesia on rehabilitation and pain after ambulatory orthopedic surgery. Anesthesiology 2006;105(3):566–73.
3. Rawal N, Hylander J, Nydahl PA, et al. Survey of postoperative analgesia following ambulatory surgery. Acta Anaesthesiol Scand 1997;41(8):1017–22.
4. Chung F, Mezei G. Factors contributing to a prolonged stay after ambulatory surgery. Anesth Analg 1999;89(6):1352–9.
5. Pavlin DL, Chen C, Penaloza DA, et al. Pain as a factor complicating recovery and discharge after ambulatory surgery. Anesth Analg 2002;95(3):627–34.

6. Hadzic A, Arliss J, Kerimoglu B, et al. A comparison of infraclavicular block versus general anesthesia for hand and wrist day-case surgeries. Anesthesiology 2004;101(1):127–32.

7. McCartney CJ, Brull R, Chan VW, et al. Early, but no long-term benefit of regional compared to general anesthesia for ambulatory hand surgery. Anesthesiology 2004;101(2):461–7.

8. Hadzic A, Williams BA, Karaca PE, et al. For outpatient rotator cuff surgery, nerve block anesthesia provides superior same-day recovery over general anesthesia. Anesthesiology 2005;102(5):1001–7.

9. Williams BA, Kentor ML, Vogt MT, et al. Economics of nerve block pain management after anterior cruciate ligament reconstruction: potential hospital cost savings via associated postanesthesia care unit bypass and same-day discharge. Anesthesiology 2004;100(3):697–706.

10. Koh AL, Levin SD, Chehab EL, et al. Neer award 2012: cerebral oxygenation in the beach chair position: a prospective study on the effect of general anesthesia compared with regional anesthesia sedation. J Shoulder Elbow Surg 2013; 22(10):1325–31.

11. Richman JM, Liu SS, Courpass G, et al. Does continuous peripheral nerve block provide superior pain control to opioids: a meta-analysis. Anesth Analg 2006; 102(1):248–57.

12. Ilfeld BM. Continuous peripheral nerve blocks: a review of the published evidence. Anesth Analg 2011;113(4):904–25.

13. Binhgham AE, Fu R, Horn JL, et al. Continuous peripheral nerve blocks compared with single-injection peripheral nerve block: a systemic review and meta-analysis of randomized controlled trials. Reg Anesth Pain Med 2012; 37(6):583–94.

14. Ilfeld BM. Continuous peripehral nerve blocks in the hospital and home. Anaesthesiol Clin 2011;29(2):193–211.

15. Swenson JD, Cheng GS, Axelrod DA, et al. Ambulatory anesthesia and regional catheters: when and how. Anaesthesiol Clin 2010;28(2):267–80.

16. Swenson JD, Bay N, Loose E, et al. Outpatient management of continuous peripehral nerve catheters using ultrasound: an experience with 602 patients. Anesth Analg 2006;103(6):1436–43.

17. Abrahams MS, Aziz MF, Fu RF, et al. Ultrasound guidance compared with electrical neurostimulation for peripheral nerve blocks: a systemic review and meta-analysis of randomized controlled trials. Br J Anaesth 2009;102(3):408–17.

18. Liu SS, Ngeow J, John RS. Evidence basis for ultrasound-guided block characteristics: onset, quality, and duration. Reg Anesth Pain Med 2010;35(Suppl 2): S26–53.

19. McCartney CJ, Lin L, Shastri U. Evidence basis for ultrasound-guided upper extremity blocks. Reg Anesth Pain Med 2010;35(Suppl 2):S10–5.

20. Salinas FV. Ultrasound and review of the evidence for lower extremity peripheral nerve blocks. Reg Anesth Pain Med 2010;35(Suppl 2):S16–25.

21. Gelfand HJ, Quanes JP, Lesley MR, et al. Analgesic efficacy of ultrasound-guided regional anesthesia: a meta-analysis. J Clin Anesth 2011;23(2):90–6.

22. Schnabel A, Meyer-Freibem CH, Zahn PK, et al. Ultrasound compared with nerve stimulation guidance for peripheral nerve catheter placement: a meta-analysis of randomized controlled trials. Br J Anaesth 2013;111(4):564–72.

23. Mariano ER, Brodsky JB. Comparison of procedural times for ultrasound-guided perineural catheter insertion in obese and nonobese patients. J Ultrasound Med 2011;301(10):1357–61.

24. Sites BD, Taenzer AH, Herrick MD, et al. Incidence of local anesthetic systemic toxicity and postoperative neurological symptoms associated with 12,668 ultrasound-guided nerve blocks: a prospective clinical registry. Reg Anesth Pain Med 2012;37(5):478–82.

25. Orebaugh SL, Kentor ML, Williams BA. Adverse outcomes associated with nerve stimulator guided and ultrasound-guided peripheral nerve blocks by supervised trainees: update of a single-site database. Reg Anesth Pain Med 2012; 37(6):577–82.

26. Barrington MJ, Kluger R. Ultrasound guidance reduces the risk of local anesthetic systemic toxicity following peripehral nerve blockade. Reg Anesth Pain Med 2013;38(4):289–99.

27. Laur JJ, Weinberg GL. Comparing safety in surface landmarks versus ultrasound-guided peripheral nerve blocks: an observational study of a transition in practice. Reg Anesth Pain Med 2012;37(6):569–70.

28. Neal JM. Local anesthetic systemic toxicity: improving patient safety one step at a time. Reg Anesth Pain Med 2013;38(4):259–61.

29. Helwani MA, Saied NN, Asaad B, et al. The current role of ultrasound use in teaching regional anesthesia: a survey of residency programs in the United States. Pain Med 2012;13(10):1342–6.

30. Neal JM, Gerancher JC, Hebl JR, et al. Upper extremity regional anesthesia: essentials of our current understanding, 2008. Reg Anesth Pain Med 2009;34: 134–70.

31. Madison SJ, Humsi J, Loland VJ, et al. Ultrasound-guided root/trunk (interscalene) block for hand and forearm anesthesia. Reg Anesth Pain Med 2013;38: 226–32.

32. Gadsden J, Hadzic A, Gandhi K, et al. The effect of mixing 1.5% mepivacaine and 0.5% bupivacaine on duration of analgesia and latency of block onset in ultrasound-guided interscalene block. Anesth Analg 2011;112:471–6.

33. Borgeat A, Perschak H, Bird P, et al. Patient-controlled interscalene analgesia with ropivacaine 0.2% versus patient-controlled intravenous analgesia after major shoulder surgery: effects on diaphragmatic and respiratory function. Anesthesiology 2000;91(1):102–8.

34. Ilfeld BM, Morey TE, Wright TW, et al. Continuous interscalene brachial plexus block for postoperative pain control at home: a randomized, double-blind, placebo-controlled study. Anesth Analg 2003;96(4):1089–95.

35. Fredrickson MJ, Ball CM, Dalgleish AJ. Analgesic effectiveness of continuous versus single-injection interscalene brachial plexus block for minor arthroscopic shoulder surgery. Reg Anesth Pain Med 2010;35(1):28–33.

36. Riazi S, Carmichael N, Awad I, et al. Effect of anaesthetic volume on the efficacy and respiratory consequences of ultrasound-guided interscalene block. Br J Anaesth 2008;101(4):549–56.

37. McNaught A, Shastri U, Carmichael N, et al. Ultrasound reduces the minimum effective local anaesthetic volume compared with peripheral nerve stimulation for interscalene block. Br J Anaesth 2011;106(6):124–30.

38. Falcão LF, Perez MV, de Castro I, et al. Minimum effective volume of 0.5% bupivacaine with epinephrine in ultrasound-guided interscalene brachial plexus block. Br J Anaesth 2013;110(3):450–5.

39. Thackery EM, Swenson JD, Gertsch MC, et al. Diaphragm function after interscalene brachial plexus block: a doubled-blind, randomized comparison of 0.25% and 0.125% bupivacaine. J Shoulder Elbow Surg 2013;22(3): 381–6.

40. Borgeat A, Ekatodramis G, Kalberer F, et al. Acute and nonacute complications with interscalene block and shoulder surgery. Anesthesiology 2001;95(4): 875–80.
41. Liu SS, Gordon MA, Shaw PM, et al. A prospective clinical registry of ultrasound-guided regional anesthesia for ambulatory shoulder surgery. Anesth Analg 2010;111(3):617–23.
42. Singh A, Kelly C, O'Brien T, et al. Ultrasound-guided interscalene block anesthesia for shoulder arthroscopy: a prospective study of 1319 patients. J Bone Joint Surg 2012;94(22):2040–6.
43. Soares LG, Brull R, Lai J, et al. Eight ball, corner pocket: the optimal needle position for ultrasound-guided supraclavicular block. Reg Anesth Pain Med 2007; 32:94–5.
44. Perlas A, Lobo G, Lo N, et al. Ultrasound-guided supraclavicular block: outcome of 510 consecutive cases. Reg Anesth Pain Med 2009;34(2):171–6.
45. Murata H, Sakai A, Hadzic A, et al. The presence of cervical and transverse cervical arteries at three ultrasound probe positions commonly used in supraclavicular brachial plexus bloc. Anesth Analg 2012;115(2):470–3.
46. Tran DQ, Dugani S, Correa JA, et al. Minimum effective volume of lidocaine for ultrasound-guided supraclavicular block. Reg Anesth Pain Med 2011;36(5): 466–9.
47. Kant A, Gupta PK, Zohar S, et al. Application of continual reassessment method to dose-finding studies in regional anesthesia: an estimate of the ED95 dose for 0.5% bupivacaine for ultrasound-guided supraclavicular block. Anesthesiology 2013;119(1):29–35.
48. Tran DQ, Clemente A, Tran DQ, et al. A comparison between ultrasound-guided infraclavicular block using the "double bubble" sign and neurostimulation-guided axillary block. Anesth Analg 2008;107(3):1075–8.
49. Desgagnés MC, Lévesque S, Dion N, et al. A comparison of a single or triple injection technique for ultrasound-guided infraclavicular block: a prospective randomized controlled study. Anesth Analg 2009;109(2):668–72.
50. De Tran QH, Bertini P, Zaouter C, et al. A prospective randomized comparison between single- and double-injection ultrasound-guided infraclavicular block. Reg Anesth Pain Med 2010;35(1):16–21.
51. Fredrickson MJ, Wolstencroft P, Kejriwal R, et al. Single versus triple injection ultrasound-guided infraclavicular block: confirmation of the effectives of a single injection technique. Anesth Analg 2010;111(5):1325–7.
52. Chin KJ, Alakkad H, Adhikary SD, et al. Infraclavicular brachial plexus block for regional anaesthesia of the lower arm. Cochrane Database Syst Rev 2013;(8):CD005487.
53. Mariano ER, Sandhu NS, Loland VJ, et al. A randomized comparison of infraclavicular and supraclavicular continuous peripheral nerve blocks for postoperative analgesia. Reg Anesth Pain Med 2011;36(1):26–31.
54. Ruíz A, Sala X, Bargalló X, et al. The influence of arm abduction on the anatomic relations of infraclavicular brachial plexus: an ultrasound study. Anesth Analg 2009;108:364–6.
55. Auyong DB, Gonzales J, Benonis JG. The Houdini clavicle: arm abduction and needle insertion site adjustment improves needle visibility for the infraclavicular nerve block. Reg Anesth Pain Med 2010;35(4):403–4.
56. Christophe JL, Bertheir F, Boillot F, et al. Assessment of topographical brachial plexus nerves variations at the axillar using ultrasonography. Br J Anaesth 2009; 103(4):606–12.

57. Gray AT. The conjoint tendon of the latissimus dorsi and teres major: an important landmark for ultrasound-guided axillary block. Reg Anesth Pain Med 2009; 34(2):179–80.

58. Remerand F, Lailan J, Couvret C, et al. Is the musculocutaneous nerve really in the coracobrachialis muscle when performing an axillary block? An ultrasound study. Anesth Analg 2010;110(6):1729–34.

59. Imasogie N, Ganapathy S, Singh S, et al. A prospective, randomized, double-blind comparison of ultrasound-guided axillary brachial plexus blocks using 2 versus 4 injections. Anesth Analg 2010;110(4):1222–6.

60. Bergman BD, Hebl JR, Kent J, et al. Neurologic complications of 405 consecutive continuous axillary catheters. Anesth Analg 2003;96(1):247–52.

61. Salonen MH, Haasio J, Bachmann M, et al. Evaluation of efficacy and plasma concentrations of ropivacaine in continuous axillary brachial plexus block: high dose for surgical anesthesia and low dose for postoperative analgesia. Reg Anesth Pain Med 2000;25(1):47–51.

62. Scheffel PT, Clinton J, Lynch JR, et al. Glenohumeral chrondrolysis: a systemic review of 100 cases from the English language literature. J Shoulder Elbow Surg 2010;19(6):944–9.

63. Wiater BP, Neradilek MB, Polissar NL, et al. Risk factors for chrondrolysis of the glenohumeral joint: a study of three hundred and seventy-five shoulder arthroscopic procedures in the practice of an individual community surgeon. J Bone Joint Surg 2012;93(7):615–25.

64. Stein BE, Srikumaran U, Tan EW, et al. Lower-extremity peripheral nerve blocks in the perioperative pain management of orthopaedic patients. J Bone Joint Surg 2012;94:e167.

65. Enneking FK, Chan V, Greger J, et al. Lower-extremity peripehral nerve blocks: essentials of our current understanding. Reg Anesth Pain Med 2005;30(1):4–35.

66. Mariano ER, Loland VJ, Sandhu NS, et al. Ultrasound guidance versus electrical stimulation for femoral perineural stimulation. J Ultrasound Med 2009;28(11):1453–60.

67. Ward JP, Albert DB, Altman R, et al. Are femoral nerve blocks effective for early postoperative pain management after hip arthroscopy? Arthroscopy 2012;28(8):1064–9.

68. Mulroy MF, Larkin KL, Batra MS, et al. Femoral nerve block with 0.25% or 0.5% bupivacaine improves postoperative analgesia following outpatient anterior cruciate ligament reconstruction. Reg Anesth Pain Med 2001;26(1):24–9.

69. Williams BA, Kentor ML, Vogt MT, et al. Reduction of verbal pain scores after anterior cruciate ligament reconstruction with 2-day continuous femoral nerve block. Anesthesiology 2006;104(2):315–27.

70. Dauri M, Fabbi E, Mariani P, et al. Continuous femoral nerve block provides superior analgesia compared with continuous intra-articular and wound infusion after anterior cruciate ligament reconstruction. Reg Anesth Pain Med 2009; 34(2):95–9.

71. Mall NA, Wright RW. Femoral nerve block use in anterior cruciate ligament reconstruction surgery. Arthroscopy 2010;26(3):404–16.

72. Bushnell BD, Sakyrd G, Noonan TJ. Hamstring donor-site block: evaluation of pain control after anterior cruciate ligament reconstruction. Arthroscopy 2010; 26(7):894–9.

73. Johnson RL, Kopp SL, Hebl JR, et al. Falls and major orthopaedic surgery with peripheral nerve blocks: a systematic review and meta-analysis. Br J Anaesth 2013;110(40):518–28.

74. Lund J, Jenstrup MT, Jaeger P, et al. Continuous adductor-canal-blockade for adjuvant post-operative analgesia after major knee surgery: preliminary results. Acta Anaesthesiol Scand 2011;55:14–9.

75. Hsu LP, Oh S, Nuber GW, et al. Nerve block of the infrapatellar branch of the saphenous nerve in knee arthroscopy: a prospective, double-blinded, randomized, placebo-controlled trial. J Bone Joint Surg 2013;95(16):1465–72.

76. Hanson NA, Derby RE, Auyong DA, et al. Ultrasound-guided adductor canal block for arthroscopic medial menisectomy: a randomized, double-blind trial. Can J Anaesth 2013;60(9):874–80.

77. Jaeger P, Grevstad U, Henningsen MH, et al. Effect of adductor-canal-blockade on established, severe pain after total knee arthroplasty: a randomized study. Acta Anaesthesiol Scand 2012;56(8):1013–9.

78. Jaeger P, Nielsen ZJ, Henningsen MH, et al. Adductor canal block versus femoral nerve block and quadriceps strength: a randomized, double-blind, placebo-controlled, cross-over study. Anesthesiology 2013;118(2):409–15.

79. Kwofie MK, Shastri UD, Gadsden JC, et al. The effects of ultrasound-guided adductor canal block versus femoral nerve block on quadriceps strength and fall risk: a randomized trial of volunteers. Reg Anesth Pain Med 2013;38(4):321–5.

80. Blumenthal S, Borgeat A, Neudorfer C, et al. Additional femoral catheter in combination with popliteal catheter for analgesia after major ankle surgery. Br J Anaesth 2011;106(30):387–93.

81. Green JS, Dilalne D, Tsui BC. Adductor canal nerve for postoperative management of medial ankle pain following ankle fusion. Acta Anaesthesiol Scand 2013;57(2):264.

82. Chen J, Lesser J, Hadzic A, et al. The importance of the proximal saphenous nerve for foot and ankle surgery. Reg Anesth Pain Med 2013;38(4):372.

83. Ilfeld BM, Morey TE, Wang RD, et al. Continuous popliteal sciatic nerve block for postoperative pain control at home: a randomized, double-blind, placebo-controlled study. Anesthesiology 2002;97(4):959–65.

84. White PF, Issioui T, Skrivanek GD, et al. The use of continuous popliteal sciatic nerve block after surgery involving the foot and ankle: does it improve the quality of recovery? Anesth Analg 2003;97(5):1303–9.

85. Hunt KJ, Higgins TF, Carlston VC, et al. Continuous peripheral nerve blockade as postoperative analgesia for open treatment of calcaneal fractures. J Orthop Trauma 2010;24(3):148–55.

86. Buys MJ, Arndt CD, Vagh F, et al. Ultrasound-guided sciatic nerve block in the popliteal fossa using lateral approach: onset time comparing separate tibial and common peroneal nerve injections versus injecting proximal to the bifurcation. Anesth Analg 2010;110(2):635–7.

87. Prasad A, Perlas A, Ramlogan R, et al. Ultrasound-guided popliteal block distal to the sciatic nerve bifurcation shortens onset time: a prospective randomized double-blind study. Reg Anesth Pain Med 2010;35(3):267–71.

88. Tran de QH, Dugani S, Pham K, et al. A randomized comparison between subepineural and conventional ultrasound-guided popliteal sciatic nerve block. Reg Anesth Pain Med 2011;36(6):548–52.

89. Perlas A, Wong P, Abdallah F, et al. Ultrasound-guided popliteal block through a common paraneural sheath versus conventional injection: a prospective, randomized, double-blind study. Reg Anesth Pain Med 2013;38(3):218–25.

Neuraxial Anesthesia for Outpatients

Elizabeth A. Alley, MD*, Michael F. Mulory, MD

KEYWORDS

- Local anesthetics • Neuraxial anesthesia • Spinal anesthesia • Epidural anesthesia
- Ambulatory anesthesia

KEY POINTS

- Spinal anesthesia with preservative-free 2-chloroprocaine offers a favorable side-effect profile and discharge times for certain ambulatory surgery procedures lasting less than 60 minutes.
- For procedures of longer duration, epidural or combined spinal epidural anesthesia may provide longer anesthesia without prolonged recovery.
- Choosing shorter-acting agents with favorable side-effect profiles will allow for a successful anesthetic plan and timely discharge in the ambulatory setting.

INTRODUCTION

Neuraxial anesthesia can be an outstanding choice for appropriate ambulatory surgery patients undergoing procedures of 60- to 90-minute duration, such as knee arthroscopy, hernia repair, and extracorporeal shock wave lithotripsy (ESWL).[1] Spinal anesthesia with short-acting agents has been shown to have a favorable side-effect profile and discharge times[2] compared with general anesthesia in the outpatient setting (**Table 1**).[3,4] Neuraxial anesthetics are associated with reduced pain scores and a decreased need for postanesthesia care unit (PACU) analgesics (**Table 2**).[5]

SELECTION OF AGENTS

Lidocaine has been used for short spinal anesthetics for decades.[6] Although lidocaine provides reliable results for outpatient anesthesia (**Table 3**),[7,8] ito uoo hao decreased in the outpatient setting because of transient neurologic symptoms (TNS).[9] Alternative agents have been studied.[10]

Bupivacaine has been used as one alternative to lidocaine for some outpatient procedures. Bupivacaine in as low of a dose as 4 mg intrathecally provides an average

No financial support or relationships were involved in the production of this article.
Department of Anesthesia, Virginia Mason Medical Center, B2-AN, 1100 Ninth Avenue, Post Box 900, Seattle, WA 98101, USA
* Corresponding author.
E-mail address: Elizabeth.Alley@vmmc.org

Table 1
Anesthetic-related side effects and patient satisfaction in the ilioinguinal hypogastric nerve block–monitored anesthesia care, general anesthesia, or spinal anesthesia for inguinal herniorrhaphy procedures

	IHNB-MAC (Group 1)	General Anesthesia (Group 2)	Spinal Anesthesia (Group 3)
Postoperative side effects (n [%])			
Backache	0	0	6 (24)[ab]
Drowsiness	4 (14)	15 (54)[a]	3 (12)[b]
Headache	2 (7)	4 (14)	3 (12)
Knee weakness	3 (11)	1 (4)	3 (12)
Muscle aches	0	2 (7)	0
Nausea and/or vomiting	2 (7)	17 (61)[a]	3 (12)[b]
Pruritus	0	0	6 (24)[ab]
Sore throat	0	6 (22)[a]	2 (8)[b]
Urine retention	0	0	5 (20)[ab]
Maximum nausea VAS (mm)	1 ± 5	27 ± 27[a]	4 ± 1[b]
Maximum pain VAS (mm)	15 ± 14	39 ± 28[a]	34 ± 32[b]
Oral analgesia after discharge (n [%])	16 (57)	18 (64)	17 (68)
Satisfaction with anesthetic technique			
Poor	0	0	0
Good	7 (25)	18 (64)[a]	9 (36)
Excellent	21 (75)	10 (36)[a]	16 (64)

Abbreviations: IHNB-MAC, ilioinguinal hypogastric nerve block–monitored anesthesia care; n, numbers; VAS, visual analog scale.
  [a] P<.05 versus IHNB-MAC group.
  [b] P<.05 versus general anesthesia group.
From Song D, Greilich N, White P, et al. Recovery profiles and costs of anesthesia for outpatient unilateral inguinal herniorrhaphy. Anesth Analg 2000;91(4):879; with permission.

PACU discharge time of 65 to 98 minutes (**Fig. 1**), which is reasonable for an outpatient setting but is associated with 4% failure rates.[11] Other researchers have studied patients receiving 5.0 mg and 7.5 mg bupivacaine in the lateral position as to provide a unilateral block.[12] Researchers have reported a wide variation of recovery profiles for bupivacaine spinals (greater than 300 minutes), which makes bupivacaine not suitable for outpatient anesthesia (**Fig. 2**).[13] The failure rate of a low dose combined with the erratic discharge of higher doses makes bupivacaine a less desirable choice for outpatients.

Preservative-free 2-chloroprocaine (2-CPC) spinal anesthesia has been increasing in use over the past decade despite concern about possible neurotoxicity based on case reports with previous preservative-containing preparations. Preservative-free 2-CPC has now been approved for use as an intrathecal anesthetic in Europe. Forty milligrams of 2-CPC has shown a reliable anesthetic time of 60 minutes, with 120 minutes to discharge ready with a very narrow range of variability.[14] A review of more than 4000 patients at one institution revealed no signs of nerve damage and a rare incidence of TNS (**Fig. 3**). In this review, patients receiving 2-CPC were ready for discharge close to an hour before patients receiving lidocaine 60 mg (171 vs 224).[15]

Table 2
Effects of central neuraxial block versus general anesthesia on ambulatory surgical patients

Outcome	n	Number of Trials	Central Neuraxial Block[a] (Mean)	General Anesthesia[a] (Mean)	OR or WMD[b] (95% Confidence Interval)	P Value
Anesthesia induction time (min)	384	7	17.8	7.8	8.1 (4.1–12.1)	.0001
PACU time (min)	476	10	56.1	51.9	0.42 (−7.1 to −7.9)	.91
VAS in PACU (mm)	563	7	12.7	24.4	−9 (−15.5 to −2.6)	.006
Nausea	637	12	5%	14.7%	0.40 (0.15–1.06)	.06
Phase 1 bypass	218	4	30.8%	13.5%	5.4 (0.6–53.6)	.15
Need for postoperative analgesics	716	11	31%	56%	0.32 (0.18–0.57)	.0001
Time until discharge from ASU (min)	839	14	190	153	34.6 (13–56.1)	.002
Excellent patient satisfaction	709	11	81%	78%	1.5 (0.8–23.1)	.45

Fifteen randomized controlled trials with 1003 patients were included for meta-analyses.
Abbreviations: ASU, ambulatory surgical unit; OR, odds ratio; POD, postoperative day; VAS, visual analog scale; WMD, weighted mean difference.
[a] Weighted by subject number.
[b] Weighted by inverse variance.
From Spencer L, Strodtbeck W, Richman J, et al. A comparison of regional versus general anesthesia for ambulatory anesthesia: a meta-analysis of randomized controlled trials. Anesth Analg 2005;101(6):1634–42; with permission.

Table 3
Postoperative follow-up

	LA/PI (%)	SAB$_{MLF}$ (%)
Evening after discharge		
Difficulty voiding[a]	2	2
Pain	88	76
Nausea	32	24
Pruritus	16	46[b]
Headache	20	12
Dizziness	12	8
Evening of postoperative day 2		
Headache[c]	8	10
Backache[d] (%) none-mild-moderate-severe	84–12–4–0	82–12–6–0
Satisfaction[e] (%)	2–8–26–64	4–6–30–60
Choose same anesthetic?	90	92

Abbreviations: LA/PI, local anesthetic + titrated propofol infusion; SAB$_{MLF}$, minidose lidocaine-fentanyl spinal anesthesia.
[a] One patient per group, both patients had mild difficulty initiating voiding (first void only).
[b] P<.05 compared with LA/PI group.
[c] None were characteristic of spinal headaches.
[d] Two cases (4%) of transient neurologic symptoms, mild-moderate in severity, duration 3 days or less.
[e] Satisfaction scale: dissatisfied-moderately satisfied-satisfied-very satisfied.
From Bruce BD, DeMeo P, Lucyk C, et al. A comparison of minidose lidocaine-fentanyl spinal anesthesia and local anesthesia/propofol infusion for outpatient knee arthroscopy. Anesth Analg 2001;93(2):323; with permission.

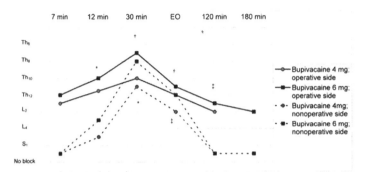

Fig. 1. The median upper limit of sensory block on the operative and nonoperative side at times shown after spinal anesthesia with hyperbaric bupivacaine 4 mg or hyperbaric bupivacaine 6 mg. The bandage obstructed the evaluation of the sensory block on the operative side after the operation. * P P P<.001 between the groups. EO, end of operation; *$P \leq 0.05$; [†]$P<0.01$; [‡]$P<0.001$. (*From* Valanne J, Korhonen AM, Jokela R, et al. Selective spinal anesthesia: a comparison of hyperbaric bupivacaine 4 mg vs 6 mg for outpatient knee arthroscopy. Anesth Analg 2001;93(6):1378; with permission.)

EPIDURAL ANESTHESIA

Epidural anesthesia can be useful for longer ambulatory surgery cases or situations of unclear case duration. Epidural anesthesia has used in ambulatory procedures involving lower-extremity surgery, hernia repair, and lower-abdomen laparoscopy.[16–18] Operating room turnover time, postanesthesia recovery and time to discharge, the need to demonstrate the ability to void before discharge, lower backache, and other procedure-related complications have been discussed as challenges

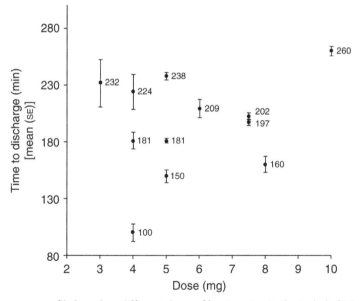

Fig. 2. Recovery profile based on different doses of bupivacaine in the included trials. (*From* Nair GS, Abrishami A, Lernitte J, et al. Systematic review of spinal anesthesia using bupivacaine for ambulatory knee arthroscopy. Br J Anaesth 2009;102:310; with permission.)

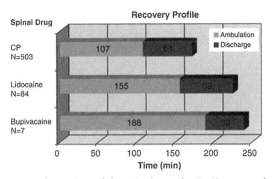

Fig. 3. Time 0 is the time of injection of the spinal anesthetic. Time to ambulation is the time of block resolution. Time to discharge (minutes) is release from PACU and is 171, 224, and 238 for chloroprocaine (CP), lidocaine, and bupivacaine, respectively. (*From* Hejtmanek MR, Pollock JE. Chloroprocaine for spinal anesthesia: a retrospective analysis. Acta Anaesthesiol Scand 2011;55:269; with permission.)

Table 4
Results

	General ($n = 16$)	Epidural ($n = 16$)	Spinal ($n = 16$)
Turnover time (min)[a]	24 ± 6 ($n = 8$)	23 ± 6 ($n = 5$)	28 ± 9 ($n = 3$)
Time to void[b] (min)[a]	NA	80 ± 16[c]	135 ± 51[c]
Time to discharge (min)[a]	104 ± 31	92 ± 18	146 ± 52[c]
Hypotension/bradycardia in the operating room[d]	2	2	2
PACU			
IV narcotics	5	2	2
Antiemetics	0	0	3[c]
Antiemetics	0	0	3[c]
Antipruritic	0	0	7[c]
Follow-up			
Headache	1	3	3[e]
Pain control	1	1	1
Back/leg pain	0	2	1
Satisfaction scores			
5 (very satisfied)	12	12	8
4 (satisfied)	3	3	6
3 (neutral)	1	1	1
2 (dissatisfied)	0	—	1

Abbreviations: HR, heart rate; IV, intravenous; NA, not applicable.
[a] Average ± SD.
[b] Time from PACU admission to void.
[c] $P<.05$.
[d] One patient had a positional headache; none required treatment.
[e] HR less than 60; systolic blood pressure less than 100 mm Hg requiring treatment.
From Mulroy M, Larkin K, Hodgson P, et al. A comparison of spinal, epidural, and general anesthesia for outpatient knee arthroscopy. Anesth Analg 2000;91(4):863; with permission.

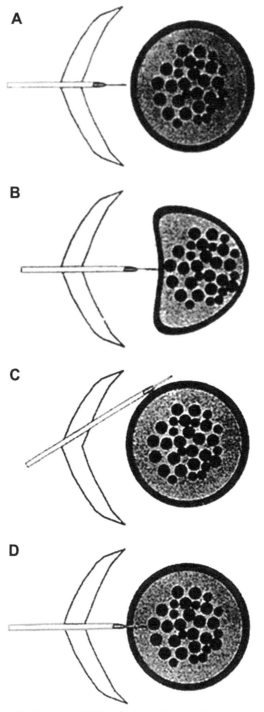

Fig. 4. CSE technique. Various possibilities for CSE block failure caused by incorrect technique. (*A*) Length of spinal needle is too short or epidural needle is not far enough into the epidural space. (*B*) Spinal needle tents the dura without puncture (possibly greater risk with pencil-point needles). (*C*) Epidural needle deviated from midline. (*D*) Correct technique with successful dural puncture. (*From* Rawal N, Van Zundert A, Holmstrom B, et al. Combined spinal-epidural technique. Reg Anesth 1997;22:416; with permission.)

	3% 2-Chloroprocaine (n = 13)	1.5% Lidocaine (n = 14)	P Value
Time to discharge—all patients (min)	130 ± 17	191 ± 32	<.0001
Time to discharge—patients not given epidural reinjection (min)	125 ± 14 (n = 11)	206 ± 14 (n = 5)	<.0001
Time to discharge—patients given epidural reinjection (min)	155 ± 6 (n = 2)	200 ± 37 (n = 9)	.02
Patients requiring epidural reinjection before incision	1	1	
Time to preoperative reinjection (min)	15	20	
Patients requiring intraoperative epidural reinjection	2	8	
Time to intraoperative reinjection (min)	56 ± 16	59 ± 24	.88
Administered volume (including test dose) (mL)	27 ± 4	31 ± 5	.03

NOTE. Data are expressed as mean ± standard deviation.

Fig. 5. Hospital discharge after knee arthroscopy. (*From* Neal J, Deck J, Kopacz D, et al. Hospital Discharge After Ambulatory Knee Arthroscopy: A Comparison of Epidural 2-Chloroprocaine Versus Lidocaine. Regional Anesthesia & Pain Medicine 2001;26(1):38; with permission.)

to using epidural anesthesia in an outpatient setting. Researchers have found similar operating room turnover times for epidural and general anesthesia when the epidural was administered in a separate induction area. Conversely, the slower onset of action after epidural administration of a local anesthetic as compared with a subarachnoid block may prevent sudden hemodynamic changes; the dose of anesthetic can be gradually titrated to the desired dermatome and level of sensory and motor blockade. In this study, PACU discharge times have been shown to be similar for epidural and general anesthesia, whereas spinal anesthesia was linked to a longer PACU discharge time and a higher incidence of side effects (**Table 4**).[1]

Combined spinal epidural (CSE) can be used in the outpatient setting.[19] This technique may take longer to place than a single-shot spinal but allows for redosing in procedures of uncertain length.[20] CSE may have a 5% failure rate of the spinal anesthetic; **Fig. 4** demonstrates several reasons. If the epidural supplementation is used, delayed postoperative recovery times are likely as shown in **Fig. 5** in outpatients for knee arthroscopy using lidocaine who were supplemented for intraoperative pain.

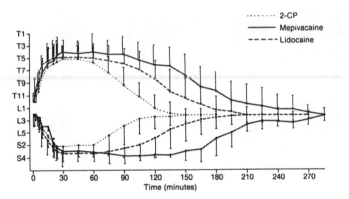

Fig. 6. Sensory dermatomal blockade level (± SD) versus time following incremental injection of 20 mL of 2-chloroprocaine (2-CP), lidocaine, and mepivacaine with 1:200,000 epinephrine. Time to 2-segment regression for 2-CP = 78 ± 15 (SD), lidocaine = 101 ± 25, and mepivacaine = 122 ± 27 minutes. L, Lumbar; S, Sacral; T, Thorasic. (*From* Kopacz DJ, Mulroy MF. Chloroprocaine and lidocaine decrease hospital stay and admission rate after outpatient epidural anesthesia. Reg Anesth 1990;15:21; with permission.)

Table 5 Overnight admission rate after outpatient lithotripsy			
	Overnight Admissions[a]	Number of ESWL Shocks[b] (18–24 kV)	Time out of ESWL Tank[b] (Minutes After 8 AM)
2-Chloroprcaine	29/412 (7.0%)	1703 ± 890	399 ± 175
Lidocaine	35/389 (9.0%)	1441 ± 596	360 ± 214
Mepivacaine	180/1699 (10.6%)	1669 ± 818	312 ± 150
Bupivacaine	11/76 (14.5%)	1632 ± 87	321 ± 167
Total	255/2576 (9.9%)	—	—

[a] $P = .08$ by chi-square.
[b] $P > .05$ by analysis of variance.
From Kopacz DJ, Mulroy MF. Chloroprocaine and lidocaine decrease hospital stay and admission rate after outpatient epidural anesthesia. Reg Anesth 1990;15:23; with permission.

A combined technique may include the risk for spinal headache, and patient choice as noted earlier for sub-arachnoid block will decrease this risk.

SELECTION OF AGENTS

The anesthetic 2-CPC may be useful for knee arthroscopy and ESWL.[19] Three percent 2-CPC provides a much shorter time to discharge than 1.5% lidocaine (120 minutes vs 191 minutes) (**Fig. 6**, **Table 5**).[21] Lidocaine epidurals may be a better choice for procedures when a 60- to 90-minute duration is anticipated. Bupivacaine epidurals do not allow for a reasonable discharge time for ambulatory procedures.

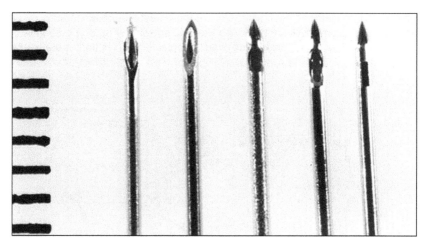

Fig. 7. The configurations of different spinal needle tips used in the study. From the left: Atraucan, Quincke, Gertie Marx (International Medical Development, Huntsville, UT), Sprotte, and Whitacre needles. Note the cutting points on the Atraucan (Atraucan B Braun Medical Melsungen, Germany) and Quincke needles. Also, note the differences in the configurations of the lateral eyes of the pencil-point needles. The eye of the Gertie Marx needle is the smallest and situated closest to the needle tip. The left horizontal markings are in 2-mm increments. (*From* Vallejo M, Mandell G, Sabo D, et al. Postdural puncture headache: a randomized comparison of five spinal needles in obstetric patients. Anesth Analg 2000;91(4):917; with permission.)

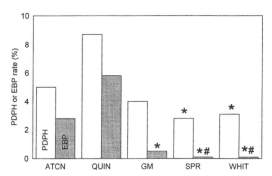

Fig. 8. Postdural puncture headache (PDPH) and epidural blood puncture (EBP) rates (%) with Atraucan (ATCN), Quincke (QUIN), Gertie Marx (GM; International Medical Development, Huntsville, UT), Sprotte (SPR), and Whitacre (WHIT) needles. * Significantly different from the Quincke group. # Different from the Atraucan group. (*From* Vallejo M, Mandell G, Sabo D, et al. Postdural puncture headache: a randomized comparison of five spinal needles in obstetric patients. Anesth Analg 2000;91(4):919; with permission.)

SIDE EFFECTS

The complication profile for spinal anesthetics in the outpatient setting is favorable. Postdural puncture headache is the most common complication at 0.8% to 1.9%. Using blunt-tipped needles as Sprotte needle has 2.8% and Whitacher has 3.1% report rate of postdural puncture headache.[22] Researchers have reported that avoiding younger patients (<18 years of age) decreases the risk (**Figs. 7** and **8**).[23]

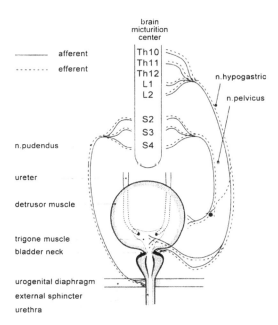

Fig. 9. The anatomy and nerve supply of the lower urinary tract. L, lumbar; S, Sciatic; TH, Thoracic. (*From* Gosling JA. The structure of the bladder and urethra in relation to function. Urol Clin North Am 1979;6:35; with permission.)

Table 6
Discharge times by subgroups resulting from protocol compliance

Group	N	Discharge Time (min) ± SD
Standard	70	153 ± 49
Accelerated		
Discharged without voiding	46	120 ± 42[a]
Voided spontaneously	62	127 ± 41[a]
Held for BUS >400, voided spontaneously	20	162 ± 45
Held for BUS >400, catheterized	3	186 ± 61

Abbreviations: BUS, bladder ultrasound; N, number.
[a] *P*<.05, compared with standard.
From Mulroy M, Salinas F, Larkin K, et al. Ambulatory surgery patients may be discharged before voiding after short-acting spinal and epidural anesthesia. Anesthesiology 2002;97(2):317; with permission.

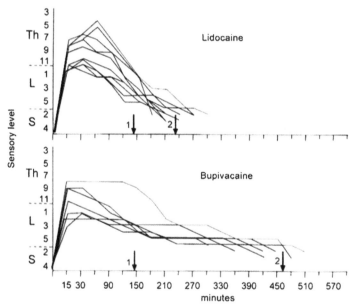

Fig. 10. (*Top*) Time course of segmental level of analgesia in 10 patients after spinal anesthesia with 2 mL lidocaine, 5% hyperbaric, until spontaneous voiding. (*Bottom*) Time course of segmental level of analgesia in 10 patients after spinal anesthesia with 2 mL bupivacaine, 0.5% hyperbaric, until spontaneous voiding. Seven patients in each group, in whom the segmental analgesia had regressed to the second sacral segment, experienced urge at cystometric capacity and could empty their bladders. The last 6 patients could void urine spontaneously when segmental analgesia had reached the third sacral segment. (*Arrow 1*) Average motor block time in the lidocaine (144 ± 35 minutes) and in the bupivacaine (148 ± 76 minutes) groups. (*Arrow 2*) Average detrusor time block in the lidocaine (233 ± 31 minutes) and in the bupivacaine (462 ± 61 minutes) groups. L, Lumbar; S, Sacral; TH, Thorasic. (*From* Kamphuis E, Ionescu T, Kuipers P, et al. Recovery of storage and emptying functions of the urinary bladder after spinal anesthesia with lidocaine and with bupivacaine in men. Anesthesiology 1998;88(2):315; with permission.)

Spinal anesthesia interrupts the micturition reflex; bladder function is impaired until the block regresses below the third sacral segment (**Fig. 9**).[24,25] Thus, prolonged blockade such as with bupivacaine or high-dose lidocaine may allow bladder overdistension, which can interfere with normal voiding. Certain risk factors increase the likelihood of urinary retention after spinal anesthesia, including age, male sex, pelvic surgery, prolonged surgery, and history of previous urologic dysfunction.[26] Shorter-acting agents for lower-risk surgery do not seem to create any increase in urinary retention (**Table 6**).[27,28] Unfortunately, unilateral low-dose spinal anesthesia (6 mg bupivacaine) does not decrease the incidence of urinary retention in high-risk patients.[29] The time from injection to voiding was also shorter in the epidural versus the spinal group. Researchers have suggested that predischarge voiding after outpatient epidural anesthesia with short-acting drugs for low-risk procedures was not necessary (**Fig. 10**).[24,28]

TNS can occur with almost any spinal anesthetic. Lidocaine has the highest incidence of TNS (>15%), which is not dependent on the dose. Bupivacaine has also been reported to have a low incidence of TNS.[30] Bupivacaine has a reported incidence of 3%, and 2-CPC has no reported incidences. Certain surgical procedures confer a higher risk of TNS (knee arthroscopy and lithotomy positions) (**Table 7**).[30,31]

Backache after epidural anesthesia, although not a common problem, seems to be related to the local anesthetic used and patient age, occurring more often in young patients.[32] 2-CPC with ethylenediaminetetraacetic acid (EDTA) in doses of 40 mg and greater has been associated with severe bilateral lower back pain, which is not at the injection site in up to 40% of patients.[33] This back pain is described as severe, deep back pain unrelieved by mechanical relaxation. EDTA-free 2-CPC seems to have similar rates of deep back pain as lidocaine (around 2%).[34,35]

Table 7
Typical incidences of TNS with outpatient spinal anesthesia

Local Anesthetic (%)	Patient Position	TNS (%)
Lidocaine 2–5	Supine	6
Lidocaine 3	Prone	0.4
Lidocaine 0.5	Knee arthroscopy	17
Lidocaine 5	Knee arthroscopy	16
Lidocaine 5	Lithotomy	24
Bupivacaine 0.25–0.75	Supine Knee arthroscopy Lithotomy	0–1 0–1 0–1
Mepivacaine 1.5	Knee arthroscopy	8
Mepivacaine 4	Mixed	30
Ropivacaine 0.25	Supine	1
Ropivacaine 0.2–0.35	Knee arthroscopy	0
Procaine 5	Knee arthroscopy	6
Prilocaine 2–5	Mixed	3–4

Bupivacaine and ropivacaine consistently result in low incidences of TNS, whereas lidocaine typically results in the highest incidences. Other local anesthetics are intermediate in incidence of TNS.
From Liu S, McDonald S. Current issues in spinal anesthesia. Anesthesiology 2001;94(5):894; with permission.

SUMMARY

Spinal anesthesia with preservative-free 2-CPC offers a favorable side-effect profile and discharge times for certain ambulatory surgery procedures lasting less than 60 minutes. For procedures of longer duration, epidural or CSE anesthesia may provide longer anesthesia without prolonged recovery. Choosing shorter-acting agents with favorable side-effect profiles will allow for a successful anesthetic plan and timely discharge in the ambulatory setting.

REFERENCES

1. Mulroy MF, Larkin KL, Hodgson PS, et al. A comparison of spinal, epidural, and general anesthesia for outpatient knee arthroscopy. Anesth Analg 2000;91:860–4.
2. Pavlin DJ, Rapp SE, Polissar NL, et al. Factors affecting discharge time in adult outpatients. Anesth Analg 1998;87(4):816–26.
3. Vaghadia H, McLeod DH, Mitchell GW, et al. Small-dose hypobaric lidocaine-fentanyl spinal anesthesia for short duration outpatient laparoscopy. I. A randomized comparison with conventional dose hyperbaric lidocaine. Anesth Analg 1997;84:59–64.
4. Song D, Greilich N, White P, et al. Recovery profiles and costs of anesthesia for outpatient unilateral inguinal herniorrhaphy. Anesth Analg 2000;91:876–81.
5. Liu SS. A comparison of regional versus general anesthesia for ambulatory anesthesia: a meta-analysis of randomized controlled trials. Anesth Analg 2005;101: 1634–42.
6. Schneider M, Ettlin T, Kaufmann M, et al. Transient neurologic toxicity after hyperbaric subarachnoid anesthesia with 5% lidocaine. Anesth Analg 1993;76:1154–7.
7. Liu S. Optimizing spinal anesthesia for ambulatory surgery. Reg Anesth 1997; 22(6):500–10.
8. Ben-David B, DeMeo PJ, Lucyk C, et al. A comparison of minidose lidocaine-fentanyl spinal anesthesia and local anesthesia/propofol infusion for outpatient knee arthroscopy. Anesth Analg 2001;93:319–25.
9. Zaric D, Christiansen C, Pace NL, et al. Transient neurologic symptoms after spinal anesthesia with lidocaine versus other local anesthetics: a systematic review of randomized, controlled trials. Anesth Analg 2005;100:1811–6.
10. Pollock JE. Transient neurologic symptoms: etiology, risk factors, and management. Reg Anesth Pain Med 2002;(6):581–6.
11. Valanne JV, Korhonen AM, Jokela RM, et al. Selective spinal anesthesia: a comparison of hyperbaric bupivacaine 4 mg versus 6 mg for outpatient knee arthroscopy. Anesth Analg 2001;93:1377–9.
12. Lacasse MA, Roy JD, Forget J, et al. Comparison of bupivacaine and 2-chloroprocaine for spinal anesthesia for outpatient surgery: a double-blind randomized trial. Can J Anaesth 2011;58:384–91.
13. Nair GS, Abrishami A, Lermitte J, et al. Systematic review of spinal anaesthesia using bupivacaine for ambulatory knee arthroscopy. Br J Anaesth 2009;102:307–15.
14. Kouri ME, Kopacz DJ. Spinal 2-chloroprocaine: a comparison with lidocaine in volunteers. Anesth Analg 2004;98:75–80.
15. Hejtmanek MR, Pollock JE. Chloroprocaine for spinal anesthesia: a retrospective analysis. Acta Anaesthesiol Scand 2011;55:267–72.
16. Dahl V, Gierloff C, Omland E, et al. Spinal, epidural or propofol anesthesia for outpatient knee arthroscopy. Acta Anaesthesiol Scand 1997;41:1341–5.
17. Labas P, Ohradka B, Cambal M, et al. Haemorrhoidectomy in outpatient practice. Eur J Surg 2002;168:619–20.

18. Schuricht AL, McCarthy CS, Wells WL, et al. A comparison of epidural versus general anesthesia for outpatient endoscopic preperitoneal herniorrhaphy. JSLS 1997;1:141–4.
19. Kopacz DJ, Mulroy MF. Chloroprocaine and lidocaine decrease hospital stay and admission rate after outpatient epidural anesthesia. Reg Anesth 1990;15:19–25.
20. Urmey WF, Stanton J, Peterson M, et al. Combined spinal-epidural anesthesia for outpatient surgery: dose response characteristics of intrathecal isobaric lidocaine using a 27-gauge Whitacre spinal needle. Anesthesiology 1996;84:481–2.
21. Neal JM, Deck JJ, Kopacz DJ, et al. Hospital discharge after ambulatory knee arthroscopy: a comparison of epidural 2-chloroprocaine versus lidocaine. Reg Anesth Pain Med 2001;26:35–40.
22. Vallejo MC, Mandell GL, Sabo DP, et al. Postdural puncture headache: a randomized comparison of five spinal needles in obstetric patients. Anesth Analg 2000; 91:916–20.
23. Pittoni G, Toffoletto F, Calcarella G, et al. Spinal anesthesia in outpatient knee surgery: 22-gauge versus 25-gauge Sprotte needle. Anesth Analg 1995;81:73–9.
24. Kamphuis ET, Lonescu TI, Kuipers PW, et al. Recovery of storage and emptying functions of the urinary bladder after spinal anesthesia with lidocaine and with bupivacaine in men. Anesthesiology 1998;88(2):310–6.
25. Gosling JA. The structure of the bladder and urethra in relation to function. Urol Clin North Am 1979;6:31–8.
26. Pavlin DJ, Pavlin EG, Gunn HC, et al. Voiding in patients managed with or without ultrasound monitoring of bladder volume after outpatient surgery. Anesth Analg 1999;89:90–7.
27. Nishikawa K, Yoshida S, Shimodate Y, et al. A comparison of spinal anesthesia with small-dose lidocaine and general anesthesia with fentanyl and propofol for ambulatory prostate biopsy procedures in elderly patients. J Clin Anesth 2007; 19:25–9.
28. Mulroy MF, Salinas FV, Larkin KL, et al. Ambulatory surgery patients may be discharged before voiding after short-acting spinal and epidural anesthesia. Anesthesiology 2002;97:315–9.
29. Voelckel WG, Kirchmair L, Rehder P, et al. Unilateral anesthesia does not affect the incidence of urinary retention after low-dose spinal anesthesia for knee surgery. Anesth Analg 2009;109:986–7.
30. Zaric D, Pace NL. Transient neurologic symptoms (TNS) following spinal anaesthesia with lidocaine versus other local anaesthetics. Cochrane Database Syst Rev 2009;(2):CD003006. http://dx.doi.org/10.1002/14651858.CD003006.pub3.
31. Liu S, McDonald S. Current issues in spinal anesthesia. Anesthesiology 2001;94: 888–906.
32. Seeberger MD, Lang ML, Drewe J, et al. Comparison of spinal and epidural anesthesia for patients younger than 50 years of age. Anesth Analg 1994;78:667–73.
33. Fibuch EE, Epper SE. Back pain following epidurally administered Nesacaine-MPF. Anesth Analg 1989;69:113–5.
34. Hynson JM, Sessler DI, Glosten B. Back pain in volunteers after epidural anesthesia with chloroprocaine. Anesth Analg 1991;72:253–6.
35. Drolet P, Veillette Y. Pack pain following epidural anesthesia with 2-chloroprocaine (EDTA-free) or lidocaine. Reg Anesth 1997;22(4):303–7.

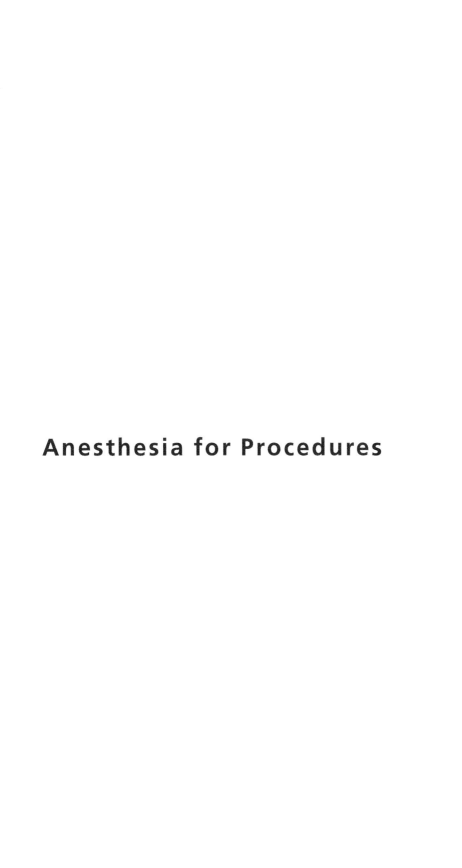

Anesthesia for Procedures

Anesthesia for Ambulatory Diagnostic and Therapeutic Radiology Procedures

Daniel Rubin, MD

KEYWORDS

• Ambulatory • Radiology • Anesthesia • Interventional radiology

KEY POINTS

- Protection from ionizing radiation is achieved with appropriate shielding with aprons and acrylic shields, along with maintaining distance from the source.
- The magnet creates projectile risks and may cause interference with the electrocardiogram, whereas the generation of electromagnetic energy may cause significant thermal injury in coiled wires.
- Iodinated contrast may cause severe cardiorespiratory compromise and should be immediately stopped, followed by an assessment of the severity/progression of the reaction and the potential need for supplemental oxygen, fluids, epinephrine, and intubation.
- A discussion should occur between the anesthesiologist and radiologist about potential concerns including length of procedure, level of procedural stimulation, positioning, need for patient cooperation, and recovery.
- There is currently no anesthetic technique that is clearly superior, and the same procedure may be performed under light sedation or a general anesthetic depending on patient characteristics or procedural concerns.

INTRODUCTION

Moderate sedation administered by nurses under the supervision of radiologists is used for most radiology procedures.[1,2] The presence of anesthesiologists is increasing because of the increasing complexity of the procedures and comorbidities of the patients. The radiology suite poses unique challenges to the anesthesiologist because of the physical obstacle of the imaging equipment, the distance from the patient, and the hazards of ionizing radiation or magnetic fields.

Disclosure: The author has no relationships with any with any companies that have any direct financial interest in any of the material provided in this article.
Department of Anesthesia and Critical Care, University of Chicago, 5841 South Maryland Avenue, MC-4028, Chicago, IL 60637, USA
E-mail address: drubin@dacc.uchicago.edu

Anesthesiology Clin 32 (2014) 371–380
http://dx.doi.org/10.1016/j.anclin.2014.02.015 **anesthesiology.theclinics.com**

CONTRAST

Intravascular ionized contrast reactions can result in chemotoxic reactions because of the physical properties of the contrast agent. The high osmolality of the contrast results in intravascular fluid shifts and may exacerbate congestive heart failure. In addition, molecular binding, particularly of calcium, may decrease inotropy. Because these reactions are secondary to the properties of the contrast, the severity of the reaction depends on dose and concentration. Patients with congestive heart failure, acute/chronic kidney disease, chronic obstructive pulmonary disease (COPD), and other critical illnesses are at increased risk for intravascular volume shifts, decreased inotropy and contrast-induced nephropathy (**Table 1**).

Contrast-induced nephropathy is likely another chemotoxic reaction resulting from renal artery vasospasm or direct action on renal tubules. Preexisting renal dysfunction is the greatest risk factor, because no reports have been described with normal function. The risk of injury may be diminished by adequate hydration with crystalloids, N-acetylcysteine, and sodium bicarbonate.[3,4]

Anaphylactoid reactions result from an undefined immune-mediated reaction.[5] The cause of these reactions is not clear but likely involves the kinin and complement systems, resulting in direct histamine release.[5] Symptoms include hives, nausea, vomiting, pruritus, angioedema, bronchospasm, hypotension, and cardiovascular collapse. The severity of symptoms is not dose dependent and may be triggered by even small amounts of contrast. Treatment includes discontinuing the contrast and may require antihistamines, fluids, supplemental oxygen, steroids, epinephrine, and airway management. A history of asthma or previous anaphylactoid reactions are risk factors and pretreatment with diphenhydramine and steroids should be considered. There is no evidence to suggest that an allergy to seafood or shellfish increases the risk (**Table 2**).[6]

OTHER CONTRAST MEDIA

Gadolinium contrast for a magnetic resonance (MR) imaging study may lead to nephrogenic systemic fibrosis in patients with either acute or chronic kidney disease or injury.[7] Ultrasonography contrast involves the intravenous administration of echogenic microbubbles, and patients with pulmonary hypertension or unstable cardiopulmonary conditions should be closely monitored during and for at least 30 minutes after administration.[8]

MRI
Magnet Safety

The magnetic field poses hazards from static magnetic fields, gradient magnetic fields, and radiofrequency (RF) energy. The American College of Radiology (ACR) guidelines require patients and non-MR personnel to have a safety screening performed by authorized MR personnel before entering zone 3 (**Fig. 1**).[9] The constant static magnetic field of the MR scanner poses the most obvious danger if ferromagnetic objects are within range.[10] Gradient magnetic fields occur with the rapidly changing magnetic fields during image acquisition and may cause excitation of peripheral nerves or cardiac arrhythmias if external leads are present. RF energy produced during image acquisition may be focused by metallic materials such as electrocardiography leads, pulmonary artery catheters, and external pacemaker leads, leading to excessive concentration of RF energy and thermal burns (**Table 3**).[11]

Anesthetic Considerations for MRI

Moderate to severe claustrophobia, anxiety, and fear of the MRI machine occur in 37% of patients, with 5% to 10% of these choosing to abort the scan.[12] Most proceed

Table 1	
Selected chemotoxic effects of intravascular contrast media	
Effects	**Responsible Physicochemical Properties**
Vascular Changes	
Increase in plasma osmolality	Hyperosmolality
Hypervolemia	—
Increase in cardiac output	—
Alteration in vascular permeability	Hyperosmolality
Inflammation or pain	—
Formation of microthrombus	—
Dilatation of vessels	Hyperosmolality
Increase in blood flow	—
Decrease in blood pressure	—
Pain	—
Cerebral Changes	
Dilatation of external carotid artery	Hyperosmolality
Stimulation of chemoreceptors	Hyperosmolality and sodium ion concentration
Alterations in systemic blood pressure	—
Alterations in heart rate	—
Tachypnea	—
Alterations in permeability of the blood-brain barrier	Hyperosmolality
Alteration in neuroelectrical activity (with disruption of blood-brain barrier)	Presence and concentration of ions
Cardiac Changes (During Coronary Angiography)	
Dilatation of coronary artery	Hyperosmolality
Electrocardiographic alterations	Hyperosmolality
Bradycardia	—
Conduction delays	—
Ventricular fibrillation	Calcium binding
Depression of myocardial contractility	Calcium binding
Renal Changes	
Renovascular constriction (sustained)	Hyperosmolality
Decrease in renal blood flow	—
Alteration in glomerular permeability	Hyperosmolality
Proteinuria	—
Osmotic diuresis	Concentration of nonresorbable solutes
Renal tubular toxic effects	Possible molecular toxicity

From Bush WH, Swanson DP. Acute reactions to intravascular contrast media: types, risk factors, recognition, and specific treatment. AJR Am J Roentgenol 1991;157:1154; with permission.

under light sedation (eg, oral or intranasal midazolam) but some require deeper sedation or even general anesthesia.[13] The anesthesiologist should take into account the severity of the anxiety, the ability to maintain a patent airway, the ability to lie supine and motionless for extended periods of time, and any comorbid conditions. Upper body examinations present the greatest challenge because access to the airway is

Table 2
Frequency and type of mild and moderate reaction to intravascular contrast media from 84,928 injections

Mild Manifestations	No. of Reactions
Urticaria	286
Pruritus	131
Erythema or rash	114
Scratchy throat	28
Nasal congestion	25
Sneezing	24
Localized facial swelling	15
Chest discomfort[a]	14
Transient cough	8
Rigors or chills	5
Tachycardia or palpitations	5
Thickened tongue[b]	2
Injected eye	1

Moderate Manifestations	No. of Reactions
Shortness of breath	55
Cardiaclike symptoms[c]	48
Laryngeal edema	38
Facial edema	14
Bronchospasm	10
Rigors	7
Hypotension	4
Diaphoresis	2
Tongue swelling	2
Hypertension	1

Many patients had more than one manifestation. Many patients also had mild manifestations, including cutaneous symptoms (n = 66), as well as moderate manifestations.

[a] Thought to not be cardiac.
[b] Patient reported a subjective sensation.
[c] Chest pain or pressure, jaw pain, left arm numbness, or a combination of these symptoms.

Data from Wang CL, Cohan RH, Ellis JH, et al. Frequency, outcome, and appropriateness of treatment of nonionic iodinated contrast media reactions. AJR Am J Roentgenol 2008;191:409–15.

severely limited during the examination and choosing a general anesthetic with a secure airway may be prudent. The airway should be secured outside zone 4 if more advanced airway techniques become necessary. If problems occur during the examination, emergency resuscitative equipment (oxygen, suction, ventilator, defibrillator, and medication) should be readily available outside zone 4 and basic life support and relocation should happen immediately and concurrently.

Monitoring/patient access
Patients should be monitored in a manner that is consistent with the American Society of Anesthesiologists (ASA) Standards for Basic Anesthetic Monitoring[14] and must be labeled MR safe/conditional before applying them to patients in zone 3 or 4. Even

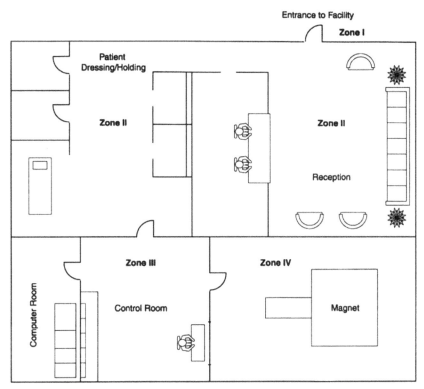

Fig. 1. Zoning layout for MRI scanner. (*From* Kanal E, Borgstede JP, Barkovich AJ, et al. American College of Radiology white paper on MR safety. AJR Am J Roentgenol 2002;178(6):1336; with permission.)

MR-conditional electrocardiography leads may display interference during the scan and interpretation of arrhythmias or ischemia may be limited during these times. The patient and monitors must be easily viewable either directly or with a monitor in a location outside zone 4. A test run using the full length of the scanner should be performed to ensure adequate length and unrestricted travel of intravenous and ventilator tubing and monitor leads. Intravenous lines and stopcocks should be easily accessible in case a medication needs to be given.

Ear safety

The noise generated by an MR machine can reach greater than 110 dB and may cause hearing loss. Ear protection (eg, foam ear plugs) should be placed in all patients, including those under general anesthesia.[15]

INTERVENTIONAL RADIOLOGY
Radiation Safety

The 3 primary sources of ionizing radiation are direct (ie, from the radiation beam); radiation leakage from the source; and, most significantly, radiation scatter from the patient. Increasing distance reduces exposure by the square of the distance, so intravenous and breathing circuit extension tubing should be used to provide for this. Lead aprons, including a thyroid collar, reduce exposure by a factor of 10 and transparent

Table 3	
New and old terminology describing MR safety of implanted devices	
Old Terminology	
MR safe	The device, when used in the MR environment, has been shown to present no additional risk to the patient or other individuals but may affect the quality of the diagnostic information. The MR conditions in which the device was tested should be specified in conjunction with the term MR safe, because a device that is safe under one set of conditions may not safe under more extreme MR imaging conditions
MR compatible	A device shall be considered MR compatible if it is MR safe and, when used in the MR environment, has been shown to neither significantly affect the quality of the diagnostic information nor have its operations affected by the MR system. The MR imaging conditions in which the device was tested should be specified in conjunction with the term MR compatible, because a device that is safe under one set of conditions may not be safe under more extreme MR conditions
New Terminology	
MR safe	An item that poses no known hazards in any MR environment. Using the new terminology, MR-safe items include nonconducting, nonmetallic, nonmagnetic items, such as a plastic Petri dish
MR conditional	An item that has been shown to pose no known hazards in a specified MR imaging environment with specified conditions of use. Conditions that define the MR environment include static magnetic field strength, spatial magnetic gradient dB/dt (time-varying magnetic fields), RF fields, and SAR. Additional conditions, including specific configurations of the item (eg, the routing or leads used for a neurostimulation system), may be required
MR unsafe	An item that is known to pose hazards in all MR environments. MR unsafe items include magnetic items such as a pair of ferromagnetic scissors

Abbreviations: db/dt, time rate of change of magnetic field (tesla/second); SAR, specific absorption rate (Watts/kg).

From Levine GN, Gomes AS, Arai AE, et al. Safety of magnetic resonance imaging in patients with cardiovascular devices: an American Heart Association scientific statement from the Committee on Diagnostic and Interventional Cardiac Catheterization, Council on Clinical Cardiology, and the Council on Cardiovascular Radiology and Intervention: endorsed by the American College of Cardiology Foundation, the North American Society for Cardiac Imaging, and the Society for Cardiovascular Magnetic Resonance. Circulation 2007;116:2880; with permission.

leaded acrylic eyeglasses can help prevent premature cataracts.[16] Pausing the study while making an intervention should be requested, as should inserting a transparent leaded shield between the anesthesia provider and the patient. Digital subtraction angiography exposes providers to high levels of radiation so remote monitoring is best during the study. Another caveat is that biplane fluoroscopy often directs the radiation toward the side of the anesthesia provider (**Fig. 2**).

ANESTHETIC CONSIDERATIONS FOR INTERVENTIONAL RADIOLOGY
Anesthetic

Anesthetic technique depends on the procedure and the patient's comorbidities. Considerations include the ability to access and secure the airway during the procedure; risk of aspiration; ability to remain supine and motionless for extended periods of time; and conditions such as obstructive sleep apnea, COPD, and congestive heart failure. There is no definitive evidence to suggest that one anesthetic agent or technique is

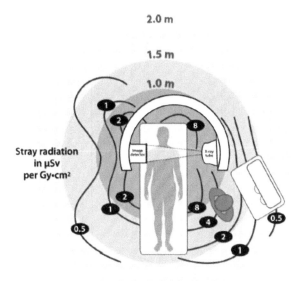

Fig. 2. Distribution of scatter radiation from a lateral C-arm with the radiation source on the same side as the anesthesiologist. Note the significantly higher amount of radiation exposure that the anesthesiologist encounters when a lateral C-arm is used with the radiation source on the same side as the anesthesiologist. (*From* Anastasian ZH, Strozyk D, Meyers PM, et al. Radiation exposure of the anesthesiologist in the neurointerventional suite. Anesthesiology 2011;114:517; with permission.)

superior to others. There should be a discussion between anesthesiologist and proceduralist to determine the optimal anesthetic. The discussion should also include the expected length of the procedure, expected level of procedural stimulation, positioning, need for patient cooperation, and goals for any physiologic parameters such as arterial blood pressure.

Monitoring/Equipment

All anesthetics should comply with the ASA Standards for Basic Anesthetic Monitoring.[14] In some patients it may be appropriate to use end-tidal carbon dioxide monitoring even under light sedation because of the difficulty of monitoring adequacy of ventilation In patients once the imaging equipment and drapes have been positioned.[17] Because most procedures are performed without an anesthesia team, suites are seldom anesthesiologist friendly, and patient access and visual monitoring are often challenging because of the significant distance from the patient and the obstruction by the imaging equipment. The anesthesia machine must be far enough away to not interfere with the movement of equipment, so extensions on the intravenous tubing, oxygen supply, and ventilator tubing are commonly required. Backup equipment, especially adjunct airway devices, oxygen, and other resources, should be readily available in the event of an unexpected difficult airway.

PROCEDURES

Some of the more common and more challenging ambulatory procedures that anesthesiologists may be used to perform sedation are presented in **Table 4**.

Table 4
Anesthetic implications for commonly performed ambulatory procedures in IR

Procedure Name	Patient Position	Anesthetic Most Commonly Performed	Complications	Special Considerations
CT/Ultrasonography guided: Abscess drainage (eg, abdominal abscess) Fluid drainage (eg, ascites) Biopsy (eg, liver)	Supine	Light-moderate sedation	Perforation Peritonitis Pneumothorax Hemorrhage Contrast reaction	May require breath holding GA required if unable to lie supine
Biliary: Biliary drainage (eg, acute cholecystitis) Biliary stent placement Cholecystostomy tube (eg, tumor obstruction)	Supine with right arm raised above the head	Moderate sedation	Hemorrhage Peritonitis Contrast reaction	Patients may have failed ERCP Hepatic dilation can be stimulating
Genitourinary: Nephrostomy (eg, obstructive uropathy) Nephrolithotomy (eg, nephrolithiasis) Abscess drainage (eg, pyelonephritis with abscess formation)	Prone	Moderate sedation/GA	Pneumothorax Hemorrhage Contrast reaction Hydrothorax	Prone positioning Dilutional anemia Blood loss can be significant Pneumothorax if supracostal approach is taken Breath holding CXR after procedure
Angiography: Diagnostic angioplasty Stent placement Arthrectomy (eg, peripheral vascular disease)	Supine	Light-moderate sedation	Hemorrhage Vascular injury Contrast reaction	Minimal stimulation once vascular access has been obtained
Venous procedures: Catheter placement (eg, end-stage renal disease) IVC filter (eg, thromboembolic risk) AV fistulagram (eg, stenosis of AV fistula)	Supine	Light-moderate	Hemorrhage Pneumothorax VAE Vascular injury	Breath holding to decrease risk of VAE

Abbreviations: AV, arteriovenous; CT, computed tomography; CXR, chest radiograph; ERCP, endoscopic retrograde cholangiopancreatography; GA, general anesthetic; IVC, inferior vena cava; VAE, venous air embolism.

POSTPROCEDURE CARE

The recovery of patients undergoing conscious sedation and general anesthesia in the radiology suite should be consistent with the standards of postanesthesia care set forth by the ASA.[18] Patients who have undergone straightforward and uncomplicated procedures may be recovered in the radiology suite if the appropriate nursing and physician staff are available. Patients who have undergone complicated or physiologically taxing procedures, general or regional anesthesia, or who have significant comorbidities may benefit from recovery in a dedicated postanesthesia care unit or intensive care unit. A discussion between the anesthesia provider and the radiologist about the patient's recovery needs should take place before the procedure so appropriate arrangements can be in place before the procedure ends.

SUMMARY

The radiology suite presents the anesthesia provider with a unique set of challenges such as ionizing radiation, intravascular contrast, magnetic fields, physical separation and barriers from the patient, so-called borrowed space, and the large range of procedures performed. Most of these procedures will continue to be performed without the presence of an anesthesia team but, because of the ever-increasing complexity of the procedures being performed and the increasing comorbidities of patients, the anesthesia provider will likely be called more often to provide care. A thorough understanding of these challenges is essential to providing a safe anesthetic in a difficult environment.

REFERENCES

1. Haslam PJ, Yap B, Mueller PR, et al. Anesthesia practice and clinical trends in interventional radiology: a European survey. Cardiovasc Intervent Radiol 2000; 23:256–61.
2. Mueller PR, Wittenberg KH, Kaufman JA, et al. Patterns of anesthesia and nursing care for interventional radiology procedures: a national survey of physician practices and preferences. Radiology 1997;202:339–43.
3. Tepel M, van der Giet M, Schwarzfeld C, et al. Prevention of radiographic-contrast-agent-induced reductions in renal function by acetylcysteine. N Engl J Med 2000;343:180–4.
4. Morton CJ, Burgess WP, Gray LV, et al. Prevention of contrast-induced nephropathy with sodium bicarbonate: a randomized controlled trial. JAMA 2004;291: 2328–34.
5. American College of Radiology manual on contrast media. Version 9. 2013. Available at: http://www.acr.org/~/media/ACR/Documents/PDF/QualitySafety/Resources/Contrast%20Manual/2013_Contrast_Media.pdf. Accessed September 10, 2013.
6. Beaty AD, Lieberman PL, Slavin RG. Seafood allergy and radiocontrast media: are physicians propagating a myth? Am J Med 2008;121:158.e1–4.
7. Sadowski EA, Bennett LK, Chan MR, et al. Nephrogenic systemic fibrosis: risk factors and incidence estimation. Radiology 2007;243:148–57.
8. http://www.fda.gov/Drugs/DrugSafety/PostmarketDrugSafetyInformationforPatients andProviders/ucm125574.htm. Acceesed September 5, 2013.
9. Kanal E, Borgstede JP, Barkovich AJ, et al. American College of Radiology white paper on MR safety. AJR Am J Roentgenol 2002;178:1335–47.

10. Chaljub G, Kramer LA, Johnson RF 3rd, et al. Projectile cylinder accidents result-ing from the presence of ferromagnetic nitrous oxide or oxygen tanks in the MR Suite. AJR Am J Roentgenol 2001;177:27–30.

11. Friedstat JS, Moore ME, Goverman J, et al. An unusual burn during routine mag-netic resonance imaging. J Burn Care Res 2013;34:e110–1.

12. Katz RC, Wilson L, Frazer N. Anxiety and its determinants in patients undergoing magnetic resonance imaging. J Behav Ther Exp Psychiatry 1994;25:131–4.

13. Tschirch FT, Gopfert K, Frohlich JM, et al. Low-dose intranasal versus oral mida-zolam for routine body MRI of claustrophobic patients. Eur Radiol 2007;17: 1403–10.

14. American Society of Anesthesiologists. Standards for basic anesthetic monitoring. Last amended October 20, 2010. Available at: http://www.asahq.org/For-Members/Standards-Guidelines-and-Statements.aspx. Accessed September 9, 2013.

15. Price DL, De Wilde JP, Papadaki AM, et al. Investigation of acoustic noise on 15 MRI scanners from 0.2 T to 3 T. J Magn Reson Imaging 2001;13:288–93.

16. Anastasian ZH, Strozyk D, Meyers PM, et al. Radiation exposure of the anesthe-siologist in the neurointerventional suite. Anesthesiology 2011;114:512–20.

17. Lightdale JR, Goldmann DA, Feldman HA, et al. Microstream capnography im-proves patient monitoring during moderate sedation: a randomized, controlled trial. Pediatrics 2006;117:e1170–8.

18. American Society of Anesthesiologists. Standards for postanesthesia care. Last amended October 1, 2009. Available at: http://www.asahq.org/For-Members/Standards-Guidelines-and-Statements.aspx. Accessed September 9, 2013.

Ambulatory Anesthesia for the Cardiac Catheterization and Electrophysiology Laboratories

J. Devin Roberts, MD

KEYWORDS

- Anesthesia • Cardiology • Electrophysiology • Intervention • Radiation safety
- TAVR

KEY POINTS

- The cardiac catheterization laboratory (CCL) and electrophysiology laboratory (EPL) environments present unique clinical challenges, including unfamiliar work areas and staff, limited space with physical barriers separating the patient from the care provider, remote locations, and procedures with rare but potentially catastrophic clinical complications.
- Ambulatory anesthesiologists must familiarize themselves with these new surroundings and practice vigilant preoperative planning and continual communication with the proceduralist and team.
- In the future, the need for anesthesiologists in the CCL and EPL will continue to grow as procedures increase in complexity and duration.

INTRODUCTION

The cardiac catheterization laboratory (CCL) and electrophysiology laboratory (EPL) present many clinical and logistical challenges to the ambulatory anesthesiologist. These challenges have been increased over the past decade with the introduction of new therapeutic procedures and a wider scope of pathology and acuity.

CONSULTATION: A MULTIDISCIPLINARY APPROACH

Effective use of clinical resources is critical to the success of a busy ambulatory surgery center. In the multidisciplinary team approach, the anesthesiologist is the one who can best manage significant patient pathology or procedures associated with significant hemodynamic instability, allowing the cardiologist to focus on the procedure.[1] Although some patients do not significantly benefit from being evaluated at least a day before the procedure, cardiology patients typically do. Patients may have a history of

Department of Anesthesia and Critical Care, University of Chicago, 5841 South Maryland Avenue MC4028, Chicago, IL 60637, USA
E-mail address: jroberts@dacc.uchicago.edu

Anesthesiology Clin 32 (2014) 381–386
http://dx.doi.org/10.1016/j.anclin.2014.02.017
1932-2275/14/$ – see front matter © 2014 Elsevier Inc. All rights reserved.

recent myocardial infarction, uncontrolled arrhythmias, heart failure, serious structural cardiac disorders, or other noncardiac morbidities not commonly encountered in the ambulatory setting, making a thorough and timely preanesthesia assessment essential. Additionally, in order to trigger appropriate anesthesia consultation, we should encourage our cardiology colleagues to perform a basic airway exam and consider the potential hazards of over sedation, aspiration and airway obstruction (**Box 1**).

GENERAL STRATEGIES FOR THE AMBULATORY ANESTHESIOLOGIST

CCLs and EPLs are generally not designed with the anesthesiologist in mind. Space for anesthesia equipment can be limited, whereas the fluoroscopy equipment and table can interfere with airway management. Extensions on intravenous tubing and breathing circuits are helpful because the fluoroscopy table is highly mobile and is usually controlled by the cardiologist. The anesthesia supply room may often be in a distant location, necessitating the use of a well-stocked anesthesia cart with emergency airway equipment and additional supplies.[1]

Avoiding common complications requires an understanding of the unique aspects of CCL and EPL procedures. Vascular access–related complications occur frequently (3%–4%)[2] and careful postoperative monitoring of access sites and appropriate vascular closure techniques are critical. It is also important to keep in mind that, as procedures increase in complexity and duration, deeper sedation is often required. Increasing the levels of sedation has implications for patient safety and regulatory compliance (institutional and state policies and non–anesthesia provider credentialing), further necessitating the anesthesiologist's increasing role in the CCL and EPL. It has been reported that oversedation, airway intervention, or conversion to general anesthesia occur in 40% of electrophysiology procedures scheduled for nongeneral anesthesia.[3]

HIGHER RISK PROCEDURES IN THE AMBULATORY SURGERY SETTING
Complex Catheter Ablation

Radiofrequency ablation is a therapeutic alternative to pharmacologic therapy for refractory atrial and ventricular arrhythmias.[4] Many of these procedures are performed under moderate sedation with standard monitors, but the increasing complexity of electrophysiology techniques has made these procedures significantly more time consuming. Partial airway obstruction, coughing, or an inability to remain supine and motionless can all interfere with both intracardiac mapping and ablation. With significant airway obstruction, swinging intra-atrial septum movement can make transseptal catheter placement by the cardiologist difficult.[5] General anesthesia may be best for some patients. Despite anecdotal practice and opinion, the literature remains sparse and unclear regarding the effects of anesthetic agents on cardiac conducting pathways relevant to electrophysiology procedures, but most anesthetic agents have some effect on cardiac conduction pathways.[6,7]

Box 1
Anesthesia comorbidities for the non–anesthesia provider
Morbid obesity
History of obstructive sleep apnea
History of severe gastroesophageal reflux disease
Inability to lie flat or still for extended periods of time
Known or suspected difficult airway (Mallampati class III or IV)

Patients undergoing ablation procedures can experience unstable arrhythmias, complete heart block, and wide shifts in hemodynamics, all of which require immediate therapy. Standard resuscitation drugs as well as additional antiarrhythmic medications should be available. Transcutaneous defibrillation pads with pacing capability should be applied and their monitoring ability tested before administering anesthesia. Many different medications may be used to induce and terminate tachyarrhythmias, such as isoproterenol, dopamine, epinephrine, adenosine, atropine, β-blockers, ibutilide, procainamide, and verapamil.[4] During long procedures the cardiology team often administers large volumes of fluid, necessitating urinary catheter placement and careful monitoring for volume overload. Particularly for transarterial or transseptal ablation catheters, patients receive heparin to prevent catheter thrombus formation and to reduce thromboembolic stroke risk. Before beginning the procedure, the patient care team should clearly identify the members responsible for heparin administration and anticoagulation monitoring.

Significant complications include thermal injury to the esophagus and formation of an atrioesophageal fistula (0.01%–0.2%), so an esophageal temperature probe is often used to monitor for esophageal thermal injury. Cardiac perforation with tamponade occurs in less than 1% to 2% of cases but often requires echocardiography, reversal of anticoagulation, and placement of a percutaneous pericardial drain for effective treatment (**Table 1**).[2,8]

Lead Extractions for Cardiovascular Implantable Electronic Devices

Indications for lead or device extraction are infection, lead fracture, and device malfunction or recall. Moderate sedation or general anesthesia may be appropriate, depending on procedure risk and the amount of hardware being removed. Leads

Table 1 Catheter mapping and ablation complications	
Complications	**Comments**
Vascular access, hemorrhage, hematoma or arteriovenous fistula	Most common, maintain vigilant postprocedure monitoring
Hypotension/arrhythmias	—
Pulmonary vein thrombus	4%–10% for AF ablations
Phrenic nerve injury	More common in AF ablation procedures; may present with shortness of breath and elevated diaphragm
Damage to cardiac valves	Echocardiographic assessment helpful
Cerebral or systemic embolism	ACT target usually maintained greater than 300 s. Greater risk with instrumentation of left heart
Esophageal injury/atrioesophageal fistula	0.01%–0.2%. Use esophageal temperature probe for additional monitoring
Cardiac tamponade	1%–2%. Assess with echocardiography; may necessitate pericardial drain or cardiac surgery. Treat hypotension aggressively with vasopressors and volume

Abbreviations: ACT, activated clotting time; AF, atrial fibrillation.

Data from Patel KD, Crowley R, Mahajan A. Cardiac electrophysiology procedures in clinical practice. Int Anesthesiol Clin 2012;50:90–110; and Dagres N, Hindricks G, Bode K, et al. Complications of atrial fibrillation ablation in a high-volume center in 1000 procedures: still cause for concern? J Cardiovasc Electrophysiol 2009;20:1014–9.

less than 12 months old can often be removed by simple traction.[9] Beyond this period, leads become fixed by fibrotic tissue and may require more advanced extraction techniques such as laser sheath removal or incremental venous mechanical dilation. With increasing frequency, high-risk procedures are performed in hybrid operating rooms that allow emergency cardiac surgery and access to cardiopulmonary bypass (CPB) in case complications occur. Because these resources are rarely found in the ambulatory surgery setting, the cardiologist and anesthesiologist must perform careful preoperative risk assessment before proceeding.

Complications include vascular avulsion resulting in massive hemorrhage, hemothorax, cardiac tamponade, valvular damage, and pneumothorax.[10] With injury to the superior vena cava or the subclavian or innominate veins, upper torso peripheral or central venous access may prove ineffective for resuscitation. Although a femoral venous introducer is necessary for placement of a temporary pacemaker during the procedure, this access may be lost during emergent femoral cannulation for CPB. Placing additional femoral or other lower extremity venous access in high-risk patients, as well as having invasive monitors such as an arterial line, may be prudent.

TRANSCATHETER AORTIC VALVE REPLACEMENT

Transcatheter aortic valve replacement (TAVR) is a new treatment of aortic stenosis and was developed as an alternative to open heart surgery in high-risk patients. Although initial clinical trials have been confined to major medical centers, it is likely that the percutaneous retrograde transfemoral approach will be performed at ambulatory surgical centers in the near future. Current indications include patients with severe aortic stenosis who are nonsurgical candidates.[11,12]

Two different types of stent-valve devices have been successfully implanted in humans: balloon-expandable valves (Edwards SAPIEN and SAPIEN XT), and a self-expanding valve (Medtronic CoreValve)[1,12] The SAPIEN valve received US Food and Drug Administration approval in November 2011.

Patients usually require general anesthesia, central intravenous access, and invasive monitoring. After induction, the proceduralist places a right ventricular pacing lead via the femoral vein. Balloon aortic valvuloplasty is performed with rapid ventricular pacing to prevent balloon migration. It is important to preserve adequate coronary blood flow during this period. A mean arterial pressure of greater than 75 mm Hg has been recommended before rapid pacing.[13] Rapid ventricular pacing may cause acute myocardial ischemia, severe hypotension, and ventricular fibrillation, necessitating external defibrillation and administration of vasoactive agents. Fluoroscopy and intraoperative transesophageal echocardiography are used to guide proper valve positioning and additional rapid ventricular pacing may be required during device deployment (not required for the Medtronic CoreValve).

Complications include stroke, abnormal valve placement (perivalvular leaks or aortic insufficiency, valve embolization into the left ventricle or aorta), coronary occlusion, atrioventricular nodal block, and cardiovascular collapse requiring emergent CPB support.[11,14]

RADIATION SAFETY

Growing involvement of anesthesiology in the CCL and EPL work environments has led to significantly increased radiation exposure.[15] During some procedures the dose of radiation received by the anesthesiologist can be greater than that received by the proceduralist.[16] Anesthesia providers should be familiar with the effects of ionized radiation and, most importantly, know how to reduce exposure (**Table 2**).

Table 2
Minimizing radiation exposure

Recommendations	Comments
Maximize distance from source	During fluoroscopy, the main source of radiation is scattered, not direct, radiation from the x-ray tube. The radiation beam attenuates according to the inverse square law ($1/d^2$). Hence doubling the distance from the source reduces the exposure by a factor of 4. Exposure is usually minimal at a distance greater than 90 cm from the source
Decrease exposure time	Anesthesia providers who are frequently in the CCL or EPL environments should wear personal dosimeters
Use maximum barrier protection	Front and back coverage via lead aprons, thyroid shield, and leaded glasses. Use stationary barriers for additional protection. The eye is the most sensitive organ for radiation injury and is rarely protected by anesthesia providers

Data from Bashore TM, Bates ER, Berger PB, et al. American College of Cardiology/Society of Cardiac Angiography and Interventions Clinical Expert Consensus Document on cardiac catheterization laboratory standards. A report of the American College of Cardiology Task Force on Clinical Expert Consensus Documents. J Am Coll Cardiol 2001;37:2170–214; and Mehlman CT, DiPasquale TG. Radiation exposure to the orthopedic surgical team during fluoroscopy: "how far away is far enough?" J Orthop Trauma 1997;11:392–8.

SUMMARY

The CCL and EPL environments present unique clinical challenges. These challenges include unfamiliar work areas and staff, limited space with physical barriers separating the patient from the care provider, remote locations, and procedures with rare but potentially catastrophic clinical complications. Ambulatory anesthesiologists must familiarize themselves with these new surroundings and practice vigilant preoperative planning and continual communication with the proceduralist and team. In the future, the need for anesthesiologists in the CCL and EPL will continue to grow as procedures increase in complexity and duration.

REFERENCES

1. Gross WL, Faillace RT, Shook DC, et al. New challenges for anesthesiologists outside of the operating room: the cardiac catheterization and electrophysiology laboratories. In: Urman RD, Gross WL, Philip BK, editors. Anesthesia outside of the operating room. Oxford (United Kingdom): Oxford University Press; 2011. p. 179–97.
2. Patel KD, Crowley R, Mahajan A. Cardiac electrophysiology procedures in clinical practice. Int Anesthesiol Clin 2012;50:90–110.
3. Trentman TL, Fassett SL, Mueller JT, et al. Airway intervention in the cardiac electrophysiology laboratory: a retrospective review. J Cardiothorac Vasc Anesth 2009;23:841–5.
4. ACC/AHA/HRS Writing Committee. ACC/AHA/HRS 2006 key data elements and definitions for electrophysiological studies and procedures: a report of the American College of Cardiology/American Heart Association Task Force on Clinical Data Standards (ACC/AHA/HRS Writing Committee to Develop Data Standards on Electrophysiology). Circulation 2006;114:2534–70.

5. Kumar S, Morton JB, Halloran K, et al. Effect of respiration on catheter-tissue contact force during ablation of atrial arrhythmias. Heart Rhythm 2012;9:1041–7.

6. Kang J, Reynolds WP, Chen XL, et al. Mechanisms underlying the QT interval-prolonging effects of sevoflurane and its interactions with other QT-prolonging drugs. Anesthesiology 2006;104:1015–22.

7. Lai LP, Lin JL, Wu MJ. Usefulness of intravenous propofol anesthesia for radiofrequency catheter ablation in patients with tachyarrhythmias: infeasibility for pediatric patients with ectopic atrial tachycardia. Pacing Clin Electrophysiol 1999;22:1358–64.

8. Dagres N, Hindricks G, Bode K, et al. Complications of atrial fibrillation ablation in a high-volume center in 1,000 procedures: still cause for concern? J Cardiovasc Electrophysiol 2009;20:1014–9.

9. Farooqi FM, Talsania S, Hamid S, et al. Extraction of cardiac rhythm devices: indications, techniques and outcomes for the removal of pacemaker and defibrillator leads. Int J Clin Pract 2010;64:1140–7.

10. Elsik M, Fynn S. Permanent pacemakers and implantable defibrillators. In: Mackay JH, Arrowsmith JE, editors. Core topics in cardiac anesthesia. 2nd edition. Cambridge (England): Cambridge University Press; 2012. p. 241–8.

11. Holmes DR Jr, Mack MJ, Kaul S, et al. 2012 ACCF/AATS/SCAI/STS expert consensus document on transcatheter aortic valve replacement. J Am Coll Cardiol 2012;59:1200.

12. Rajagopal V, Kapadia SR, Tuzcu EM. Advances in the percutaneous treatment of aortic and mitral valve disease. Minerva Cardioangiol 2007;55:83–94.

13. Fassl J, Walther T, Groesdonk HV, et al. Anesthesia management for transapical transcatheter aortic valve implantation: a case series. J Cardiothorac Vasc Anesth 2009;23:286–91.

14. Zajarias A, Cribier AG. Outcomes and safety of percutaneous aortic valve replacement. J Am Coll Cardiol 1829;2009:53.

15. Katz JD. Radiation exposure to anesthesia personnel: the impact of an electrophysiology laboratory. Anesth Analg 2005;101:1725–6.

16. Anastasian ZH, Strozyk D, Meyers PM, et al. Radiation exposure of the anesthesiologist in the neurointerventional suite. Anesthesiology 2011;114:512–20.

Nonoperating Room Anesthesia for the Gastrointestinal Endoscopy Suite

John E. Tetzlaff, MD[a],*, John J. Vargo, MD, MPH[a],
Walter Maurer, MD[b]

KEYWORDS

- Anesthesia • Sedation • Monitoring • Propofol • Gastrointestinal endoscopy

KEY POINTS

- Anesthesia service participation in sedation for gastrointestinal (GI) endoscopy is increasing.
- Advanced GI endoscopy presents many challenges for the anesthesia service.
- The pre- and postprocedure care of these patients is dictated by the unique circumstances found in the GI endoscopy suite.

The trend for anesthesia services has been defined by increasing demand for coverage for procedures outside the operating room. This is particularly evident in the demand for anesthesia services for gastrointestinal (GI) endoscopy. Diagnostic colonoscopy and esophagogastroduodenoscopy (EGD) in the United States have traditionally included moderate sedation directed by the endoscopist.[1] In fact, the GI community is moving in the direction of teaching sedation techniques to GI fellows[2] and using capnography for safety.[3] For a variety of reasons, there is increasing use of anesthesia-directed sedation for routine GI endoscopy.[4] In addition, the techniques and technology for GI endoscopy are evolving rapidly, allowing endoscopic interventional procedures for an increasing array of conditions, some of which previously required a surgical approach. These technical innovations have created the need for deep sedation or general anesthesia provided by the anesthesia team to increase patient safety and improve the endoscopic outcome.[5,6] This has created the need for unique anesthesia services for the advanced GI endoscopy suite.

Disclosures: J.E. Tetzlaff has nothing to disclose; J.J. Vargo is a consultant for Boston Scientific, Inc., Cook Medical, Inc., Ethicon EndoSurgery, Inc., and Olympus America, Inc.; W. Maurer has received honoraria from Ethicon EndoSurgery.
a Cleveland Clinic Lerner College of Medicine of Case Western Reserve University, 9500 Euclid Avenue, Cleveland, OH 44195, USA; b Department of General Anesthesia, Anesthesiology Institute, Cleveland Clinic, 9500 Euclid Avenue, Cleveland, OH 44195, USA
* Corresponding author. Department of General Anesthesia, Anesthesiology Institute, Cleveland Clinic, E-30, 9500 Euclid Avenue, Cleveland, OH 44195.
E-mail address: tetzlaj@ccf.org

Anesthesiology Clin 32 (2014) 387–394
http://dx.doi.org/10.1016/j.anclin.2014.02.006
1932-2275/14/$ – see front matter © 2014 Elsevier Inc. All rights reserved.

THE PATIENTS

Most diagnostic endoscopy patients are healthy ambulatory patients. However, there are an increasing number of patients requiring endoscopy related to inflammatory bowel diseases (eg, Crohn or ulcerative colitis), in whom anesthesia services are requested, particularly after surgery. Many of these routine procedures are being ordered for patients being considered for major surgery or organ transplantation, with significant comorbidity. The various common coexisting diseases encountered in the GI endoscopy[7] suite are listed in **Box 1**.

THE PROCEDURES

Most GI endoscopy procedures are still colonoscopy or EGD for cancer screening or diagnosis of various benign conditions. When upper or lower GI bleeding is the indication, therapeutic options include banding and coagulation. The number and complexity of advanced endoscopic procedures (**Box 2**) are rapidly increasing.[8] The traditional limits of the length of the endoscope have been reduced by double balloon endoscopy (DBE), in which the combination of a balloon-tipped enteroscope and overtube can be used to telescope the gut, allowing much greater depth of penetration. With upper and lower DBE, access to the entire GI tract is possible, as is biopsy, or interventions for bleeding. Ultrasound has been added to the endoscope, allowing diagnosis of many lesions previously accessible only by surgery, including the biliary tree and the pancreas. Combined with fine needle aspiration (FNA) for tissue, endoscopic ultrasound (EUS) has an increasing role in guiding further treatment of many difficult malignancies, including chemotherapy, radiation, or surgery. With the increasingly aggressive treatment of inflammatory or malignant diseases of the GI tract, there is an increasing indication for dilation of post-treatment strictures and obstructions.

Box 1
Common coexisting disease in GI endoscopy patients

Anemia

Bacteremia

Cholangitis

Chronic obstructive pulmonary disease

Coagulopathy

Congestive heart failure

Coronary artery disease

Gastroesophageal reflux

Gastroparesis

GI bleeding

Inflammatory bowel disease

Intestinal obstruction

Liver failure

Obstructive sleep apnea

Renal insufficiency/failure

Valvular heart disease

Box 2
Advanced endoscopic techniques

Closure of tracheo-esophageal fistula

Double-balloon endoscopy

Endoscopic-assisted fine needle aspiration (biopsy)

Endoscopic dilation of stricture or anastomosis

Endoscopic drainage of pancreatic pseudocyst

Endoscopic mucosal ablation

Endoscopic mucosal resection

Endoscopic removal of common bile duct or pancreatic duct stones

Endoscopic retrograde cholangiopancreatography

Endoscopic treatment of acute GI bleeding

Endoscopic ultrasound

GI tract stenting

Percutaneous endoscopic gastrostomy tube placement

Stenting of the GI tract is possible with the aid of EGD and EUS techniques for the entire length of the GI tract from the proximal esophagus to the rectum, and it can include ligation of tracheoesophageal fistula or esophageal perforation (**Figs. 1** and **2**) with clips or a stent. The options for surgical nutrition have expanded with the availability of percutaneous endoscopic gastrostomy (PEG) tube placement. Finally, the rapidly expanding endoscopic technique of endoscopic retrograde cholangiopancreatography (ERCP) has created the option to diagnose and treat stone or stricture in the common bile duct or pancreatic duct, and to decompress infectious cholangitis or pancreatic pseudocyst in very sick patients.

ANESTHESIA TECHNIQUES FOR GI ENDOSCOPY

The work of anesthesia in the GI endoscopy suite is unique from the operating room practice in 3 key areas. There is preanesthesia preparation, the anesthetic techniques, and care of the patients immediately after the procedure.

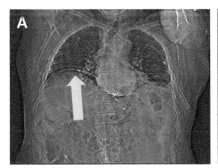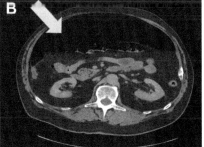

Fig. 1. 78-year-old woman transferred for management of iatrogenic esophageal perforation seen by GI and anesthesia teams. There was evidence of pneumoperitoneum without pneumothorax on chest radiograph (*A*) as well as computed tomography scan (*B*). *Arrows* indicates pneumothorax.

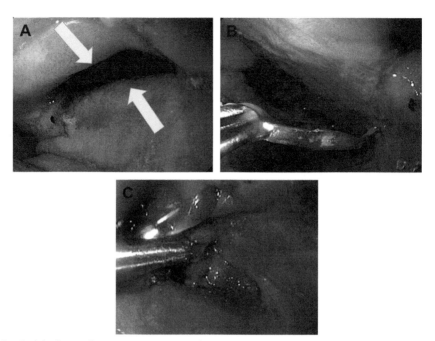

Fig. 2. (*A*) The perforation at the time of endoscopy using carbon dioxide insufflation to minimize the risk of exacerbating the pneumoperitoneum. (*B, C*) The perforation was closed with the application of metallic clips. *Arrows* indicates colon perforation.

PREANESTHESIA PREPARATION FOR THE GI ENDOSCOPY SUITE

An important distinction is practice management that creates issues for the anesthesia service in patient preparation (**Box 3**).[9] In most operating room settings, scheduling is closed, and cases are booked only by the primary surgeon, who is also the primary care physician (PCP) for the patient. In contract, most GI endoscopy suites are ambulatory units with open scheduling, and the endoscopists are consultants. The procedures are scheduled by a wide array of physicians including gastroenterologists, but also internists, cardiologists, colorectal surgeons, and others. As a consequence, there is limited if any responsibility for preparation, since the endoscopist is rarely the PCP for the patient. Because endoscopists do not perform these procedures, there is a limited understanding of the environment and what is needed. Simple things like the physician responsible for the history and physical or nothing by mouth status must be defined in an environment where this is not a routine. Consent can be handled by the assigned endoscopist, but any other preparation may become the responsibility of the anesthesia team. Getting complex patients or those with severe comorbidity to be seen by the anesthesiologist prior to the procedure can also be a challenge. Electronic health screening is an option to reduce some of this uncertainty for ambulatory patients. Although obvious, it is surprising for in-patients how often highly complex patients are scheduled for GI endoscopy[10] without ever having been seen by a gastroenterologist. Many centers have made this a requirement.

ANESTHETIC TECHNIQUE

There are a variety of anesthetic technique issues unique to the advanced GI endoscopy suite (**Box 4**). Premedication is an important element of the anesthesia technique for GI

Box 3
Preanesthetic issues with preparation for anesthesia in the GI suite

Variable PCP

Open scheduling

Who optimizes the patient?

Electronic health screening

The Endoscopist often has not Previously Met the Patient

Preparation for Anesthesia is not part of the Routine

NPO status must be defined

Many patients have an abnormal GI tract and are at risk for aspiration

Routine endoscopy for critically ill patients

High level of comorbidity in patients for advanced endoscopy

Obtaining informed consent in the setting of altered mental status

Management of automated implantable cardiac defibrillators

---

endoscopy. For upper endoscopy, glycopyrrolate can reduce secretions and improve the effectiveness of topical anesthesia. Anxiolysis with midazolam[11] is often chosen as an element of any balanced technique. Topical anesthesia is important to reduce the stimulus of upper endoscopic intubation, and this can be accomplished with benzocaine or lidocaine spray. The decision of whether to choose endotracheal intubation is important. Because many of the techniques (EGD, EUS, ERCP) are frequently performed in the lateral or semiprone positions, some providers routinely intubate. Others strive to maintain spontaneous ventilation, and use minimally invasive airway maneuvers including chin lift, jaw thrust, and nasal trumpet to supplement nasal cannula oxygen

---

Box 4
Anesthetic technique issues in the GI endoscopy suite

Glycopyrrolate

Topical anesthesia

Anxiolysis

Lateral or prone position

Endotracheal intubation or not?

Bleeding

Long procedure

Stomach or intestinal obstruction

Pancreatic pseudocyst

Sepsis

Propofol

Propofol with opioid, ketamine, or dexmedetomidine

Nausea prophylaxis

Ketorolac

Carbon dioxide insufflation via endoscope

---

delivery without adverse events for advanced endoscopy.[12] The presence of an infectious process or planned pseudocyst drainage is a relative indication to choose endotracheal intubation, as are lengthy procedures (DBE), intestinal or stomach obstruction, Zenker diverticulum with retained food, or morbid obesity. Propofol is particularly appropriate when spontaneous ventilation is chosen because of the ease of titration. Propofol can be mixed with synthetic opioids, ketamine, or dexmedetomidine when analgesia is needed. When endotracheal intubation is selected, inhalation anesthetics can be selected, although there is a report of GI endoscopy with low-dose inhaled agent as a sedative technique.[13] Ketorolac has a role in these cases because of the inflammatory nature of postprocedure pain[14] as well as decrease in the need for narcotics. Prophylaxis of nausea and vomiting is critical because of the emetogenic properties of endoscopy and insufflation of the GI tract with air or water. Decadron and a 5-HT3 antagonist are routinely chosen. Some improvement has been reported with the use of carbon dioxide insufflation,[15] which is safe from the anesthesia standpoint[16] with the few obvious exceptions including chronic obstructive pulmonary disease (COPD) and intestinal obstruction.[17,18] This accentuates the already obvious need for universal use of capnography during procedural sedation.[19]

POSTANESTHESIA CARE

The anesthesia team has the same role as with any postanesthesia patient to manage the airway, oxygenation, hemodynamics, pain control, and treatment of nausea. Things are different when there are issues that arise from endoscopy (**Box 5**). Direct issues, such as perforation, will be managed by the endoscopist, often in the endoscopy suite. On the other hand, when ERCP results in acute pancreatitis or when ERCP for cholangitis or infected pancreatic cyst contributes to sepsis, the management is less clear. Arranging for admission and acute management can fall to the anesthesia team, at least initially. A gray zone for who is in charge can occur when there is a medical issue in a high-risk patient (eg, pre-heart or lung transplant) scheduled for a screening endoscopy. Another gray area is the management of pain in patients with chronic pain of a GI origin. Admission can be indicated, but the issue is again who is responsible.

AN INCREASING ROLE FOR ANESTHESIA IN THE GI ENDOSCOPY SUITE OF THE FUTURE

There is some evidence that anesthesia care improves the outcome for some GI endoscopic procedures, especially advanced techniques. As the technology

---

Box 5
Anesthesia issues during recovery from GI endoscopy

Airway

Oxygenation

Hemodynamic instability

Respiratory insufficiency

Nausea

Bleeding

Acute pancreatitis after ERCP

Acute pain control

Acute sepsis

advances, so will the demand for anesthesia services. With the advent of natural orifice transluminal endoscopic surgery (NOTES),[8] a new patient population with need for anesthesia services will present itself, as endoscopic techniques are developed to accomplish surgery in the abdomen, pelvis, and perhaps even the thorax. The technology for sedation also presents an opportunity for anesthesia guidance with the introduction of computer-assisted, patient-demand sedation devices,[20] as their safety and efficacy can well be established by the traditional supervision of the anesthesia team.[21,22]

REFERENCES

1. Aisenberg J, Cohen LB. Sedation in endoscopic practice. Gastrointest Endosc Clin N Am 2006;16:695–708.
2. Vargo JJ, DeLegge MH, Feld AD, et al. Multisociety sedation curriculum for gastrointestinal endoscopy. Gastrointest Endosc 2012;76:e1–25.
3. Gerstenberger PD. Capnographic monitoring for endoscopic sedation: coming soon to an endoscopy unit near you? ASGE News 2011;18:1–4.
4. Alharbi O, Rabeneck L, Paszat LF, et al. A population-based analysis of outpatient colonoscopy in adults assisted by an anesthesiologist. Anesthesiology 2009;111:734–40.
5. Chelazzi C, Consales G, Boninsegni P, et al. Propofol sedation in a colorectal cancer screening outpatient cohort. Minerva Anestesiol 2009;75:677–83.
6. Ootaki C, Stevens T, Vargo J, et al. Does general anesthesia increase the diagnostic yield of endoscopic ultrasound-guided fine needle aspiration of pancreatic masses? Anesthesiology 2012;117:1044–50.
7. Martindale SJ. Anesthetic considerations during endoscopic retrograde cholangiopancreatography. Anaesth Intensive Care 2006;35:202–9.
8. DeVilliers WJ. Anesthesiology and gastroenterology. Anesthesiol Clin North America 2009;27:57–70.
9. Cohen LB, DeLegge MH, Aisenberg J, et al. AGA Institute review of endoscopic sedation. Gastroenterology 2007;133:675–701.
10. Ross C, Frishman WH, Peterson SJ, et al. Cardiovascular considerations in patients undergoing gastrointestinal endoscopy. Cardiol Rev 2008;16:76–81.
11. Padmanabian U, Leslie K, Eer AS, et al. Early cognitive impairment after sedation for colonoscopy: the effect of adding midazolam and/or fentanyl to propofol. Anesth Analg 2009;109:1448–55.
12. Cote GA, Hovis RM, Ansstas MA, et al. Incidence of sedation-related complications with propofol use during advanced endoscopic procedures. Clin Gastroenterol Hepatol 2010;8:137–42.
13. Lahoud GY, Hopkins PM. Balanced conscious sedation with intravenous induction and inhalation maintenance for patients requiring endoscopic and/or surgical procedures. Eur J Anaesthesiol 2007;24:116–21.
14. De Oliveira GS, Agarwal D, Benzon HT. Perioperative single dose ketorolac to prevent postoperative pain: a meta analysis of randomized trials. Anesth Analg 2012;114:424–33.
15. Bretthauer M, Seip B, Aasen S, et al. Carbon dioxide insufflation for more comfortable endoscopic retrograde cholangiopancreatography: a randomized, controlled, double-blind trial. Endoscopy 2007;39:58–64.
16. Suzuki T, Minami H, Komatsu T, et al. Prolonged carbon dioxide insufflation under general anesthesia for endoscopic submucosal dissection. Endoscopy 2010;42:1021–9.

17. Dellon ES, Hawk JS, Grimm IS, et al. The use of carbon dioxide for insufflation during GI endoscopy: a systematic review. Gastrointest Endosc 2009;69:843–9.
18. Takano A, Kobayashi M, Takeuchi M, et al. Capnographic monitoring during endoscopic submucosal dissection with patients under deep sedation: a prospective, crossover trial of air and carbon dioxide insufflations. Digestion 2011; 84:193–8.
19. Kodali BS. Capnography outside the operating rooms. Anesthesiology 2013;118: 192–201.
20. Pambianco DJ, Vargo JJ, Pruitt RE. Computer-assisted personalized sedation for upper endoscopy and colonoscopy: a comparative, multicenter randomized trial. Gastrointest Endosc 2011;73:765–72.
21. Gross JB, Bailey PL, Connis RT, et al. Practice guidelines for sedation and analgesia by non-anesthesiologists. Anesthesiology 2002;96:1004–17.
22. Trummel J. Sedation for gastrointestinal endoscopy: the changing landscape. Curr Opin Anaesthesiol 2007;20:359–64.

Chronic Pain: Anesthesia for Procedures

Magdalena Anitescu, MD, PhD

KEYWORDS

- Interventional pain-relieving procedures • Anesthesia for pain interventions
- Complications in pain management

KEY POINTS

- Pain management is an evolving field of medical specialty that uses increasingly complex procedures to diagnose and treat refractory and unrelenting chronic pain.
- To increase patient satisfaction and relieve anxiety associated with advanced pain-relieving procedures, physicians use anesthetic techniques ranging from local anesthetic infiltrations to general anesthesia.
- Balancing patient safety and comfort during anesthesia for pain-relieving procedures is becoming essential for the successful treatment of various and difficult pain conditions.

INTRODUCTION

Whether pain is chronic or arises immediately after a surgical intervention, it is the symptom most feared by patients. In particular, patients suffering from chronic pain are often afraid of embracing interventional procedures fearing aggravation of their symptoms. Therefore, in order to alleviate anxiety associated with various pain techniques and to improve patient satisfaction while treating chronic pain syndromes, pain physicians may use various anesthetic techniques for interventional pain-relieving procedures. This article describes the anesthesia techniques commonly used in pain practices.

HISTORY OF INTERVENTIONAL PAIN MANAGEMENT

Although medical management of pain has been used for thousands of years, interventional techniques to treat chronic, refractory, or unrelenting pain are much more recent, concomitant with the discovery, development, and advances in neural blockade and regional analgesia. Koller's discovery in 1884 that cocaine numbs the tongue[1,2] prompted physicians to use this product in a variety of interventional techniques aimed to relieve pain, such as caudal epidural injections (Cushing,[3] 1902), trigeminal ganglion block (Schloesser,[4] 1903), spinal anesthesia, and epidural analgesia using loss of resistance techniques. Identifying specific pain generators was the next step in the evolution of interventional pain management as a medical subspecialty.

Disclosure: The author has no financial interest in any of the materials discussed.
Pain Management Fellowship Program, Department of Anesthesia and Critical Care, University of Chicago Medical Center, 5841 South Maryland Avenue, MC 4028, Chicago, IL, USA
E-mail address: manitescu@dacc.uchicago.edu

Anesthesiology Clin 32 (2014) 395–409
http://dx.doi.org/10.1016/j.anclin.2014.02.001

Diagnostic blockade by administering a low dose of local anesthetic in a specific region via an interventional procedure to pinpoint the source of pain was first introduced in 1924 by von Gaza[5] who tried to identify pain arising from sympathetic or sensory nerves. Others attempted to identify specific sources of pain using procaine.[6] Bonica's extensive experience with diagnostic blockade and his and others' constant quest for multidisciplinary interventional pain treatments, coupled with advances in the understanding of clinical anatomy and the structural basis of pain through Bogduk and colleagues'[7] more recent studies, made pain interventions develop into complex, more advanced, lengthy procedures. Often those complex procedures required deep levels of sedation or occasionally general anesthesia.

ANESTHESIA TECHNIQUES IN OFF-SITE LOCATIONS

The anesthetic techniques that are used for interventional pain-relieving procedures range from minimal or no sedation to general anesthesia. With the increase in the number and complexity of pain-relieving procedures, more are now performed in offices and freestanding ambulatory surgery centers where anesthesiologists are available for care. Although anesthesia is not needed for simple pain interventions, a constant trend to improve patient satisfaction with pain relief prompts physicians to use sedation more often than in previous decades.[8] In an already ailing patient population, anxiolysis and amnesia offered by sedation may distinguish one physician's practice from another. Sedation analgesia for a procedure relies on anxiolytics, sedatives, hypnotics, or dissociative medications to decrease anxiety, pain, or movement in patients.[9] Although practice guidelines may differ in different regions,[10] the American Society of Anesthesiologists (ASA) and The Joint Commission consider sedation a continuum and recognize 3 levels of sedation plus general anesthesia (**Table 1**). The most common agents used for sedation are opioids and benzodiazepines for their anxiolytic and amnesic effects. Sedation can relax muscles and maintain analgesia (**Table 2**).[11]

INTERVENTIONAL PAIN-RELIEVING PROCEDURES

Following an ascending trend in complexity and difficulty, interventions performed by trained pain physicians can range from a simple procedure in the office to a surgical case in an operating room. To align a patient's expectations with the complexity of interventional pain-relieving procedures, physicians administer anesthesia to limit the anxiety, pain or emotional distress in patients who suffer from chronic pain. A brief

Table 1 Description of levels of sedation	
Type of Sedation	**Definition**
Minimal sedation	Patients are in drug-induced state of anxiolysis Patients respond normally to verbal commands
Moderate sedation (conscious sedation)	Patients have drug-induced depression of consciousness Patients respond purposefully to voice or tactile stimulation No interventions are needed to maintain patients' airway
Deep sedation	Patients have drug-induced depression of consciousness Patients cannot be easily aroused Patients respond purposefully after repeated or painful stimulation Ventilatory function may be impaired

From Jones DR, Salgo P, Meltzer J. Videos in clinical medicine. Conscious sedation for minor procedures in adults. N Engl J Med 2011;364:e54; with permission.

Table 2
Comparative spectrum of pharmacologic effects

Drug	Anxiolysis[a]	Sedation	Hypnosis	Analgesia	Amnesia	Anesthesia	Dependency
Methohexital	0	+	+	0	+	+	+
Diazepam	+	+	+	0	+	+	+
Midazolam	+	+	+	0	+	+	+
Propofol	0	+	+	0	+	+	+
Ketamine	0	0	0	+	+	+/D	0
Fentanyl	0	+	0	+	0	+	+
Remifentanil	0	+	+	+	0	+	+
Dexmedetomidine	0	+	+	+	+	S	0/A

Abbreviations: A, attenuates withdrawal symptoms from barbiturates, benzodiazepines, opioids; D, dissociative anesthetic state; S, anesthetic sparing effect; +, produces effect; 0, no effect.

[a] Possessing receptor specificity for effect.

Data from Smith HS, Colson J, Sehgal N. An update of evaluation of intravenous sedation on diagnostic spinal injection procedures. Pain Physician 2013;16(Suppl 2):SE217–28.

description of common pain procedures and their anesthetic requirements is shown in **Table 3**.

Most in-office procedures (trigger points, joint injections, bursa injections) can be tolerated easily by patients without sedation and sometimes without skin infiltration by local anesthetic. Infusion treatments with lidocaine or ketamine may simply require ASA standard monitoring because of their side effects.

Intravenous lidocaine, which blocks sodium channels indiscriminately, has been effective for several conditions: trigeminal neuralgia, diabetic neuropathy, fibromyalgia, cancer pain resistant to opioid therapy, and pain from spinal cord injury or central pain.[12] Because lidocaine is a potent antiarrhythmic and can be associated with seizure activity, those procedures are performed by an anesthesiologist according to the ASA standards for monitored anesthesia care. Monitoring takes place for the duration of the infusion and recovery period. The author's institutional protocol is described in **Box 1**.

Ketamine, once a battlefield anesthetic, interacts with a variety of receptor subtypes, including opioid, N-methyl-D-aspartic acid (NMDA), γ-aminobutyric acid type A and alpha-amino-3-hydroxy-5-methyl-4- isoxazole propionate, that act in chronic pain states. Acting as an antagonist on centrally located NMDA receptors, ketamine is effective against neuropathic pain, cancer pain, fibromyalgia, opioid tolerance, diabetic neuropathy, and headache.[13,14] Because ketamine can produce hallucinations,

Table 3
Common Interventional pain procedures and their Anesthetic Management

Locations	Procedures	Additional Imaging/ Fluoroscopy	Additional Imaging/ Ultrasound	Types of Sedation/ Anesthesia
Office	Trigger points	No	No/yes	None
	Major/minor joint injections/ bursa injections	No	No/yes	None/local skin infiltration
	Infusions (lidocaine/ketamine)	No	No	None/minimal/ moderate sedation
Pain clinic procedure room/ ambulatory surgery center	Routine procedures: Epidural steroid injections, transforaminal epidural steroid injections, medial branch nerve blocks, and so forth	Yes	Yes/no	Local skin infiltration, $\pm$ minimal sedation
	Complex procedures: sympathetic chain blocks, discographies, gasserian ganglion blocks and RF, minimally invasive lumbar decompression	Yes	No	Local infiltration, $\pm$ minimal-moderate sedation
Surgery center	Kyphoplasty, spinal cord stimulator, drug delivery system insertion	Yes	No	Local infiltration, deep sedation, general anesthesia, regional anesthesia

Abbreviation: RF, radiofrequency.

Box 1
University of Chicago protocol for lidocaine infusion

Consultation

- Obtain baseline electrocardiogram (EKG) and cardiac history.
- Evaluate patients for arrhythmias before scheduling the procedure.

Day of Procedure

- Assess patients for fasting and alertness.
- Determine effects of previous infusion, if any on
  - Pain reduction
  - Duration of effects
  - Patient function after infusion
  - Decrease in use of pain medication since infusion
- Verify that patients have companion to accompany them home.
- Obtain signed consent on the consent form.

Procedure

- Apply the standard monitors: blood pressure, EKG, pulse oximeter, capnograph.
- Start IV access and administer 1-mg/kg lidocaine bolus over 3 to 5 minutes.
- Follow with 4 mg/kg lidocaine (or 2–4 mg) administered slowly over 30 minutes (or 20–30 minutes).
- Record the following at 1, 5, 10, 15, 20, 25, and 30 minutes:
  - Time of administration
  - Blood pressure
  - Heart rate
  - Pulse oximetry
  - Pain score
- Stop the infusion in the event of seizure activity or cardiac instability.

Recovery

- Patients recover within 30 to 60 minutes after the procedure.
- Vital signs are monitored over 15 minutes during recovery.
- At the end of the recovery period, patients are discharged from the clinic to the accompanying caregiver.

Follow-up

- In 4 weeks, patients return for the evaluation of treatment or repeat infusion.
- The dose of lidocaine is not increased if the initial infusion was performed with 4 mg/kg over 20 minutes.

pretreatment with midazolam and sometimes with fentanyl are indicated to reduce these side effects. With these medications, most patients are mildly to moderately sedated during infusion and may take up to 1 hour to recover after treatment. These infusions may be administered in the office or in an ambulatory surgery center under the direct care of an anesthesiologist who applies ASA standard monitors. The author's clinic protocol is described in **Box 2**.

Box 2
University of Chicago protocol for ketamine infusion

Consultation

- Obtain baseline electrocardiogram (EKG) and cardiac history.
- Evaluate patients for arrhythmias before scheduling the procedure.

Day of Procedure

- Assess patients for fasting and alertness.
- Determine effects of previous infusion, if any on
  - Pain reduction
  - Duration of effects
  - Patient function after infusion
  - Decrease in use of pain medication since infusion
- Verify that patients have a companion to accompany them home.
- Obtain signed consent on the consent form.

Procedure

- Apply the standard monitors: blood pressure, EKG, pulse oximeter, capnograph.
- Start IV access and pretreat with
  - Midazolam 2 mg IV
  - Ondansetron 4 mg IV
- Begin ketamine infusion with 0.3 mg/kg in 100-mL bag for 30 to 45 minutes.
- Record the following at 1, 5, 10, 15, 20, 25, and 30 minutes:
  - Time of administration
  - Blood pressure
  - Heart rate
  - Pulse oximetry
  - Pain score
- Depending on the patients' vital signs and pain scores, the infusion may be extended to 60 minutes.
- Stop the infusion in the event of the following adverse effects:
  - Hallucinations
  - Blood pressure increase more than 20% of baseline
  - Severe anxiety
  - Nausea
  - Unmanageable, symptomatic nystagmus
- Most adverse effects disappear when infusion is stopped.
- Assess patients for urgent management.

Recovery

- Patients recover within 30 to 60 minutes after the procedure.
- Vital signs are monitored every 5 to 15 minutes during recovery.

- At the end of the recovery period, patients are discharged from the clinic to the accompanying caregiver.

Follow-up

- In 4 weeks, patients return for the evaluation of treatment or repeat infusion.
- Infusion doses may be increased to 0.6 mg/kg to 1.0 mg/kg, depending on the effect of the infusion on pain scores and the patients' function or satisfaction with pain relief.

Sedation for pain interventions that are performed in ambulatory surgery centers or in freestanding office pain clinics is inconsistent across interventional pain settings.[9] In the United States, approximately 46% of interventional pain physicians recently surveyed use intravenous (IV) sedation for patients during routine lumbar steroid injections; up to 53% of the same responders use it in cervical epidural steroid injections.[15] In many office anesthetizing locations, deep sedation is discouraged for routine pain-relieving procedures. For diagnostic procedures, such as discography, selective nerve root block, or medial branch nerve blocks, the added effect of opioids and benzodiazepines may alter the accuracy of the results and expose patients to unnecessary, more invasive procedures, such as radiofrequency ablation or spine surgery.

Some interventional pain-relieving procedures may be performed in the operating room with patients under deep sedation, regional or general anesthesia. Among such procedures are the placement of a spinal cord stimulator and generator, implantation of an intrathecal drug delivery device, and vertebral body augmentation (VBA) with kyphoplasty (KP) or vertebroplasty (VP).

The choice of anesthetic often depends on the presence or absence of serious patient comorbidities. Patients undergoing VBA are usually frail. Care is taken in positioning patients for the procedure, and neurologic status is evaluated immediately after the procedure.[16–19] There is no consensus on the type of anesthesia to be used for the VBA. The number of vertebrae to be treated in addition to the consideration of patients' comorbidities typically affect the decision.

Active distention with the balloon during KP can be painful, and general anesthesia may be an option. VP may be performed with patients under sedation; however, if the number of vertebrae treated exceeds 3, a long operating time for patients in an uncomfortable position may make general anesthesia preferable. Patients' comorbidities and age favor local anesthesia and conscious sedation. In patients with advanced chronic obstructive pulmonary disease and carbon dioxide retention, deep sedation can aggravate respiratory depression, worsen oxygenation, and increase the right ventricular afterload because of hypercapnia and pulmonary vasoconstriction. Regional anesthesia and analgesia may be a reasonable alternative for these cases. With neuraxial short-acting local anesthetic agents and small doses of neuraxial opioids, a VBA can be performed with light systemic sedation and maximum patient comfort.[20–23] In the author's institution, balloon KP is performed in the operating room to treat vertebral compression fractures. Patients are given mild sedation, and the vertebral pedicles are infiltrated with lidocaine 2% and bupivacaine 0.5%.

The most feared complication of VBA is cement extravasation. With patients pain free from a general or regional anesthetic, cement leakage toward a nerve root or in a vessel can be easily masked. Using a slow injection with pastelike cement under direct fluoroscopic views from both posteroanterior and lateral positions may decrease the risk of devastating complications.

COMPLICATIONS RELATED TO ANESTHETIC TECHNIQUES IN INTERVENTIONAL PAIN PROCEDURES

With the constant growth in complexity and duration of interventional pain-relieving procedures, patients are often immobile for long periods. Although minimal or moderate sedation does not offer an additional risk, deep sedation techniques have produced adverse events with devastating results for patients.

Despite a perfect fluoroscopic image, paresthesia from needle placement in the neuraxium may alert the physician to needle malposition. The needle is redirected or the procedure is aborted. Patients under deep sedation, however, cannot trigger this safety signal and may awaken from the procedure gravely injured. That is the reason that certain procedures benefit from patient feedback (**Table 4**).

Airway Compromise

Among the most serious complications from conscious sedation that progress to deep sedation are respiratory and cardiovascular depression or collapse. Aggressive rescue measures are necessary immediately when such situations occur.[9] For patients who are in the prone position, the ability to regain airway control is compromised, especially when sedation is administered with hypnotic agents, such as propofol, by non–anesthesia trained personnel.[24] Airway compromise associated with unrecognized high doses of hypnotics during sedation can induce a seizurelike phenomenon often associated with apnea and rapid desaturation.[25] If propofol is administered during a procedure, minimal to moderate sedation states should be maintained with appropriate IV doses to prevent complications (**Table 5**).[8]

Disinhibition and Agitation

No cases of paradoxic agitation and hyperactivity during minimal sedations have been described. These states are not infrequently seen during deep sedation.[26] Uncontrolled movements that appear with disinhibition during neuraxial needle placement can be associated with severe and devastating permanent complications, such as cord puncture, cord compression, or worsening of an already serious spinal stenosis. Agitation caused by a benzodiazepine can be quickly reversed with flumazenil[27]; the so-called propofol hyperexcitable state is controlled only by awakening patients or inducing general anesthesia. In those situations, more damage can be done making propofol a poor choice for these procedures.

Table 4	
Interventional procedures in which patient feedback is valuable	
Procedure	
Therapeutic	**Diagnostic**
Epidural injections (especially cervical)	Selective nerve root block
Intrathecal catheter placement	Facet joint injections (especially cervical)
Spinal cord stimulator placement	Discography
Sympathetic blocks	
Intradiscal ablations	

Adapted from Prager JP, April C. Complications related to sedation and anesthesia for interventional pain therapies. Pain Med 2008;9(Suppl 1):S121–7; with permission.

Table 5	
Uses and dosages of propofol	
Clinical Use	**Dose**
Induction of general anesthesia	Bolus: 1.0–2.5 mg/kg IV; dose reduced in elderly
Maintenance of general anesthesia	Infusion: 50–150 mcg/kg/min IV, combined with opiates or nitrous oxide
Sedation	Infusion: 25–75 mcg/kg/min IV
Antiemetic	Bolus: 10–20 mg IV; can repeat q 5–10 min Infusion: 10 mcg/kg/min

Adapted from Prager JP, April C. Complications related to sedation and anesthesia for interventional pain therapies. Pain Med 2008;9(Suppl 1):S121–7; with permission.

Predisposition to Neural Injury

Despite the safety of needle placement under fluoroscopic visualization during pain interventions, complications from malpositioning the needle within the spinal cord continue. An analysis of closed claims in anesthesiology showed that claims associated with chronic pain cases are increasing, surpassing obstetric anesthesia claims (**Fig. 1**). Among interventional pain procedures, cervical epidural steroid injections are associated with the most severe outcomes from needle malposition. In an analysis of the closed claims data from 2005 to 2008, Rathmell and colleagues[28] found that unfavorable outcomes from cervical interventions were more severe than adverse outcomes from all other interventions (**Fig. 2**).

In-depth analysis of the cases in malpractice claims showed that a traumatic spinal cord injury was present more often when patients had received deep sedation or general anesthesia or were unresponsive during the procedure.[29]

Many patients undergoing interventional pain-relieving procedures, especially neuraxial injections, have spinal stenosis and are at risk for a severe neurologic deficit if epidural pressure is increased. In awake patients, pain on epidural injection alerts the physician to decrease the amount of medication or to deliver the injectate more slowly while constantly communicating with patients. In profound sleep states

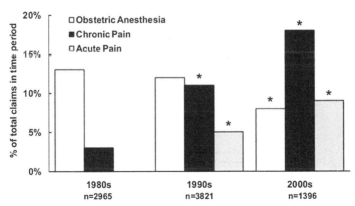

Fig. 1. Proportion of obstetric, chronic pain, and acute pain claims by decade. Claims for surgical anesthesia not shown. * $P<.01$ compared with 1980s by z test. (*From* Metzner J, Posner KL, Lam MS, et al. Closed claims' analysis. Pract Res Clin Anaesthesiol 2011;25:263–76; with permission.)

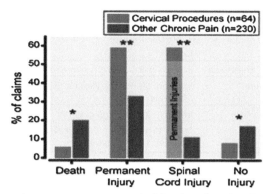

Fig. 2. Cervical procedure outcomes compared with other chronic pain treatment. Patients who underwent cervical procedures were more likely to have spinal cord injury and less likely to die than other chronic pain claim patients. Most spinal cord injuries (87%) were permanent; one patient with a spinal cord injury after a cervical procedure died. * P<0.01 ** P<.001. (*From* Rathmell JP, Michna E, Fitzgibbon DR, et al. Injury and liability associated with cervical procedures for chronic pain. Anesthesiology 2011;114:918–26; with permission.)

associated with deep sedation, however, patients are unable to communicate discomfort. Devastating injuries, such as more severe pain, loss of sensation, and sometimes paralysis, may result.[24]

The ability to perform a technically correct procedure may be blunted in deeply sedated patients. When radiofrequency denervation is planned after diagnostic medial branch nerve blocks, correct placement of the needle is confirmed with sensory and motor stimulation. Although motor response from the multifidus muscle is possible in patients under deep sedation, radicular pain from a malpositioned needle may not be

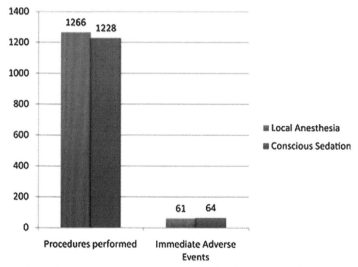

Fig. 3. Immediate adverse event rates: comparison of local anesthesia alone versus conscious sedation (odds ratio value of 0.813; 95% confidence intervals, 0.57–1.15). (*From* Schaufele MK, Marin DR, Tate JL, et al. Adverse events of conscious sedation in ambulatory spine procedures. Spine J 2011;11:1093–100; with permission.)

Table 6

Descriptive characteristics of sedation for interventional techniques

Study/Methods	Participants	Interventions	Outcomes	Results	Conclusions
Manchikanti et al, 2004 randomized, double blind	180 patients with cervical facet joint pain	Randomization into 3 equal groups (60 per group); titration of agent 1 mL at a time; relaxed or 5 mL max given Group I: NaCl Group II: midazolam Group III: fentanyl	80% pain relief and ability to perform previously painful movements	Pain relief of >80% was noted in 5% of the patients in group I, 8% in group II, and 8% in group III. However, >50% relief was noted in 8% of the patients in group I, 13% of the patients in group II, and 27% of the patients in group III. Overall, 8% of the patients in group I, 13% in group II, and 27% in group III were able to perform movements that were painful before injection.	The administration of sedation with midazolam or fentanyl is a confounding factor in the diagnosis of cervical facet joint pain in patients with chronic neck pain. However, if >80% pain relief with the ability to perform prior painful movements is used as the standard for evaluating the effect of controlled local anesthetic blocks, the diagnostic validity of cervical facet joint nerve blocks may be preserved.
Manchikanti et al, 2004 randomized, double blind	180 patients with lumbar facet joint pain	Randomization into 3 equal groups (60 per group); titration of agent 1 mL at a time; relaxed or 5 mL max given Group I: NaCl Group II: midazolam Group III: fentanyl	80% pain relief and ability to perform previously painful movements	Pain relief of >80% was noted in 2% of the patients in group I, 5% of the patients in group II, and 7% in group III. Pain relief of >50% was noted in 7% of the patients in group I, 5% of the patients in group II, and 13% of the patients in group III. There were no significant differences among the groups.	The administration of sedation with midazolam or fentanyl is a confounding factor in the diagnosis of lumbar facet joint pain in patients with chronic low back pain. However, this study suggests that if strict criteria, including pain relief and the ability to perform prior painful movements, are used as the standard for evaluating the effect of controlled local anesthetic blocks, the diagnostic validity of lumbar facet joint nerve blocks may be preserved.

(continued on next page)

Table 6 (continued)					
Study/Methods	Participants	Interventions	Outcomes	Results	Conclusions
Manchikanti et al, 2006 randomized, double blind	60 patients with combined cervical facet joint pain and lumbar facet joint pain	Randomization into 3 equal groups (20 per group); titration of agent 1 mL at a time; relaxed or 5 mL max given Group I: NaCl Group II: midazolam Group III: fentanyl	80% pain relief and ability to perform previously painful movements	Overall, 50% of the patients were relaxed or sedated in the placebo group, whereas 100% of the patients in the midazolam and fentanyl groups were relaxed or sedated. As many as 10% of the patients reported significant relief (2 reported 80%) with the ability to perform prior painful movements.	Perioperative administration of sodium chloride, midazolam, or fentanyl can confound results in the diagnosis of combined cervical and lumbar facet joint pain. False-positive results with placebo or sedation may be seen in a small proportion of patients.

Abbreviations: max, maximum; NaCl, sodium chloride.
Adapted from Manchikanti L, Boswell MV, Cash KA, et al. Influence of prior opioid exposure on diagnostic facet joint nerve blocks. J Opioid Manage 2008;4:351–60.

recognized. Injury to the nerve root during radiofrequency lesioning in deeply sedated patients can go undiagnosed until patients are awakened.[24]

Opioids, although essential in moderate sedation for their excellent analgesic effects, should be used rarely in diagnostic interventional procedures. The addition of IV fentanyl is relatively contraindicated for diagnostic procedures, such as selective nerve root block, celiac plexus block, or discography. With fentanyl added, it is unclear if pain relief is present because of the local anesthetic blockade or the IV opioid.

Adding anesthetics to interventional pain-relieving procedures to relieve anxiety and to comfort patients has mixed effects. With conscious sedation, short of severe psychiatric comorbidities or a paradoxic reaction, pain-relieving interventions can be performed with significantly less risk for adverse events. In a study of 2494 patients that analyzed adverse events after conscious sedation in ambulatory spine procedures, there was no statistically significant difference in adverse events in patients who had pain-relieving procedures under local anesthetic alone or with local anesthetic and conscious sedation with midazolam (**Fig. 3**).[30]

For diagnostic procedures that require long times and immobile patients receiving moderate sedation, the proper administration of moderate sedation did not seem to influence the results of the procedure. Manchikanti and colleagues[31] evaluated the effect of sedation on pain relief after diagnostic medial branch blocks in cervical and lumbar facet joints. Using identical methodology, they found no significant difference between the sedation groups (sodium chloride, midazolam, fentanyl) or between anatomic regions treated (cervical, lumbar) and concluded that IV sedation with fentanyl or midazolam does not alter a patient's response to a diagnostic block (**Table 6**).[9]

SUMMARY

Interventional pain-relieving procedures are becoming longer and more complex. Patients with chronic, unrelenting pain are often offered interventions during which they must be motionless. Anesthetic techniques are increasingly used by pain practitioners in order to decrease patient anxiety and pain and to provide amnesia for interventional pain-relieving procedures. Varying from local anesthetic infiltrations to general anesthesia, techniques depend on the patients' comorbidities and type of procedure. In general, routine pain interventions do not require additional sedation. When sedation is necessary, moderate sedation is preferred because patients are responsive and can alert the physician to needle malpositioning. When general anesthesia is used in vertebral augmentation procedures, frequent fluoroscopic imaging limits the possible complications from cement extravasation.

As for diagnostic interventions, there is no consensus about the influence of sedation on the accuracy and validity of the diagnostic procedure performed.[9]

Maintaining the balance between patients' comfort and safety influences the changes in the evolving field of pain management.

REFERENCES

1. Brown DL, Fink BR. The history of neural blockade and pain management. In: Cousins MJ, Bridenbaugh PO, editors. Neural blockade in clinical anesthesia and management of pain. 3rd edition. Philadelphia: Lippincott Raven; 1998. p. 3–34.
2. Manchikanti L. The growth of interventional pain management in the new millennium: a critical analysis of utilization in the Medicare population. Pain Physician 2004;7:465–82.

3. Cushing H. On the evidence of shock in major amputations by cocainization of large nerve-trunks preliminary to their division. Ann Surg 1902;36:36–321.

4. Schloesser H. Heilung periphar Reizzustande sensibler und motorischer Nerven. Klin Monbl Augenheilkd 1903;41:255.

5. Von Gaza W. Die Resektion der Paravertebralen Nervenund die isolierte-Durchschneidung des Ramus communicans. Arch Klin Chir 1924;133:479.

6. Steindler A, Luck JV. Differential diagnosis of pain in the low back: allocation of the source of the pain by the procaine hydrochloride method. JAMA 1938;110:106–13.

7. Bogduk N, Christoforidis N, Cherry D, et al. Epidural use of steroids in the management of back pain. Report of working party on epidural use of steroids in the management of back pain. National Health and Medical Research Council. Canberra (Australia): Commonwealth of Australia; 1994. p. 1–76.

8. Prager JP, April C. Complications related to sedation and anesthesia for interventional pain therapies. Pain Med 2008;9(Suppl 1):S121–7.

9. Smith HS, Colson J, Sehgal N. An update of evaluation of intravenous sedation on diagnostic spinal injection procedures. Pain Physician 2013;16(Suppl 2):SE217–28.

10. Jones DR, Salgo P, Meltzer J. Videos in clinical medicine. Conscious sedation for minor procedures in adults. N Engl J Med 2011;364(25):e54.

11. Colson JD. The pharmacology of sedation. Pain Physician 2005;8:297–308.

12. Marmura M, Rosen N, Abbas M, et al. Intravenous lidocaine in the treatment of refractory headache: a retrospective case series. Headache 2009;49:286–91.

13. Krusz JC. Intravenous treatment of chronic daily headaches in the outpatient headache clinic. Curr Pain Headache Rep 2006;10:47–53.

14. Patil SK, Anitescu M. Efficacy of outpatient ketamine infusions in refractory chronic pain syndromes: a 5 year retrospective analysis. Pain Med 2012;13:263–9.

15. Ahmed SU, Tonidandel W, Trella J, et al. Peri-procedural protocols for interventional pain management techniques: a survey of U.S. pain centers. Pain Physician 2005;8:182–5.

16. Kasperk C, Ingo A, Grafe IA, et al. Three-year outcomes after kyphoplasty in patients with osteoporosis with painful vertebral fractures. J Vasc Interv Radiol 2010;21:701–9.

17. McGirt MJ, Parker SL, Wolinsky JP, et al. Vertebroplasty and kyphoplasty for the treatment of vertebral compression fractures: an evidenced-based review of the literature. Spine 2009;9:501–8.

18. Liu JT, Liao WJ, Tan WC, et al. Balloon kyphoplasty versus vertebroplasty for treatment of osteoporotic vertebral compression fracture: a prospective, comparative, and randomized clinical study. Osteoporos Int 2010;21:359–64.

19. Pflugmacher R, Taylor R, Agarwal A, et al. Balloon kyphoplasty in the treatment of metastatic disease of the spine: a 2-year prospective evaluation. Eur Spine J 2008;17:1042–8.

20. Krueger A, Bliemel C, Zettl R, et al. Management of pulmonary cement embolism after percutaneous vertebroplasty and kyphoplasty: a systematic review of the literature. Eur Spine J 2009;18:1257–65.

21. Elshaug AG, Garber AM. How CER could pay for itself –insights from vertebral fracture treatments. N Engl J Med 2011;364:1390–3.

22. Burton AW, Hamid B. Kyphoplasty and vertebroplasty. Curr Pain Headache Rep 2008;12:22–7.

23. Schofer MD, Efe T, Timmesfeld N, et al. Comparison of kyphoplasty and vertebroplasty in the treatment of fresh vertebral compression fractures. Arch Orthop Trauma Surg 2009;129:1391–9.

24. Abram SE, Francis MC. Hazards of sedation for interventional pain procedures. Anesthesia Patient Safety Foundation Newsletter; 2012.
25. Walder B, Tramer MR, Seeck M. Seizure-like phenomena and propofol: a systematic review. Neurology 2002;58:1327–32.
26. Braidy HF, Singh P, Ziccardi VB. Safety of deep sedation in an urban oral and maxillofacial surgery training program. J Oral Maxillofac Surg 2011;69:2112–9.
27. McKenzie WS, Rosenberg M. Paradoxical reaction following administration of a benzodiazepine. J Oral Maxillofac Surg 2010;68:3034–6.
28. Rathmell JP, Michna E, Fitzgibbon DR, et al. Injury and liability associated with cervical procedures for chronic pain. Anesthesiology 2011;114:918–26.
29. Metzner J, Posner KL, Lam MS. Domino KB closed claims analysis. Best Pract Res Clin Anaesthesiol 2011;25:263–76.
30. Schaufele MK, Marin DR, Tate JL, et al. Adverse events of conscious sedation in ambulatory spine procedures. Spine J 2011;11:1093–100.
31. Manchikanti L, Boswell MV, Cash KA, et al. Influence of prior opioid exposure on diagnostic facet joint nerve blocks. J Opioid Manag 2008;4:351–60.

Pediatric Ambulatory Anesthesia

David A. August, MD, PhD[a],*, Lucinda L. Everett, MD[b]

KEYWORDS

- Upper respiratory infection • Apnea • Undiagnosed hypotonia • Anxiolysis
- Pregnancy testing • Remifentanil • Circumcision • Acetaminophen

KEY POINTS

- Risk stratification is important to determine when it is safe to proceed with anesthesia in a child with current or recent upper respiratory infection.
- Patients at risk of apnea should be admitted for overnight monitoring; these include former premature infants younger than 55 to 60 weeks postconceptual age, full-term infants younger than 44 weeks postconceptual age who demonstrate any respiratory abnormalities, and certain children with sleep apnea who are recovering from tonsillectomy.
- In children with muscular dystrophy, the risk of hyperkalemic cardiac arrest after a brief exposure to volatile anesthetics seems low. Although children with mitochondrial disease have a variable response to anesthetic drugs; propofol infusion syndrome is not definitively linked to intraoperative propofol use.
- Dorsal penile nerve block and caudal block both work well for postcircumcision pain.
- A single loading dose of rectal acetaminophen for postoperative analgesia is best used with other drugs and when a delayed response is acceptable.

INTRODUCTION

Anesthetizing children for ambulatory surgery presents continuing challenges and many are reviewed elsewhere.[1-4] This update addresses several current issues in patient selection and preparation, and intraoperative and postoperative considerations for selected procedures, with an emphasis on pain management.

In 2006, approximately 3.3 million out of 53.3 million outpatient procedures were performed on patients younger than age 15, according to the Centers for Disease Control and Prevention's National Center for Health Statistics.[5] The growth in volume over the decade occurred overwhelmingly in freestanding sites, with 43% of ambulatory procedures now being done in these settings. Ambulatory visits accounted for

Disclosure: Neither author is affiliated with companies that have a direct or competing financial interest in the material discussed in this article.

[a] Department of Anesthesia, Critical Care, and Pain Medicine, Massachusetts General Hospital, 55 Fruit Street, GRB-444, Boston, MA 02114, USA; [b] Department of Anesthesia, Critical Care, and Pain Medicine, Massachusetts General Hospital, 55 Fruit Street, GRB-415, Boston, MA 02114, USA

* Corresponding author.

E-mail address: daugust@partners.org

Anesthesiology Clin 32 (2014) 411–429
http://dx.doi.org/10.1016/j.anclin.2014.02.002
1932-2275/14/$ – see front matter © 2014 Elsevier Inc. All rights reserved.

62% of visits or admissions in which a procedure was performed. Patients younger than age 15 have the lowest rates of ambulatory surgery, at 58 per 1000 for boys and 49 per 1000 for girls. Details of case statistics for pediatric patients are shown in **Table 1**.

PATIENT SELECTION

Appropriate patient selection is critical to the success of outpatient surgery. Special areas of concern with children presenting for ambulatory anesthesia include upper respiratory tract infection (URI), apnea risk (among infants and those with sleep apnea), cardiac disease, and undiagnosed myopathy. The facility and expertise of available staff must also be considered in selecting younger or higher-risk children for outpatient surgery.

Upper Respiratory Infection

Children with URIs are at risk for perioperative respiratory adverse events (PRAEs) and risk stratification is crucial in deciding whether to postpone anesthesia. The approach to this dilemma has been refined over time. Initial reports emphasized the potentially severe consequences of anesthesia, including lung collapse, ICU admission, and even death.[6] More recently, better evidence has allowed practitioners to exclude the children who are at highest risk, make appropriate clinical decisions, and proceed when children with less severe URI are undergoing minor procedures. This decision-making process may be facilitated by algorithms (**Fig. 1**)[6] and should include consideration of the following risk factors:

- Patient factors: Three issues to consider are symptom duration, illness severity, and the presence of underlying lung disease. In terms of symptom duration, a URI that is current or within the last 2 weeks is associated with a high PRAE risk.[7,8] Waiting 4 weeks after a URI seems to provide an adequate clinical safety margin[6,9] although laboratory studies suggest that airway reactivity may persist even longer. More severe symptoms (ie, copious purulent secretions, wet cough, high fever, and systemic findings such as lethargy and poor appetite) constitute higher PRAE risk. Such patients are often excluded from anesthetic outcome studies in children with URI.[7,10-12] Finally, PRAEs are more likely in the presence of underlying respiratory problems such as asthma or prematurity-associated chronic lung disease.[11]

Table 1	
Statistics on ambulatory surgery in patients younger than 15 years of age	
Total ambulatory procedures (all ages)	53,329,000
Ambulatory procedures younger than 15 y	3,266,000
Case breakdown—patients younger than 15 y	
Myringotomy and tubes	667,000
Tonsillectomy with or without adenoidectomy	530,000
Orthopedic procedures	295,000
Operations on the male genital organs	166,000
Adenoidectomy	132,000
Hernia repair	73,000

Adapted from Centers for Disease Control and Prevention. National Survey of Ambulatory Surgery. 2006. Available at: http://www.cdc.gov/nchs/nsas.htm. Accessed January 30, 2014.

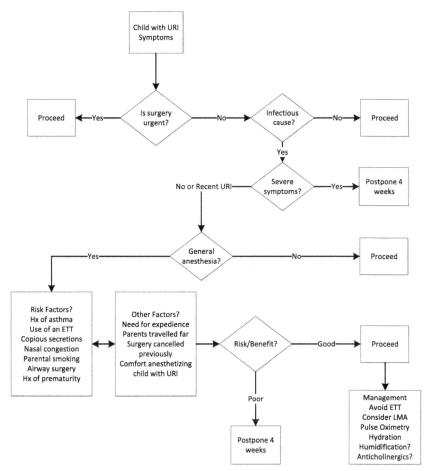

Fig. 1. Suggested algorithm for the assessment and anesthetic management of the child with an upper respiratory infection. ETT, endotracheal tube; Hx, history; LMA, laryngeal mask airway. (*From* Tait AR, Malviya S. Anesthesia for the child with an upper respiratory infection: still a dilemma? Anesth Analg 2005;100:62; with permission.)

- Anesthetic factors: Airway management is a major risk factor for PRAE. Face-mask anesthesia is associated with the lowest risk, followed by laryngeal mask airway, and finally by endotracheal intubation.[7,9,11,12] In addition to the device itself, other maneuvers may also reduce PRAE risk, such as lubricating the laryngeal mask airway with lidocaine.[13]
- Surgical factors: Airway surgery is associated with a high risk of PRAE.[7,11,14] However, simpler cases such as adenoid removal may be better tolerated, and even therapeutic, compared with more complex procedures such as palatoplasty. Myringotomy with ear tube placement seems to be quite safe,[15] likely because of its short duration and lack of airway stimulation.

Apnea Risk in Infants

Up to 55 to 60 weeks postconceptual age (PCA), ex-preterm infants are at increased risk of postanesthetic apnea and should be observed overnight.[16] Additional risk factors include lower gestational age (even at the same PCA), ongoing apnea at home, and anemia.[16,17] Recent retrospective series confirm that apnea risk is fairly low (4/331 = 1.1%), that it may not persist beyond the postanesthesia care unit (PACU),[18] and that it may be limited to patients with preexisting apnea and lower gestational ages.[17] Postanesthetic apnea remains an active research area, with the goals of increasing safety through better and more cost-effective targeted policies for overnight admission after anesthesia.

Although apnea in preterm babies has been described for decades, the risk of post-anesthetic apnea among full-term infants has received less attention. There are rare case reports of apnea in apparently healthy term infants having minor procedures. In most of these cases, some unusual clinical behavior was noted (eg, respiratory irregularities or an unexpectedly rapid induction).[19–21] One case also used clonidine in a caudal block.[22] Several of these infants were subsequently found to have an abnormal sleep study, raising the possibility that anesthesia can unmask an underlying respiratory control disorder. Use of clonidine or opioids in a patient less than 44 weeks PCA, or any clinical abnormality during anesthesia, emergence, or early recovery may warrant overnight monitoring. Because continuous pulse oximetry alone does not always detect apnea, respiratory monitoring should also include chest-wall motion (eg, impedance pneumography). Very young infants should be scheduled early in the day to allow prolonged observation if needed.

Sleep Apnea and Tonsillectomy

Tonsillectomy is frequently performed for obstructive sleep apnea (OSA). Careful patient selection is critical to safe performance of outpatient tonsillectomy. Children younger than 4 years of age have a higher incidence of unplanned admission and return to the surgery center compared with older children having ear, nose, or throat surgery.[23] The American Academy of Otolaryngology–Head and Neck Surgery recommends overnight admission for monitoring after tonsillectomy in patients younger than 3 years of age with OSA or if OSA is severe (ie, apnea-hypopnea index ≥10 events per hour or oxygen saturation <80%).[24] Children with OSA have been shown to have increased sensitivity to opioids.[25] Other conditions, such as trisomy 21, overweight, syndromes, or neurologic impairment, also increase after posttonsillectomy.[26,27] There have been numerous reports of adverse events, including death, after tonsillectomy.[28] Because a cytochrome P450 variant causing rapid metabolism of codeine may be a factor in these deaths, the Food and Drug Administration issued a warning against using codeine for posttonsillectomy analgesia in children in early 2013.[29]

Cardiac Risk

Cardiac arrest in healthy children occurs rarely. Volatile anesthetic-induced cardiac arrest has mostly disappeared because of the transition from halothane to sevoflurane, along with better awareness of this potential complication and liberalized nil per os (nothing by mouth) guidelines. The Pediatric Perioperative Cardiac Arrest Registry indicates that respiratory-related cardiac arrests still occur among otherwise healthy patients (ie, children who might present for ambulatory surgery) and that laryngospasm with hypoxia is a frequent trigger.[30]

Children with congenital heart disease with asymptomatic lesions (eg, a small ventricular septal defect) or full anatomic repairs with documented good residual function may be candidates for outpatient procedures, even in a freestanding setting. Patients with complex lesions are only candidates for outpatient status in a full-service facility with appropriate cardiology and intensive care services.

Undiagnosed Weakness or Hypotonia

Hypotonic patients presenting for diagnostic evaluation present an anesthetic challenge. In addition to usual concerns about respiratory compromise in a weak patient, the anesthesiologist must formulate a provisional diagnosis to make rational drug choices. Sources of confusion about medication safety include the limited information parents receive from health care providers about these complex diseases and the proliferation of inadequately sourced information on the Internet. One general rule is to avoid succinylcholine because of its well-known ability to produce hyperkalemia in patients with weakness and the potential danger it poses to patients in whom the cause of weakness is undiagnosed.[31] This article reviews concerns about three drug-related issues: malignant hyperthermia (MH), acute hyperkalemic cardiac arrest, and propofol infusion syndrome (PRIS).

MH

Only a few diseases are strongly associated with MH: King-Denborough syndrome (KDS), central core disease (CCD), and multiminicore myopathy.[32] Of note, mitochondrial disease is not in this category. Obviously, a trigger-free technique is necessary when anesthetizing these children and may also be considered for others with undiagnosed hypotonia who are estimated to have a small (<1.09%) MH risk during diagnostic muscle biopsy.[33]

Recognizing children with these rare diseases may not be straightforward.[34,35] Creatine kinase (CK) levels are often normal or only slightly elevated. Clues to KDS include family history (often with dominant inheritance), facial dysmorphism similar to that of Noonan syndrome (ie, webbed neck, micrognathia, low-set ears, high-arched or cleft palate), short stature, cryptorchidism, and developmental delay. Children with CCD may not have facial dysmorphism but can have skeletal anomalies such as clubfoot, scoliosis, and hip dysplasia, as well as an autosomal dominant family history. Multiminicore myopathy mostly affects axial musculature (ie, scoliosis, pelvic girdle) and exhibits recessive inheritance.

Achieving a trigger-free condition may require prolonged (ie, >60 min) high-flow flushing of the anesthesia machine. In the busy ambulatory surgery setting, it may be more efficient to place activated charcoal filters on the inspiratory and expiratory limbs of the machine, a technique that requires 10 minutes or less to reduce volatile anesthetic levels to below 5 parts-per-million.[36]

Hyperkalemic cardiac arrest

Perioperative hyperkalemic cardiac arrest and rhabdomyolysis is a recognized risk of succinylcholine administration in patients with muscular dystrophy. There are also case reports describing arrests after children awaken from a seemingly uncomplicated anesthetic using volatile agents without succinylcholine. Although these arrests share some clinical features with MH, they are a different entity. MH is a hypermetabolic state caused by failure of intracellular calcium reuptake, whereas muscular dystrophy-associated arrests are attributed to volatile anesthetic-induced destabilization of cell membranes with subsequent leakage of potassium-rich intracellular fluid, which may be enhanced by muscular activity or shivering during recovery.[37–39]

Although some investigators suggest avoiding volatile agents in muscular dystrophy,[38] this idea is not universally accepted. One recent series in which 66 of 117 muscular dystrophy patients received volatiles agents[39] suggests that they can be used safely. If acute rhabdomyolysis is dose-related rather than triggered, then brief exposure (ie, during induction to facilitate intravenous [IV] access or airway management) could be safe, but definitive evidence is lacking.

Muscular dystrophy may be suspected in children with elevated CK levels and a positive family history (ie, often but not always X-linked recessive), whose physical examination findings can include lower limb wasting, a waddling gait, Gower sign (ie, "climbing" up one's legs to move from a sitting to standing position), or pseudohypertrophy of the calves due to fibrofatty infiltration.[40,41]

PRIS

PRIS, a potentially fatal syndrome characterized by severe bradycardia, lipemic serum, metabolic acidosis, rhabdomyolysis, hepatomegaly, and cardiac and renal failure, is generally associated with lengthy, high-dose propofol infusions in the ICU (>4 mg/kg/h for >48 hours).[42] Case reports have raised the question of whether PRIS can also occur at lower doses and after shorter durations.[43] It has been suggested that patients with mitochondrial diseases may be especially susceptible to PRIS[44] because propofol acts as a mitochondrial poison, reducing the ability of these organelles to perform various functions, including fatty acid oxidation, even as its vehicle adds another fat source.[42,45] There is no definitive evidence that PRIS is linked to intraoperative use of propofol for children with mitochondrial disorders and case series demonstrate the successful use of propofol among patients with various mitochondrial diseases.[46–48] The best clinical advice may be that careful clinical titration is appropriate in patients who represent a wide spectrum of disease with variable responses to anesthetics.[44] Minimizing fasting periods, maintaining hydration, supplementing dextrose, avoiding lactate-containing fluids, as well as monitoring anesthetic depth,[49] blood sugar, acid-base status, and temperature should all be considered. Clues to the presence of mitochondrial myopathy in a child with undiagnosed weakness include other laboratory abnormalities besides elevated CK (eg, lactic acidosis, hypoglycemia), evidence of multisystem involvement (eg, encephalopathy, seizures, cardiomyopathy), normal physical features, and a pattern of acute worsening symptoms during crisis periods brought on by catabolic stress such as fever or hypoglycemia (**Table 2**).[32,44,47,50]

Preoperative Pregnancy Testing

Adolescent females presenting for anesthesia, particularly in their parents' presence, may be hesitant to give an accurate history of the possibility of pregnancy. Institutions are increasingly implementing a standing policy of routine preoperative pregnancy testing in women of childbearing age. Such a policy requires consideration of logistical, legal, and ethical issues as outlined in **Table 3**. If testing is not routine, then a careful history should be obtained, ideally in the absence of the parents.

PREOPERATIVE MANAGEMENT
Nonpharmacological Anxiolysis

Anxiolytic premedication may be problematic in a rapid-turnover ambulatory surgery setting. For example, midazolam may delay recovery and discharge, whereas clonidine may require a lengthy onset time.[51,52] There are several nonpharmacological techniques to reduce preoperative anxiety, including professional entertainers (eg, clowns and magicians), audiovisual material (eg, videos, games, music), verbal techniques (eg, humor and distraction), and parental presence during the induction of anesthesia (PPIA).[53]

Clowns and magicians

Professional clowns can alleviate anxiety in parents and children before and during inhalational induction. Although they may do so more effectively than PPIA and oral

Table 2
Anesthetic considerations for children with undiagnosed hypotonia

	KDS, CCD, Multiminicore Myopathy	Muscular Dystrophy (DMD, Becker-type)	Mitochondrial Disorders
Drug Concerns	MH	Hyperkalemic response, including rhabdomyolysis and cardiac arrest	Anesthetic effects on mitochondrial function Sensitivity to anesthetics (variable)
Laboratory Diagnosis	Normal or mildly elevated CK	Markedly elevated CK	Elevated lactate and CK Hypoglycemia
H & P Diagnosis	Syndromic facial appearance Limb anomalies Cryptorchidism Scoliosis	Male Leg wasting Gower sign Calf pseudohypertrophy	Crisis periods Multisystem involvement (encephalopathy, seizures, cardiomyopathy)
Anesthetic Considerations	Trigger-free	"Nearly" trigger-free: avoid succinylcholine Limited volatile exposure is acceptable (eg, to facilitate intravenous access)	No definitive link to PRIS from intraoperative exposure Titrate anesthetics Avoid prolonged fasting, dehydration, hypoglycemia, and lactated fluids

Abbreviations: DMD, Duchenne muscular dystrophy; H & P, history and physical examination.

Table 3
Considerations in preoperative pregnancy testing

Is it important to identify pregnancy before anesthesia or sedation? What is the risk?	Concerns include risk of congenital malformation, spontaneous abortion, medicolegal risk American Society of Anesthesiologists (ASA) Task Force on Preanesthesia Evaluation[123]: the literature is inadequate to inform patients or physicians on whether anesthesia causes harmful effects on early pregnancy Pregnancy testing may be offered to female patients of childbearing age and for whom the result would alter the patient's management
What is the incidence of undiagnosed pregnancy?	Kahn et al[124]: 5 positive tests per 2588; 3 unrecognized pregnancies, 1 asymptomatic ectopic, 1 false positive Wheeler & Cote[125]: 3 positive tests per 235 (2 were adults); all denied possibility Malviya et al[126]: test results correlated with history (n ~ 500)
What constitutes adequate informed consent?	ASA Committee on Ethics[127]: Routine pregnancy testing of all women and/or testing in the absence of informed consent is inconsistent with the privacy and autonomy rights of women making health care decisions about these sensitive issues "Mature minor" status may apply if patient believes herself to be pregnant Generally, parents need to consent for routine testing
Who can be informed if the test is positive?	Varies by state; essential to know local law Law may either require or prohibit informing parents Support structure (social work) and referral ability should be available if testing is performed
Logistical questions	Accuracy of test, turnaround time, cost, point-of-care credentialing requirements Most centers use urine testing unless unable to obtain sample Laboratory medicine notes lack of sensitivity early

midazolam,[53–55] the availability of clowns specially trained and vetted for pediatric hospital work and who have undergone health screening, background checks, and instruction in engaging children who have physical limitations may be limited. Additionally, they may be perceived as disrupting normal routine and causing delays.[55] Interactive magic also reduces anxiety in hospitalized children.[56] When professional magicians are not available, anesthesiologists may perform simple tricks (eg, the "magic ball") to reduce anxiety during inhalational induction.[57]

Audiovisual material and games
Children who view a preselected funny video streamed into the OR on a large screen are less anxious on entry into the OR and during inhalational induction.[58] Videos can also be brought into the OR via hand-held devices.[59] Interactive music therapy for children can reduce anxiety preoperatively and during separation from parents but its effect during inhalational induction is inconsistent and probably therapist-dependent.[53] Hand-held video games limit the increase in or even reduce anxiety during induction better than midazolam or PPIA[53,60] and may also be combined with nitrous oxide.[61]

Humor and verbal methods
During PPIA, certain adult-child interactions may reduce children's anxiety and improve coping.[62] Although emotion-based behavior (eg, reassurance, empathy, or apology) seems more natural, it seems to be less effective than distracting behavior (eg, humor, distracting talk, or medical reframing). To use humor effectively, the anesthesiologist must understand what is funny to a child of a particular age.[63] Babies smile and laugh before their sixth month; however, these actions may reflect other feelings besides amusement, such as joy, pleasure, excitement, or even fear.[64,65] Although psychologists generally agree that children do not fully understand humor before age two, even very young children can still enjoy certain styles of humor.[65,66] For teenagers, the challenge is not deciding what will be funny so much as the ability to quickly form an emotional bond which will allow shared humor to be effective. **Table 4** provides suggestions for using humor at these two age extremes.

INTRAOPERATIVE MANAGEMENT
Intubation Without Neuromuscular Blockade: Remifentanil
Tracheal intubation without neuromuscular blockade (NMB) has become increasingly common in pediatric anesthesia,[67] even though NMB use may actually be associated with lower PRAE risk.[14] In the ambulatory surgical setting, there are several reasons to avoid NMB: there are no truly short-acting nondepolarizers; emergence may be delayed if the NMB is not reversible in time; and incomplete NMB reversal may produce subtle findings such as difficulty swallowing and visual changes, which delay street readiness.[68] NMB reversal may be associated with side effects such as nausea or even with postoperative respiratory complications in adults.[69]

Remifentanil can provide favorable conditions for endotracheal intubation without the need for NMB. The intubating dose of remifentanil depends on its context (ie, what other drugs are given, what airway technique is used, and what endpoint is measured). In adults, the bolus dose of remifentanil for good or excellent direct laryngoscopy ranges from 1 to 8 µg/kg depending on whether it is combined with propofol, thiopental, midazolam, desflurane, or sevoflurane[70–73]; and on whether a lightwand or laryngoscope is used.[74] Lower doses of 1 to 1.5 µg/kg, remifentanil also attenuate the hemodynamic response[75,76] and increased intraocular pressure[77] associated with airway manipulation.

Table 4
Age-specific humor for infants, toddlers, and adolescents

	Humor Format	Humor Content	Play Signals
6–18 mo	Tactile, visual	Tickling; "peek-a-boo"; motionless face Simple incongruity Clowning (funny faces, silly walks) Familiar object presented in novel way	Safe environment Familiarity PPIA Smiling, laughing
18 mo–2 y	Visual, verbal Simple phrases (ie, no readymade jokes or riddles)	Symbolic play: treat an incongruous object as though it is real (eg, "talk" to a pen as though it is a phone, "comb" hair with a pen while saying "combing hair!") Simple name changes (eg, calling a cat a dog)	Smiling, laughing Simple declarations (eg, "This is only pretend," "This is funny") Humor box with jokes, cartoons, etc located in preoperative area
Teenagers	Verbal Spontaneous wit Readymade stories, jokes, and riddles	Standard humor Topical items Irony "Gross" jokes	First, establish a trusting, empathetic relationship Do not "talk down" or marginalize Use generic conversational questions (eg, "Who's your favorite comedian?") Let teenager use humor first, then follow-up

The general principles and specific examples are from McGhee's theory of childhood humor development and other sources.[64–66] The last column (Play signals) describes ways to put the child in the appropriate frame of mind (sometimes called the "playful set") for humor to be effective. Note that the ages listed here are only approximate; children pass through the stages of humor development in order but the exact ages at which these transitions occur differ between individuals.

In children, one systematic review suggested that excellent intubating conditions can be obtained 85% of the time when 4 μg/kg of remifentanil is combined with propofol, but only 29% of the time when the dose was reduced to 1 μg/kg.[78] With 8% sevoflurane, an even lower remifentanil dose of 1 to 2 μg/kg provides excellent conditions more than 75% of the time. In terms of timing, 3 μg/kg of remifentanil allows intubation of neonates as quickly as succinylcholine, but with less favorable conditions.[79] Infants may have less predictable pharmacodynamics responses than other ages. In one study, the remifentanil ED50 for ideal intubating conditions did not differ overall among age groups (ie, neonates through 3-year-olds) but infants had the most variability (95% confidence interval of 2–5.4 μg/kg).[80]

Remifentanil also has effects on heart rate, airway reactivity, and muscle tone. Its bradycardic and sympatholytic effects may be appropriate for conditions such as pulmonary hypertension or dynamic ventricular outflow obstruction, whereas remifentanil infusions reduce desflurane-associated airway irritation and bolus doses of 1 to 2 μg/kg blunt hemodynamic response to intubation.[81,82] For most infants and young children anticholinergic pretreatment (ie, glycopyrrolate 10 μg/kg or atropine 20 μg/kg) is used to maintain heart rate[79] and with this even infants can tolerate up to 6 μg/kg of remifentanil.[80] The effects of a remifentanil bolus on muscle tone and chest-wall rigidity is inconsistently reported.[79,80]

Pain Management for Circumcision

Circumcision is a common outpatient surgical procedure for which many pain management strategies have been studied, including ring blocks (either alone or combined with the dorsal penile nerve block [DPNB]), cyanoacrylate glue (instead of sutures), topical anesthesia, and pudendal nerve blocks.[83–87]

DPNB is a purely regional technique that can be used without any other anesthesia for elective circumcision. It has been shown to shorten PACU stay and reduce postoperative nausea and vomiting (PONV).[88] Ultrasound guidance improves DPNB outcomes compared with injection by anatomic landmarks, with lower pain scores on arrival to the PACU and during the next 30 minutes, a longer time-to-first-analgesia, less frequent rescue morphine, lower rescue doses, and reductions in oral codeine before PACU discharge.[89–91] The longer procedural time required for ultrasound[89,91] may limit its acceptance in busy ambulatory surgery settings. DPNB can be prolonged by mixing it with certain adjuvants, such as tramadol, clonidine, and fentanyl.[83,84] Problems with DPNB include block failure, drug errors, bupivacaine toxicity, ischial osteomyelitis, abscess, hematoma, preputial bleeding, urethral injury, hematoma, and edema.[88,92–94]

Caudal epidural analgesia does not differ from DPNB or parenteral agents with respect to the need for other analgesics, rescue analgesia, or PONV, but it does have a higher incidence of motor block and leg weakness.[95] When specifically compared with ultrasound-guided DPNB, caudal block prolonged analgesia, but did not affect overall rescue morphine requirement.[90] The effect of caudal blockade on procedural and discharge times is open to debate, with one study showing that children who received caudal blocks went home earlier than those getting penile blocks but also required more time in the operating room.[96] Other investigators have not observed an effect on recovery times.[90] Adding ketamine or clonidine to the caudal block mixture may prolong analgesia but may also lengthen arousal time, delay micturition, and enhance motor weakness.[97–99] Complications in children from neuraxial anesthesia are well described but are atypical for single-shot caudal blocks commonly used for circumcision.[100] Given that caudal blockade has similar effectiveness to other analgesic techniques but is associated with motor weakness and longer procedural times, DPNB or parenteral drugs may be preferable for ambulatory circumcision surgery, especially among patients who are old enough to walk.

Acetaminophen: Rectal Dosing

Children undergoing ambulatory surgical procedures often receive a single dose of acetaminophen per rectum (PR) shortly after induction to provide analgesia, which likely acts via inhibition of central nervous system COX-3 enzymes.[101] For very short surgeries, acetaminophen may be the sole analgesic; however, for other surgeries it may be part of a multimodal pain-control strategy. The existing literature provides a range for PR acetaminophen dosing from 15 to 45 mg/kg, depending on age, prematurity status, suppository formulation, setting (ie, perioperative vs nonsurgical), measured outcome (ie, antipyresis, clinical analgesia, reduced need for other analgesic drugs, or blood concentrations within a certain target range usually defined as 10–20 μg/mL), and other factors.[102–106] PR acetaminophen dosing in the surgical setting is summarized in **Table 5**.

Accurate dosing of acetaminophen is important for several reasons. Hepatotoxicity is a real risk, especially among children who are underweight,[107] malnourished,[108] myopathic,[109] or have preexisting liver disease. Even a limited overdose within a short time period can cause liver toxicity.[110] The recent widespread use of IV acetaminophen

Table 5 Rectal acetaminophen dosing		
	20 mg/kg PR	40 mg/kg (max 1 g) PR
Premature infants	Target range[a] likely for 28–32 wk GA, but less for 32–36 wk GA Analgesia likely Tmax 4–5 h	—
Term neonates Older term infants and children Adults	Target range[a] not achieved Analgesia unlikely Effective for antipyresis	Adequate blood levels achieved Analgesia likely Cmax has significant variability Repeated doses increase chance of Cmax reaching target range[a] Tmax 1–3 h

Summary perioperative studies of rectal acetaminophen for various age groups.

Abbreviations: Cmax, maximum serum concentration of acetaminophen; GA, gestational age; Tmax, time after drug administration at which Cmax is reached.

[a] Serum acetaminophen concentration of 10–20 µg/mL, which is frequently used to indicate adequate analgesic levels.

has led to many large (eg, tenfold) overdoses.[111] Furthermore, anesthesiologists cannot assume that dosage guidelines will be followed after surgery.[112] Limited understanding of acetaminophen label instructions by practitioners and lay people is reflected by the decision to simplify national dosing guidelines for this drug in the United Kingdom[107] and by observations that physicians, including anesthesiologists, frequently administer incorrect doses.[113] Finally, epidemiologic studies have found an association between early acetaminophen exposure and asthma.[114] Although the significance of this association is not established, caution suggests using only the minimum acetaminophen dose required.

A dose of 20 mg/kg PR can produce adequate blood levels at the lowest gestational ages 76% of the time in a group of 28-week to 32-week gestational age newborns.[106] When this dose is given to full-term newborns, infants, and children, the maximum serum concentration (Cmax) frequently falls short of desired therapeutic concentrations[105,115] and fails to provide adequate analgesia, despite producing adequate antipyresis.[116] In older infants and children, higher doses of 40 to 45 mg/kg PR more often result in therapeutic blood levels[103,117] and reduce rescue opioid requirements after outpatient surgery.[104] Even at these higher doses, Cmax is still quite variable,[103,105,106] suggesting that many patients fail to reach target blood levels. Reasons for this variability may include erratic absorption due to rectal vault contents, effects of positioning the capsule within the rectum (ie, proximal vs distal placement affects the extent of first-pass hepatic metabolism), different binding agents used in suppository manufacture, effects of temperature on suppository melting speed, variable milligram per kilogram doses administered with fixed-size suppositories, and even gender differences.[103,106,117,118] To increase the likelihood that Cmax will reach therapeutic levels despite its variability, repeated doses may be administered.[105,118,119] Importantly, repeated doses must avoid exceeding the maximum daily dose of 100 mg/kg for children, 75 mg/kg for infants, 60 mg/kg for PCA more than 32-week preterm infants, and 40 mg/kg for PCA more than 28-week preterm infants[102]; and may thus require intervals more than 8 hours in premature babies.[105,106] Of note, Cmax did not reach toxic levels in any of these studies, including those involving newborns and those who received repeated doses.[103–106,118]

Tmax, the time at which Cmax is reached, is notable for a significant delay after PR administration. For adults, Tmax is more than 80 minutes.[119] For infants and children, Tmax is 138 to 180 minutes depending on dose (15–45 mg/kg PR), age, and type of surgery.[103,117] However, one recent study reported Tmax of only 1.16 hour after a 10 to 15 mg/kg dose with vaccination.[115] For term neonates, Tmax is 90 minutes[105] and for preterm neonates, Tmax is 4 to 5 hours regardless of gestational age.[106]

These results support the conclusion of a recent meta-analysis,[120] suggesting that PR acetaminophen is best thought of as part of the overall perioperative pain management plan rather than a primary analgesic. Moreover, PR acetaminophen is most suited to cases in which a delayed and sustained analgesic effect is appropriate.[117] The ideal PR acetaminophen dose for postoperative analgesia remains unknown. Concentration-effect studies need to address several issues, including determining the desired therapeutic blood level of acetaminophen. The often quoted target range of 10 to 20 mg/L may provide analgesia after tonsillectomy in children[121] but may not be applicable to other procedures or ages. In addition, what is the relationship between acetaminophen blood level and analgesia? Some studies find no consistent relationship between serum concentration and pain score.[105,106,120] This is possibly due to ceiling effects or age-related differences in blood-brain barrier permeability.[105,122]

SUMMARY

Ambulatory anesthesia is safe for a variety of procedures in the pediatric population with careful attention to patient selection. Respiratory concerns include identifying significant upper respiratory infection, and ensuring appropriate overnight monitoring for patients at risk of apnea (ie, former premature infants or patients with significant OSA). Patients with muscular dystrophy or mitochondrial disorders must be evaluated carefully and drugs chosen to minimize the impact of anesthesia on respiratory and other muscle function. Techniques to reduce anxiety and attention to postoperative analgesia can contribute to a smooth perioperative course.

REFERENCES

1. Bryson GL, Chung F, Cox RG, et al. Patient selection in ambulatory anesthesia—an evidence-based review: part II. Can J Anaesth 2004;51:782–94.
2. Bryson GL, Chung F, Finegan BA, et al. Patient selection in ambulatory anesthesia—an evidence-based review: part I. Can J Anaesth 2004;51:768–81.
3. Collins CE, Everett LL. Challenges in pediatric ambulatory anesthesia: kids are different. Anesthesiol Clin 2010;28:315–28.
4. Bettelli G. High risk patients in day surgery. Minerva Anestesiol 2009;75:259–68.
5. Cullen KA, Hall MJ, Golosinskiy A. Ambulatory surgery in the United States, 2006. Natl Health Stat Report 2009;(11):1–25.
6. Tait AR, Malviya S. Anesthesia for the child with an upper respiratory tract infection: still a dilemma? Anesth Analg 2005;100:59–65.
7. von Ungern-Sternberg BS, Boda K, Chambers NA, et al. Risk assessment for respiratory complications in paediatric anaesthesia: a prospective cohort study. Lancet 2010;376:773–83.
8. von Ungern-Sternberg BS, Boda K, Schwab C, et al. Laryngeal mask airway is associated with an increased incidence of adverse respiratory events in children with recent upper respiratory tract infections. Anesthesiology 2007;107:714–9.

9. Rachel Homer J, Elwood T, Peterson D, et al. Risk factors for adverse events in children with colds emerging from anesthesia: a logistic regression. Paediatr Anaesth 2007;17:154–61.

10. Becke K. Anesthesia in children with a cold. Curr Opin Anaesthesiol 2012;25: 333–9.

11. Tait AR, Malviya S, Voepel-Lewis T, et al. Risk factors for perioperative adverse respiratory events in children with upper respiratory tract infections. Anesthesiology 2001;95:299–306.

12. Parnis SJ, Barker DS, Van Der Walt JH. Clinical predictors of anaesthetic complications in children with respiratory tract infections. Paediatr Anaesth 2001;11: 29–40.

13. Schebesta K, Guloglu E, Chiari A, et al. Topical lidocaine reduces the risk of perioperative airway complications in children with upper respiratory tract infections. Can J Anaesth 2010;57:745–50.

14. Mamie C, Habre W, Delhumeau C, et al. Incidence and risk factors of perioperative respiratory adverse events in children undergoing elective surgery. Paediatr Anaesth 2004;14:218–24.

15. Levy L, Pandit UA, Randel GI, et al. Upper respiratory tract infections and general anaesthesia in children. Peri-operative complications and oxygen saturation. Anaesthesia 1992;47:678–82.

16. Cote CJ, Zaslavsky A, Downes JJ, et al. Postoperative apnea in former preterm infants after inguinal herniorrhaphy. A combined analysis. Anesthesiology 1995; 82:809–22.

17. Murphy JJ, Swanson T, Ansermino M, et al. The frequency of apneas in premature infants after inguinal hernia repair: do they need overnight monitoring in the intensive care unit? J Pediatr Surg 2008;43:865–8.

18. Laituri CA, Garey CL, Pieters BJ, et al. Overnight observation in former premature infants undergoing inguinal hernia repair. J Pediatr Surg 2012;47:217–20.

19. Tetzlaff JE, Annand DW, Pudimat MA, et al. Postoperative apnea in a full-term infant. Anesthesiology 1988;69:426–8.

20. Cote CJ, Kelly DH. Postoperative apnea in a full-term infant with a demonstrable respiratory pattern abnormality. Anesthesiology 1990;72:559–61.

21. Karayan J, LaCoste L, Fusciardi J. Postoperative apnea in a full-term infant. Anesthesiology 1991;75:375.

22. Breschan C, Krumpholz R, Likar R, et al. Can a dose of 2microg.kg(-1) caudal clonidine cause respiratory depression in neonates? Paediatr Anaesth 1999;9:81–3.

23. Bhattacharyya N. Ambulatory pediatric otolaryngologic procedures in the United States: characteristics and perioperative safety. Laryngoscope 2010; 120:821–5.

24. Roland PS, Rosenfeld RM, Brooks LJ, et al. Clinical practice guideline: polysomnography for sleep-disordered breathing prior to tonsillectomy in children. Otolaryngol Head Neck Surg 2011;145:S1–15.

25. Brown KA, Laferriere A, Lakheeram I, et al. Recurrent hypoxemia in children is associated with increased analgesic sensitivity to opiates. Anesthesiology 2006; 105:665–9.

26. Kieran S, Gorman C, Kirby A, et al. Risk factors for desaturation after tonsillectomy: analysis of 4092 consecutive pediatric cases. Laryngoscope 2013; 123(10):2554–9.

27. Goldman JL, Baugh RF, Davies L, et al. Mortality and major morbidity after tonsillectomy: etiologic Factors and Strategies for Prevention. Laryngoscope 2013; 123(10):2544–53.

28. Cote CJ, Posner KL, Domino KB. Death or neurologic injury after tonsillectomy in children with a focus on obstructive sleep apnea: Houston, we have a problem! Anesth Analg 2013. [Epub ahead of print].
29. Kuehn BM. FDA: no codeine after tonsillectomy for children. JAMA 2013;309: 1100.
30. Bhananker SM, Ramamoorthy C, Geiduschek JM, et al. Anesthesia-related cardiac arrest in children: update from the Pediatric Perioperative Cardiac Arrest Registry. Anesth Analg 2007;105:344–50.
31. Sullivan M, Thompson WK, Hill GD. Succinylcholine-induced cardiac arrest in children with undiagnosed myopathy. Can J Anaesth 1994;41:497–501.
32. Saettele AK, Sharma A, Murray DJ. Case scenario: hypotonia in infancy: anesthetic dilemma. Anesthesiology 2013;119:443–6.
33. Flick RP, Gleich SJ, Herr MM, et al. The risk of malignant hyperthermia in children undergoing muscle biopsy for suspected neuromuscular disorder. Paediatr Anaesth 2007;17:22–7.
34. Klingler W, Rueffert H, Lehmann-Horn F, et al. Core myopathies and risk of malignant hyperthermia. Anesth Analg 2009;109:1167–73.
35. Dowling JJ, Lillis S, Amburgey K, et al. King-Denborough syndrome with and without mutations in the skeletal muscle ryanodine receptor (RYR1) gene. Neuromuscul Disord 2011;21:420–7.
36. Birgenheier N, Stoker R, Westenskow D, et al. Activated charcoal effectively removes inhaled anesthetics from modern anesthesia machines. Anesth Analg 2011;112:1363–70.
37. Girshin M, Mukherjee J, Clowney R, et al. The postoperative cardiovascular arrest of a 5-year-old male: an initial presentation of Duchenne's muscular dystrophy. Paediatr Anaesth 2006;16:170–3.
38. Yemen TA, McClain C. Muscular dystrophy, anesthesia and the safety of inhalational agents revisited; again. Paediatr Anaesth 2006;16:105–8.
39. Segura LG, Lorenz JD, Weingarten TN, et al. Anesthesia and Duchenne or Becker muscular dystrophy: review of 117 anesthetic exposures. Paediatr Anaesth 2013;23:855–64.
40. Gurnaney H, Brown A, Litman RS. Malignant hyperthermia and muscular dystrophies. Anesth Analg 2009;109:1043–8.
41. Mercuri E, Muntoni F. Muscular dystrophies. Lancet 2013;381:845–60.
42. Kam PC, Cardone D. Propofol infusion syndrome. Anaesthesia 2007;62: 690–701.
43. Laquay N, Pouard P, Silicani MA, et al. Early stages of propofol infusion syndrome in paediatric cardiac surgery: two cases in adolescent girls. Br J Anaesth 2008;101:880–1.
44. Niezgoda J, Morgan PG. Anesthetic considerations in patients with mitochondrial defects. Paediatr Anaesth 2013;23:785–93.
45. Wolf A, Weir P, Segar P, et al. Impaired fatty acid oxidation in propofol infusion syndrome. Lancet 2001;357:606–7.
46. Footitt EJ, Sinha MD, Raiman JA, et al. Mitochondrial disorders and general anaesthesia: a case series and review. Br J Anaesth 2008;100:436–41.
47. Driessen J, Willems S, Dercksen S, et al. Anesthesia-related morbidity and mortality after surgery for muscle biopsy in children with mitochondrial defects. Paediatr Anaesth 2007;17:16–21.
48. Gurrieri C, Kivela JE, Bojanic K, et al. Anesthetic considerations in mitochondrial encephalomyopathy, lactic acidosis, and stroke-like episodes syndrome: a case series. Can J Anaesth 2011;58:751–63.

49. Morgan PG, Hoppel CL, Sedensky MM. Mitochondrial defects and anesthetic sensitivity. Anesthesiology 2002;96:1268–70.

50. Koenig MK. Presentation and diagnosis of mitochondrial disorders in children. Pediatr Neurol 2008;38:305–13.

51. Viitanen H, Annila P, Viitanen M, et al. Premedication with midazolam delays recovery after ambulatory sevoflurane anesthesia in children. Anesth Analg 1999; 89:75–9.

52. Dahmani S, Brasher C, Stany I, et al. Premedication with clonidine is superior to benzodiazepines. A meta analysis of published studies. Acta Anaesthesiol Scand 2010;54:397–402.

53. Yip P, Middleton P, Cyna AM, et al. Non-pharmacological interventions for assisting the induction of anaesthesia in children. Cochrane Database Syst Rev 2009;(3):CD006447.

54. Vagnoli L, Caprilli S, Messeri A. Parental presence, clowns or sedative premedication to treat preoperative anxiety in children: what could be the most promising option? Paediatr Anaesth 2010;20:937–43.

55. Vagnoli L, Caprilli S, Robiglio A, et al. Clown doctors as a treatment for preoperative anxiety in children: a randomized, prospective study. Pediatrics 2005; 116:e563–7.

56. Hart R, Walton M. Magic as a therapeutic intervention to promote coping in hospitalized pediatric patients. Pediatr Nurs 2010;36:11–6 [quiz: 17].

57. Spencer RF. The magic ball induction. Anesth Analg 1994;79:395–6.

58. Mifflin KA, Hackmann T, Chorney JM. Streamed video clips to reduce anxiety in children during inhaled induction of anesthesia. Anesth Analg 2012;115:1162–7.

59. Gomes SH. YouTube in pediatric anesthesia induction. Paediatr Anaesth 2008; 18:801–2.

60. Patel A, Schieble T, Davidson M, et al. Distraction with a hand-held video game reduces pediatric preoperative anxiety. Paediatr Anaesth 2006;16:1019–27.

61. Denman WT, Tuason PM, Ahmed MI, et al. The PediSedate device, a novel approach to pediatric sedation that provides distraction and inhaled nitrous oxide: clinical evaluation in a large case series. Paediatr Anaesth 2007;17:162–6.

62. Chorney JM, Torrey C, Blount R, et al. Healthcare provider and parent behavior and children's coping and distress at anesthesia induction. Anesthesiology 2009;111:1290–6.

63. Litman RS. Allaying anxiety in children: when a funny thing happens on the way to the operating room. Anesthesiology 2011;115:4–5.

64. McGhee PE. Humor, its origin and development. San Francisco (CA): W. H. Freeman; 1979.

65. Bariaud F. Chapter 1: age differences in children's humor. In: McGhee PE, editor. Humor and children's development: a guide to practical applications. New York: Haworth Press; 1989. p. 22.

66. Dowling JS. Humor: a coping strategy for pediatric patients. Pediatr Nurs 2002; 28:123–31.

67. Simon L, Boucebci KJ, Orliaguet G, et al. A survey of practice of tracheal intubation without muscle relaxant in paediatric patients. Paediatr Anaesth 2002;12: 36–42.

68. Murphy GS, Szokol JW, Avram MJ, et al. Postoperative residual neuromuscular blockade is associated with impaired clinical recovery. Anesth Analg 2013;117: 133–41.

69. Grosse-Sundrup M, Henneman JP, Sandberg WS, et al. Intermediate acting non-depolarizing neuromuscular blocking agents and risk of postoperative

respiratory complications: prospective propensity score matched cohort study. BMJ 2012;345:e6329.

70. Demirkaya M, Kelsaka E, Sarihasan B, et al. The optimal dose of remifentanil for acceptable intubating conditions during propofol induction without neuromuscular blockade. J Clin Anesth 2012;24:392–7.

71. Bouvet L, Stoian A, Rousson D, et al. What is the optimal remifentanil dosage for providing excellent intubating conditions when coadministered with thiopental? A prospective randomized dose-response study. Eur J Anaesthesiol 2010;27: 653–9.

72. Kim WJ, Choi SS, Kim DH, et al. The effects of sevoflurane with propofol and remifentanil on tracheal intubation conditions without neuromuscular blocking agents. Korean J Anesthesiol 2010;59:87–91.

73. Lee J, Jung CW. The target concentration of remifentanil to suppress the hemodynamic response to endotracheal intubation during inhalational induction with desflurane. Korean J Anesthesiol 2011;60:12–8.

74. Jeon YT, Oh AY, Park SH, et al. Optimal remifentanil dose for lightwand intubation without muscle relaxants in healthy patients with thiopental coadministration: a prospective randomised study. Eur J Anaesthesiol 2012;29:520–3.

75. Min JH, Chai HS, Kim YH, et al. Attenuation of hemodynamic responses to laryngoscopy and tracheal intubation during rapid sequence induction: remifentanil vs. lidocaine with esmolol. Minerva Anestesiol 2010;76:188–92.

76. Alanoglu Z, Tolu S, Yalcin S, et al. Different remifentanil doses in rapid sequence anesthesia induction: BIS monitoring and intubation conditions. Adv Clin Exp Med 2013;22:47–55.

77. Hanna SF, Ahmad F, Pappas AL, et al. The effect of propofol/remifentanil rapid-induction technique without muscle relaxants on intraocular pressure. J Clin Anesth 2010;22:437–42.

78. Aouad MT, Yazbeck-Karam VG, Mallat CE, et al. The effect of adjuvant drugs on the quality of tracheal intubation without muscle relaxants in children: a systematic review of randomized trials. Paediatr Anaesth 2012;22:616–26.

79. Choong K, AlFaleh K, Doucette J, et al. Remifentanil for endotracheal intubation in neonates: a randomised controlled trial. Arch Dis Child Fetal Neonatal Ed 2010;95:F80–4.

80. Hume-Smith H, McCormack J, Montgomery C, et al. The effect of age on the dose of remifentanil for tracheal intubation in infants and children. Paediatr Anaesth 2010;20:19–27.

81. Mireskandari SM, Abulahrar N, Darabi ME, et al. Comparison of the effect of fentanyl, sufentanil, alfentanil and remifentanil on cardiovascular response to tracheal intubation in children. Iran J Pediatr 2011;21:173–80.

82. Yoon SH, Kim KH, Seo SH. Dose of remifentanil for minimizing the cardiovascular changes to tracheal intubation in pediatric patients. Korean J Anesthesiol 2010;59:167–72.

83. Naja ZA, Ziade FM, Al-Tannir MA, et al. Addition of clonidine and fentanyl: comparison between three different regional anesthetic techniques in circumcision. Paediatr Anaesth 2005;15:964–70.

84. Shrestha BR, Bista B. Tramadol along with local anaesthetics in the penile block for the children undergoing circumcision. Kathmandu Univ Med J (KUMJ) 2005; 3:26–9.

85. Irwin MG, Cheng W. Comparison of subcutaneous ring block of the penis with caudal epidural block for post-circumcision analgesia in children. Anaesth Intensive Care 1996;24:365–7.

86. Salgado Filho MF, Goncalves HB, Pimentel Filho LH, et al. Assessment of pain and hemodynamic response in older children undergoing circumcision: comparison of eutectic lidocaine/prilocaine cream and dorsal penile nerve block. J Pediatr Urol 2013;9:638–42.

87. Elemen L, Seyidov TH, Tugay M. The advantages of cyanoacrylate wound closure in circumcision. Pediatr Surg Int 2011;27:879–83.

88. Serour F, Cohen A, Mandelberg A, et al. Dorsal penile nerve block in children undergoing circumcision in a day-care surgery. Can J Anaesth 1996;43:954–8.

89. O'Sullivan MJ, Mislovic B, Alexander E. Dorsal penile nerve block for male pediatric circumcision–randomized comparison of ultrasound-guided vs anatomical landmark technique. Paediatr Anaesth 2011;21:1214–8.

90. Sandeman DJ, Reiner D, Dilley AV, et al. A retrospective audit of three different regional anaesthetic techniques for circumcision in children. Anaesth Intensive Care 2010;38:519–24.

91. Faraoni D, Gilbeau A, Lingier P, et al. Does ultrasound guidance improve the efficacy of dorsal penile nerve block in children? Paediatr Anaesth 2010;20:931–6.

92. French LK, Cedar A, Hendrickson RG. Case report: bupivacaine toxicity with dorsal penile block for circumcision. Am Fam Physician 2012;86:222.

93. Abaci A, Makay B, Unsal E, et al. An unusual complication of dorsal penile nerve block for circumcision. Paediatr Anaesth 2006;16:1094–5.

94. Soh CR, Ng SB, Lim SL. Dorsal penile nerve block. Paediatr Anaesth 2003;13:329–33.

95. Cyna AM, Middleton P. Caudal epidural block versus other methods of postoperative pain relief for circumcision in boys. Cochrane Database Syst Rev 2008;(4):CD003005.

96. Weksler N, Atias I, Klein M, et al. Is penile block better than caudal epidural block for postcircumcision analgesia? J Anesth 2005;19:36–9.

97. Margetts L, Carr A, McFadyen G, et al. A comparison of caudal bupivacaine and ketamine with penile block for paediatric circumcision. Eur J Anaesthesiol 2008;25:1009–13.

98. Sharpe P, Klein JR, Thompson JP, et al. Analgesia for circumcision in a paediatric population: comparison of caudal bupivacaine alone with bupivacaine plus two doses of clonidine. Paediatr Anaesth 2001;11:695–700.

99. Gauntlett I. A comparison between local anaesthetic dorsal nerve block and caudal bupivacaine with ketamine for paediatric circumcision. Paediatr Anaesth 2003;13:38–42.

100. Polaner DM, Taenzer AH, Walker BJ, et al. Pediatric Regional Anesthesia Network (PRAN): a multi-institutional study of the use and incidence of complications of pediatric regional anesthesia. Anesth Analg 2012;115:1353–64.

101. Berde CB, Jaksic T, Lynn AM, et al. Anesthesia and analgesia during and after surgery in neonates. Clin Ther 2005;27:900–21.

102. Berde CB, Sethna NF. Analgesics for the treatment of pain in children. N Engl J Med 2002;347:1094–103.

103. Anderson BJ, Woolard GA, Holford NH. Pharmacokinetics of rectal paracetamol after major surgery in children. Paediatr Anaesth 1995;5:237–42.

104. Dashti GA, Amini S, Zanguee E. The prophylactic effect of rectal acetaminophen on postoperative pain and opioid requirements after adenotonsillectomy in children. Middle East J Anesthesiol 2009;20:245–9.

105. van Lingen RA, Deinum HT, Quak CM, et al. Multiple-dose pharmacokinetics of rectally administered acetaminophen in term infants. Clin Pharmacol Ther 1999;66:509–15.

106. van Lingen RA, Deinum JT, Quak JM, et al. Pharmacokinetics and metabolism of rectally administered paracetamol in preterm neonates. Arch Dis Child Fetal Neonatal Ed 1999;80:F59–63.

107. Eyers S, Fingleton J, Perrin K, et al. Proposed MHRA changes to UK children's paracetamol dosing recommendations: modelling study. J R Soc Med 2012; 105:263–9.

108. Berling I, Anscombe M, Isbister GK. Intravenous paracetamol toxicity in a malnourished child. Clin Toxicol (Phila) 2012;50:74–6.

109. Ceelie I, James LP, Gijsen V, et al. Acute liver failure after recommended doses of acetaminophen in patients with myopathies. Crit Care Med 2011;39:678–82.

110. Kubic A, Burda AM, Bockewitz E, et al. Hepatotoxicity in an infant following supratherapeutic dosing of acetaminophen for twenty-four hours. Semin Diagn Pathol 2009;26:7–9.

111. Dart RC, Rumack BH. Intravenous acetaminophen in the United States: iatrogenic dosing errors. Pediatrics 2012;129:349–53.

112. Sutters KA, Holdridge-Zeuner D, Waite S, et al. A descriptive feasibility study to evaluate scheduled oral analgesic dosing at home for the management of postoperative pain in preschool children following tonsillectomy. Pain Med 2012;13: 472–83.

113. Wilson-Smith EM, Morton NS. Survey of i.v. paracetamol (acetaminophen) use in neonates and infants under 1 year of age by UK anesthetists. Paediatr Anaesth 2009;19:329–37.

114. McBride JT. The association of acetaminophen and asthma prevalence and severity. Pediatrics 2011;128:1181–5.

115. Walson PD, Halvorsen M, Edge J, et al. Pharmacokinetic comparison of acetaminophen elixir versus suppositories in vaccinated infants (aged 3 to 36 months): a single-dose, open-label, randomized, parallel-group design. Clin Ther 2013;35:135–40.

116. Karbasi SA, Modares-Mosadegh M, Golestan M. Comparison of antipyretic effectiveness of equal doses of rectal and oral acetaminophen in children. J Pediatr (Rio J) 2010;86:228–32.

117. Montgomery CJ, McCormack JP, Reichert CC, et al. Plasma concentrations after high-dose (45 mg.kg-1) rectal acetaminophen in children. Can J Anaesth 1995; 42:982–6.

118. Birmingham PK, Tobin MJ, Fisher DM, et al. Initial and subsequent dosing of rectal acetaminophen in children: a 24-hour pharmacokinetic study of new dose recommendations. Anesthesiology 2001;94:385–9.

119. Holmer Pettersson P, Jakobsson J, Owall A. Plasma concentrations following repeated rectal or intravenous administration of paracetamol after heart surgery. Acta Anaesthesiol Scand 2006;50:673–7.

120. Varela ML, Howland MA. Single high-dose rectal acetaminophen in children. Ann Pharmacother 2004;38:1935–41.

121. Anderson BJ, Woollard GA, Holford NH. Acetaminophen analgesia in children: placebo effect and pain resolution after tonsillectomy. Eur J Clin Pharmacol 2001;57:559–69.

122. Hahn TW, Mogensen T, Lund C, et al. Analgesic effect of i.v. paracetamol: possible ceiling effect of paracetamol in postoperative pain. Acta Anaesthesiol Scand 2003;47:138–45.

123. Apfelbaum JL, Connis RT, Nickinovich DG, et al. Practice advisory for preanesthesia evaluation: an updated report by the American Society of Anesthesiologists Task Force on Preanesthesia Evaluation. Anesthesiology 2012;116:522–38.

124. Kahn RL, Stanton MA, Tong-Ngork S, et al. One-year experience with day-of-surgery pregnancy testing before elective orthopedic procedures. Anesth Analg 2008;106:1127–31 [table of contents].

125. Wheeler M, Cote CJ. Preoperative pregnancy testing in a tertiary care children's hospital: a medico-legal conundrum. J Clin Anesth 1999;11:56–63.

126. Malviya S, D'Errico C, Reynolds P, et al. Should pregnancy testing be routine in adolescent patients prior to surgery? Anesth Analg 1996;83:854–8.

127. Palmer SK, Van Norman GA, Jackson SL. Routine Pregnancy Testing Before Elective Anesthesia Is Not an American Society of Anesthesiologists Standard. Anesth Analg 2009;108(5):1715–6.

Initial Results from the National Anesthesia Clinical Outcomes Registry and Overview of Office-Based Anesthesia

Fred E. Shapiro, DO[a], Samir R. Jani, MD, MPH[a], Xiaoxia Liu, MS[b], Richard P. Dutton, MD, MBA[c], Richard D. Urman, MD, MBA[b],*

KEYWORDS

- Office-base anesthesia • Ambulatory anesthesia • Patient safety • Patient outcomes
- Anesthesia Quality Institute • National Anesthesia Clinical Outcomes Registry

KEY POINTS

- Safe office-based anesthesia practices dictate proper patient and procedure selection, appropriate provider qualifications, adequately equipped facilities, and effective administrative infrastructure.
- Our analysis of the data from the Anesthesia Quality Institute National Anesthesia Clinical Outcomes Registry included patient demographics, adverse outcomes, procedure and anesthesia type and duration, and case coverage by type of anesthesia provider.
- There is increasing emphasis on continuous quality improvement, electronic health records, use of checklists, and outcomes data reporting.

INTRODUCTION

The past 3 decades have seen an impressive shift of surgical care from the hospital to the outpatient setting.[1] Initially, ambulatory surgical centers (ASC) were heavily used for elective day surgery, but further migration to physician offices is now common. The ability to perform surgery in an office strongly correlates with improvement in delivering safe and effective office-based anesthesia (OBA).[2] The remarkable numbers help illustrate this growing movement. The American Society of Anesthesiologists

[a] Beth Israel Deaconess Medical Center, 330 Brookline Avenue, Boston, MA 02215, USA; [b] Brigham and Women's Hospital, 75 Francis Street, Boston, MA 02115, USA; [c] Anesthesia Quality Institute, 520 N. Northwest Highway, Park Ridge, IL 60068, USA
* Corresponding author. Brigham and Women's Hospital, Harvard Medical School, 75 Francis Street, Boston, MA 02115.
E-mail address: urmanr@gmail.com

Anesthesiology Clin 32 (2014) 431–444
http://dx.doi.org/10.1016/j.anclin.2014.02.018
1932-2275/14/$ – see front matter © 2014 Elsevier Inc. All rights reserved.

(ASA) originally estimated that more than 10 million office procedures were performed in 2005, which doubles the approximations from just 10 years prior.[3] Current assessments show 17% to 24% of all elective ambulatory surgeries take place in an office.[4] It is apparent that this trend will continue; thus, the ability to deliver OBA must be in the repertoire of current and future anesthesiologists.

The impetus for the shift to OBA is a combination of technological improvements, financial incentives, and patient/provider preference. Improvements in technology allow for compact and portable monitors that require minimal support infrastructure, which is crucial for the office because of space and storage concerns. Additionally, this portability has made way for a previously unknown entity, the mobile anesthesia provider who brings all necessary equipment and medications to safely anesthetize patients.

Financially, the office provides opportunity for potential savings, which is well documented in the literature. For example, a recent study observed the cost of dental rehabilitation in pediatric patients is almost 13 times less in an office versus a hospital, equating to a savings of $6800 per patient.[5] This savings is caused by a minimal or nonexistent facility fee and a significantly shorter aggregate time per patient (from preoperative to recovery), emphasizing office efficiency. The potential savings for individuals, insurers, and the health care system as a whole is tremendous; payers are incentivizing doctors to perform procedures in the office. The margin of profit for the providers is the same or greater when operating in the office, which also encourages growth.[6]

Many providers and patients prefer the office over other settings.[7] Providers have greater control over scheduling, more consistent/efficient support staff, and the ability to create the optimal workflow. For patients, the appeal of office procedures includes greater privacy; perception of increased personal attention; lower risk of nosocomial infection; and less aggravation by avoiding large, confusing hospitals.[2]

ADMINISTRATIVE AND SAFETY ISSUES
Literature Review

A literature review of safety in the office setting shows there are no randomized controlled trials comparing office-based surgery with other surgical locations. Thus, most of our understanding regarding safety in the office is derived from retrospective data (**Table 1**).

The hallmark office safety study was conducted by Vila and colleagues[8] and examined 2-year data for adverse events reported to the Florida Board of Medicine. The study stated that the office setting carried a 10-fold increase in relative risk compared with ambulatory surgical centers. There was immediate criticism caused by an inherent limitation in study design because the numerator for calculating the adverse events was derived from all offices, whereas the denominator used for total number of procedures was from only accredited offices.

Several researchers were unable to corroborate Vila and colleague's findings, and a more recent study by Coldiron and colleagues[9] examined self-reported data to the Florida State Medical Board from 2000 to 2007. During this period, there were a total of 31 deaths and 143 major complications, including emergency transfer to the hospital. Most patients who experienced an adverse event were ASA class 1 patients undergoing elective cosmetic procedures. One weakness of this study is that the data represents only voluntarily reported information from a limited number of offices, which limits the conclusions that may be drawn.

Keyes and colleagues[10] analyzed data using the American Association for Accreditation of Ambulatory Surgery Facilities' (AAAASF) mandatory Internet-based

Table 1
Key studies addressing safety in OBA

Key Papers, Year	Method	Finding
Hoefflin et al,[15] 2001	23,000 cases from single plastic surgery office	No significant complications
Vila et al,[8] 2003	2 y of adverse events reported to Florida board	10-fold relative risk in office compared with ASC
Perrot et al,[16] 2003	>34,000 oral and maxillofacial surgeries	Complication rate of 0.4%–1.5% for all types of anesthesia
Byrd et al,[7] 2003	5316 cases from single plastic surgery office	Complication rate 0.7% (mostly hematoma)
Coldiron et al,[9] 2008	Self-reported data to Florida board from 2000 to 2007	174 adverse events; 31 deaths in this time frame
Soltani et al,[12] 2013	AAAASF data from 2000–2012; only reviewed plastic surgery offices	22,000 of 5.5 million cases; complication rate 0.4%; 94 deaths; 0.0017% death rate.
Failey et al,[18] 2013	2611 cases from single AAAASF facility under TIVA/conscious sedation	No deaths, cardiac events, transfers; 1 DVT

Abbreviations: AAAASF, American Association for Accreditation of Ambulatory Surgery Facilities; DVT, deep vein thrombosis; TIVA, total intravenous anesthesia.
   Data from Refs.[7–9,15,16,18]

data collection system for adverse events in AAAASF-accredited offices. This study has had 3 iterations looking at various time frames, with the first being 2001 to 2002. This initial study found the complication rate for events like hematoma, wound infection, and sepsis was approximately 0.33% and approximated a death rate of 1 in 58,810 surgeries. More importantly, the complication and mortality rates were similar to other surgical settings, supporting the notion that office surgery is just as safe.

The next study by Keyes and colleagues[11] reviewed data from 2001 to 2006 and included over 1 million outpatient procedures in plastic surgery offices. There were 23 deaths in this time period, which equates to a 0.002% mortality rate. The overwhelming cause was from pulmonary embolism (13 out of 23), which the researchers emphasize may occur in any surgical setting. Of note, most of the patients who developed this complication were undergoing abdominoplasty. Although it may be tempting to make the conclusion that office-based surgery shares the same risk profile as other surgical settings, the researchers think that this data reflect the inherent risks of the cosmetic plastic surgery procedures regardless of setting.

In the 2013 study, Soltani and colleagues[12] analyzed the AAAASF's data from 2001 to 2012, specifically focusing on accredited plastic surgery offices. This review included more than 5.5 million procedures with just less than 22,000 adverse events reported, resulting in a complication rate of 0.4%. There were 94 deaths reported in the same time period, resulting in an incidence of 0.0017%, which yields a risk of death for plastic surgery in an office setting of 1 in 41,726. The top cause of mortality was confirmed to be pulmonary embolism (40 in 94). Although this last study has helped improve our understanding of safety in the office, it is important to note that this data only included plastic surgery, so extrapolation to other procedures must be done cautiously. Although each study found similar rates of adverse events and mortality, the data were aggregated by incorporating the previous years' results into subsequent analyses, which further weakens the conclusions.

A review of the ASA's Closed Claims Database has also increased our knowledge of office anesthesia morbidity. This crucial quality-improvement database collects information about the nature of claims associated with adverse anesthesia events. Domino[13] reviewed the first closed claims report and reported that injuries in the office carried higher severity than other ambulatory claims. For instance, 40% of office claims were caused by death, whereas it was only 25% for other ambulatory settings; office claims also resulted in more frequent payments and higher reward amounts for office injuries.

The most commonly reported events were respiratory issues (29%), and many were discovered to be preventable by better monitoring. Another key point was inadequate monitoring after the procedure, leading to further morbidity. Although vigilance is imperative in every stage of the procedure, the anesthesia provider may not be present as patients recover from anesthesia; the transition of care needs to be systematic and comprehensive.

In 2010, the Society for Ambulatory Anesthesia (SAMBA) published outcomes from OBA, based on the data reported through the SAMBA Clinical Outcomes Registry (SCOR).[14] Data were collected from 7 practices from 2008 to 2009 and resulted in 37,669 cases examined for different adverse events. Case cancellation occurred 3.2% of the time, which was the most common issue. This finding may represent a proclivity toward safety in the office where the case was canceled if a patient was not optimized (medically or appropriate nil per os status for example). In all, the rates of all major complications were well less than 1%, but there were serious adverse events. Concerning airway complications, there were 31 unplanned intubations, 4 confirmed aspiration events, and 25 cases of laryngospasm. Unintended admission to the hospital occurred 24 times. There were 2 instances of wrong site surgery. Regarding medications, there were 6 documented medication errors and 17 patients required reversal of narcotics or benzodiazepines. No deaths were found in the data.

Other published studies have tried to determine the safest anesthetic technique in the office. Hoefflin and colleagues[15] reported no deaths in 23,000 general anesthetics without regard to procedure. Perrott and colleagues[16] specifically examined oral and maxillofacial surgeries done under a variety of anesthetics. They calculated a complication rate of approximately 0.4% to 1.5% for cases done under local, conscious sedation, and general anesthesia with no statistically significant differences and concluded that each option was safe. Bitar and colleagues[17] reviewed close to 5000 intravenous sedation cases and found about a dozen adverse events, with the most frequent complication being postoperative nausea and vomiting; there were no deaths. Failey and colleagues[18] published a retrospective chart analysis of 2611 plastic surgery procedures done at an AAAASF-accredited facility that showed one instance of deep vein thrombosis (DVT) and no deaths, cardiac events, or hospital transfers when total intravenous anesthesia (TIVA) or moderate sedation was administered.

Accreditation and Other Administrative Issues

As office-based surgery grows, so do concerns about patient safety. The ASA has advocated that the quality and safety of OBA be on par with hospitals and ASCs. There are several barriers to achieving this. Surgeons who operate in a hospital must have privileges to do so, which requires certification and credentials in addition to documented ongoing education. Moreover, operations in hospitals are subject to peer review in order to educate all physicians when an adverse event does occur and potentially avoid it in the future. None of this holds true for the office where the proceduralist may make the decision regarding what procedure to perform with little if any quality-improvement process.

Additionally, the anesthesia providers may vary in terms of education, training, and experience. An anesthesiologist, a certified registered nurse anesthetist (CRNA), or a nurse with little or no training who is acting under the direction of the proceduralist may be administering the anesthesia. There has been much debate regarding the role of an anesthesiologist versus another anesthesia provider. One study showed that hospital admission rates postoperatively were higher when it was a lone CRNA providing care compared with a solo anesthesiologist or the anesthesia care team model.[19] Although this is not conclusive evidence, it supports the value of an anesthesiologist in the office setting. The ASA strongly advocates that a physician should be involved in the care of all patients undergoing OBA from a patient-safety standpoint, but this is not a requirement for many state laws and may not be practical in certain areas.[20]

Another important safety issue is the lack of regulation, which creates variable levels of care.[4] Currently, there are no federal guidelines establishing a national standard. Almost 30 states have addressed the issue, but each differs significantly in many crucial aspects.[21] Some states require accreditation as a proxy to standardization through one of 3 agencies: The Joint Commission, the AAAASF, or the Accreditation Association for Ambulatory Health Care (AAAHC). Although all use a comprehensive survey of each facility's physical layout, administration, record keeping, and controlled substance policy, each of these organizations has different benchmarks for accreditation (**Table 2**), further complicating the ability to create a national standard.[22] Of the 3, the AAAASF is the only one to require adverse events reporting. The AAAHC not only accredits offices but also anesthesia practices that specialize in OBA who may travel to multiple offices. It is important to note that although accreditation provides some basic standards, true quality and safety are a daily challenge that must be an inherent and integral part of safety culture.

Facility, Patient, and Procedure Selection

Before providing the office, a thorough and detailed inspection of the location and institutional infrastructure is necessary. A comprehensive look at the physical location is absolutely essential to assess equipment; space limitations; patient flow, including designating a postanesthesia care unit (PACU) (which may be the procedure room or examination room); and availability of basic anesthesia necessities, such as supplemental oxygen and continuous suction. If the anesthesia machine is present, it must not be obsolete by the ASA's definitions and should undergo regularly scheduled maintenance.[23] Additionally, proper scavenging systems for inhaled anesthetics need to be in place if volatile agents are used. This requirement may not be practical in all offices; thus, TIVA may be the only option for general anesthesia. ASA standard monitors need to be available and require routine maintenance and testing.[24]

Table 2			
Accreditation agencies key differences			
	AAAASF	AAAHC	Joint Commission
Number of offices	>2000	~556	>500
Cost + accreditation for 3 y	$3000–$5000	$3800	$7780
Adverse-events reporting	Yes	No	No
Surgeon qualification	Yes	No	No
Anesthesia requirement	MD or supervised by MD	MD or supervised by MD	MD or CRNA

Regarding equipment, standard airway instruments in accordance with the ASA's difficult airway algorithm should be available in various sizes.[25] Crucial rescue and emergency medications must be available, such as those for reversal of narcotics and benzodiazepines; Advanced Cardiac Life Support (ACLS) medications; and, in an environment with any malignant hyperthermia triggers, dantrolene. Drugs should be checked periodically to ensure they do not expire. A defibrillator is another vital piece of equipment that should be routinely serviced and available at all times.

Having the proper administrative infrastructure is also essential. This requirement starts with a designated medical director who is responsible for reviewing and updating policies regarding clinical activities, such as each team member's role, staffing minimums, controlled substance guidelines, and infection control. Emergency contingency plans for events like fire in the procedure room or elsewhere in the building, patient transfer to a higher level of care, loss of electricity, or equipment failure need to be established and promulgated.

It is critical that each caregiver in the office setting have valid licensure or certification to perform the tasks that will be expected of him or her in accordance with each individual's training and education. For the surgeon and anesthesia provider, this includes ACLS certification (and Pediatric Advanced Life Support if the patient population includes children) and airway skills necessary for emergency situations. Nursing staff and other personnel should have Basic Life Support skills with ongoing recertification as required by law or accreditation. Lastly, the anesthesia provider should ensure that the location complies with all federal, state, and local laws with regard to controlled substances.

An additional complexity to safely providing OBA is the appropriate selection of patients. Currently, there is no universally accepted algorithm or process to determine if a patient is a good candidate for a given procedure and anesthetic plan in the ambulatory setting, let alone the office setting.[26] Until there are standard recommendations, patient selection falls under the purview of the caregivers and, thus, subject to personal discretion with assistance from guidelines. It is advisable for each facility to have an internal policy regarding unsuitable patients for each procedure. A general list of medical conditions that add an increased risk to anesthesia care should be maintained to highlight patients who are not appropriate for office-based surgery.

The first step to any OBA patient is a thorough preanesthetic assessment to minimize risk. This assessment must include a thorough history and physical examination consistent with regulatory and professional guidelines, with special attention paid to cardiopulmonary status. Although important in every setting, this is even more imperative in the office because of the inherent lack of backup. Inquiring about previous difficult intubation and personal/family history of malignant hyperthermia can be lifesaving. Risk stratification of DVT/pulmonary embolism development is also crucial to help minimize morbidity and mortality. Optimization of patients' baseline chronic medical conditions before the anesthetic is essential.

Also paramount to patient safety is the relationship between the proceduralist and anesthesiologist. A careful discussion between anesthesia and surgical personnel regarding issues such as length of procedure and anticipated blood loss is critical. This discussion needs to be frank, and any concerns must be addressed before initiating OBA. Acting in a consultant's role, the anesthesiologist's primary duty is to the patients, and he or she must stand firm if a patient is not suitable for an office procedure.

Postanesthesia recovery plans are just as critical as intraoperative plans. Confirmation of adequate transportation for patients from the office to their home should be mandatory and requires a preidentified responsible adult who will escort the patients home. Postoperative nausea and vomiting can be a significant issue that may delay discharge from the office. Therefore, high-risk patients/procedures should not be started late in the day. As a rough guideline, the American Society of Plastic Surgeons recommends that procedures should be no longer than 6 hours and the last procedure should end no later than at 15:00 in the afternoon[27] to allow ample time for recovery and discharge. Lastly, it is recommended that a formal postanesthesia discharge scoring system, along with other clinical criteria in accordance to ASA standards, should be used to determine a patient's readiness to be discharged home.[28]

The allure of office surgery is compelling, but it is not appropriate for every surgeon and anesthesia provider; it requires a uniquely different skill set. An office-based anesthetic must be quick in onset and offset to allow patient alertness and mobility once the procedure is over. Further, the lack of support personnel cannot be understated; one must be comfortable handling any and all emergency situations that may arise in this remote setting. The information presented is not an exhaustive list but rather are points to consider in making a final determination to assess if one can safely deliver anesthesia in a specific location. If adverse events occur, they should be recorded and reviewed.

DATA ANALYSIS FROM THE ANESTHESIA QUALITY INSTITUTE

The Anesthesia Quality Institute (AQI) was founded in 2008 by the ASA to enhance quality improvement. It houses the National Anesthesia Clinical Outcomes Registry (NACOR), which is the largest anesthesia database in the country with 162 practices enrolled. Although NACOR collects data about all aspects of the modern practice of anesthesiologist in the United States, the authors identified OBA as a subset in an attempt to offer a snapshot of the current state of this frontier of anesthesiology.

Data are submitted electronically and housed at the AQI headquarters in Park Ridge, Illinois. Approximately 30 AQI member practices working in 90 facilities perform OBA. Data are collected in a prospective and retrospective manner (ie, all cases from 2010 to present are submitted to AQI regardless of when the practice began participating in NACOR). There is a wide range of how much OBA each practice performs, with some exclusively performing OBA, whereas others have only performed a handful of cases since 2010. Although there are minimum data entry requirements, not all details about each case may have been recorded. This point is the principal reason the denominators differ among each characteristic. The authors included the cumulative data from NACOR because any bias in the larger data will affect their OBA statistics. Pearson chi-square tests were performed to compare the differences between the office-based data and the NACOR extract data in terms of age group, gender, anesthesia type, and explicit overage. A log-rank test was performed to evaluate the difference in duration across all time intervals. Throughout, a P value less than .05 was considered statistically significant, and all tests were 2 sided. The analyses were performed with SAS version 9.3 (SAS Institute, Cary, NC).

As stated previously, various socioeconomic forces are propelling office-based surgery. Initially thought to be a realm only for young and healthy patients, current data show that this is hardly the rule, with patients older than 65 years composing more than 13% of OBA patients and geriatric patients (aged >80 years) composing 2.5%. Minors are also represented, and 7% of OBA patients are younger than 18 years, including infants less than 12 months old (0.14% of OBA cases). The age of OBA patients is significantly different from those in the general NACOR database (**Table 3**) as is gender, with females comprising more than 61% of patients (**Table 4**).

Table 3
Age distribution of OBA and in non-OBA NACOR cases

Variable	Office Based (N = 84,461) n (%)	NACOR (N = 12,557,021) n (%)
Age group (y)		
<1	121 (0.14)	64,951 (0.52)
1–18	6024 (7.35)	1,302,276 (10.37)
19–49	35,862 (42.46)	4,397,863 (35.02)
50–64	29,362 (34.76)	3,218,552 (25.63)
65–79	10,760 (12.74)	2,682,377 (21.36)
80+	2152 (2.55)	891,002 (7.10)

P = <.0001.

An added concern for office-based anesthesiologists is patients with significant comorbidities, which coincides with increasingly older patients undergoing OBA. Evaluating ASA physical status classification from OBA data, patients ranged from ASA class 1 to 5 (**Fig. 1**). Not surprisingly, more than 75% of the patients were assigned ASA 1 or 2 physical status, which is to be expected in an ambulatory population. Individuals assigned ASA physical status 4 and 5 made up a minority of OBA patients (slightly more than 3%) yet they were still cared for in the office. These data suggest that OBA patients can present with significant comorbidities; a prudent anesthesia provider needs to be equipped to screen and handle these complicated cases appropriately.

Procedures in the office are as varied as those in the hospital setting. Using *Current Procedural Terminology* codes, the authors identified the most commonly performed procedures. Colonoscopy (including diagnostic and screening) comprised almost 11,000 cases and is the most common office procedure. Next is knee arthroscopy with meniscectomy and/or anterior cruciate ligament reconstruction, with more than 3900 cases. Finally, hysteroscopy with either endometrial ablation or sampling is the third most common at approximately 3000 cases (**Table 5**). Reviewing the most common codes highlights the diverse nature of OBA, with top specialties being gastroenterology, orthopedics, and gynecology. Additionally, each of these procedures is done with a different proceduralist/surgeon, emphasizing the need to have open communication to meet each provider's expectations.

Regarding the length of procedures, there is evidence in the ambulatory literature that the duration of greater than 1 hour is associated with higher rates of unplanned hospital admissions.[29] In the AQI non-OBA dataset, more than 76,000 cases reported the duration of procedure, with 30 minutes being most common at approximately 6500 cases. About 25% of cases lasted anywhere from 25 to 35 minutes, with nearly two-thirds reporting a duration of an hour or less. The non-OBA cases have significantly longer procedure duration (minutes) than OBA cases (P<.0001). The estimated

Table 4
Distribution of gender in OBA and non-OBA NACOR cases

Variable	Office Based (N = 85,821) n (%)	NACOR (N = 12,507,307) n (%)
Gender		
Female	52,477 (61.15)	7,479,832 (59.80)
Male	33,344 (38.85)	5,027,475 (40.02)

P = <.0001.

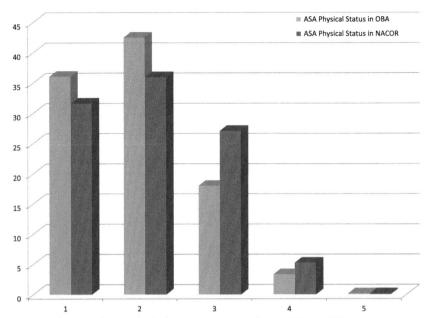

Fig. 1. Distribution of ASA physical status in OBA and non-OBA NACOR cases.

mean and standard deviation for each is 84.2 ± 60.9 and 62.1 ± 50, respectively (**Fig. 2**). More than 1100 cases lasted longer than 4 hours (1.5% of the data), which supports the notion that more complex procedures are being performed in the office. When comparing the distribution of duration (0–295 minutes) to other settings, office-based procedures are significantly different.

The authors found that OBA was overwhelmingly delivered by physicians working alone (**Table 6**), followed by the anesthesia care team model, which is a combination of attending anesthesiologists, anesthesiology residents, anesthesiologist assistants, and/or CRNAs working together to help deliver care.[30] The smallest group of providers is CRNAs working alone, composing slightly more than 1% of the cases. When compared with non-OBA data, this was significantly different than the makeup of providers in other settings.

General anesthesia, monitored anesthesia care (MAC), regional, sedation, and neuraxial (both spinal and epidural) anesthesia have all been used in the office. The most common anesthetic was general anesthesia (no differentiation between endotracheal vs supraglottic or maintenance with inhaled anesthetic vs TIVA), which was used in 68% of the 44,484 cases that provided details on the type of anesthesia. The second

Table 5 Most common office procedures in NACOR database	
Procedure	**Number of Cases**
Colonoscopy	10,918
Knee arthroscopy	3914
Hysteroscopy	3071
Oocyte retrieval	2702
Upper gastrointestinal endoscopy	1906

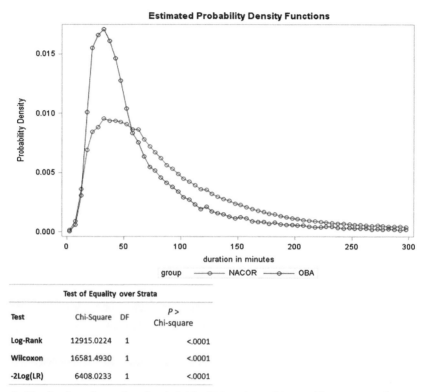

Fig. 2. Distribution of case duration (min) in OBA and non-OBA NACOR cases. DF, degrees of freedom; P, probability; LR, log-rank.

most common anesthetic was MAC, and together these 2 types composed almost 95% of the anesthetics delivered. The author's analysis showed that the type of anesthesia used in the office differed from the overall data (**Table 7**).

To date, there are minimal adverse outcomes data in NACOR that are specific to the office-based setting, with only 17 cases reported. The most common adverse event was hyperthermia in the PACU, with 5 patients reported. The most serious event was a single unplanned hospital admission and 1 prolonged PACU stay. In addition, 1 episode of noncompliance with antibiotic guidelines occurred. There were 2 episodes of postoperative nausea and vomiting (PONV) and 2 occurrences of uncontrolled pain in the PACU. There were no deaths (**Table 8**).

Table 6
Type of coverage by provider for OBA and non-OBA NACOR cases

Variable	Office Based (N = 29,735) n (%)	NACOR (N = 8,403,006) n (%)
Coverage		
CRNA ALONE	336 (1.13)	293,060 (3.49)
PHYSICIAN ALONE	22,398 (75.33)	4,333,393 (51.57)
Other	7001 (23.54)	3,776,553 (44.94)

P = <.0001.

Table 7
Anesthesia type in OBA compared with non-OBA NACOR cases

Variable	Office Based (N = 44,484) n (%)	NACOR (N = 9,365,286) n (%)
Anesthesia Type		
ESP	1241 (2.83)	853,823 (9.22)
GEN	30,638 (69.91)	6,566,028 (70.93)
LOC	4 (0.01)	10,093 (0.11)
MAC	11,600 (26.47)	1,537,381 (16.61)
OTH	56 (0.13)	96,677 (1.04)
REG	284 (0.65)	192,662 (2.08)

$P = <.0001$.
Abbreviations: ESP, epidural/spinal; GEN, general anesthesia; LOC, local anesthesia only; OTH, other; REG, regional anesthetic.

An unanticipated finding was ASA physical status 4 and 5 patients being anesthetized in the office, especially because an ASA PS 5 indicates that the individual is not expected to survive with or without the procedure.[31] The paucity of CRNAs functioning as the sole anesthesia provider was another surprising finding. This lack may be caused by an unwillingness on the part of the proceduralist/surgeon to take on a supervising role or the unwillingness of a CRNA to work in such a remote setting with no backup. Further research is warranted to determine the cause.

The duration of the procedure was also determined to be different in the office, with most procedures taking less than an hour, highlighting the need for an anesthesia provider to be able to induce, position, and reverse the anesthetics quickly and efficiently while delivering appropriate PONV prophylaxis and postoperative analgesia.

The NACOR/AQI data have limitations. All data are self-reported and, thus, subject to selection bias; it may be that participant practices are more inclined to deliver higher-quality care. Additionally, there is no mandated reporting of all information regarding patient or provider demographics, adverse events, or poor outcomes, which may lead to practices not stating all information requested in the data-reporting template. Lastly, because there are limited outcomes data, it would be important to learn from other adverse events to minimize the risk to OBA patients. One approach is stronger collaboration between NACOR and SCOR.

Table 8
OBA outcomes reported in NACOR

Outcome	Number of Occurrences
Hyperthermia in PACU	5
PONV	3
Uncontrolled pain in PACU	2
Difficult IV start	2
Unplanned hospital admission	1
Prolonged PACU stay	1
Adverse drug reaction	1
No antibiotics given	1
Cardiac arrhythmia	1

Abbreviation: IV, intravenous.

FUTURE DIRECTION OF OBA

As with the transformation that occurred in hospitals and ASCs in improving quality and safety, the office is next on the horizon. It seems that regulation and oversight will continue to grow and exert external pressure in offices performing any type of surgery. Furthermore, it can be expected that state legislatures will start to delineate what procedures are appropriate for offices or at least what qualifications are needed to perform certain procedures. As states become more involved in regulation, the federal government would be the next logical entity to create a unified national standard of quality and reporting, much like hospitals and ASCs currently have.[32] As already customary in these settings, payments from providers will most likely be tied to adhering to these rules and regulations.

With a federal mandate for electronic health records, an office-based anesthesia information management system (AIMS) is another frontier in the evolving medical software arena. Creating, installing, and updating an AIMS is a cumbersome project for many hospital systems; this is magnified in the office.[33] Nonetheless, the implementation of an AIMS will have several benefits. One major benefit is the ease in creating a database for outcomes research and quality-assurance initiatives because paper records can be lost, illegible, and can lack standard data-entry methods. Additionally, an AIMS has been shown to improve compliance by prompting practitioners for such critical events, such as DVT prophylaxis and antibiotic administration, in real time. The advent of sophisticated monitors that can communicate via both wired and wireless methods may free up the anesthesia providers' hands to care for the patients instead of taking care of documentation. Also, being able to remotely monitor patients can help an anesthesia provider ensure a patient's safety in the recovery area while still caring for a patient in the procedure room.

It is an exciting and challenging period for OBA. In such a fluid and dynamic situation, there are sure to be unforeseen issues. With quality and safety as guiding philosophies, OBA will continue to flourish, already embraced by both providers and patients.

REFERENCES

1. Cullen KA, Hall MJ, Golosinskiy A. Ambulatory surgery in the United States, 2006. National health statistics reports; no 11. Revised. Hyattsville (MD): National Center for Health Statistics; 2009.
2. Hunstad JP, Walk PH. Office-based anesthesia. Semin Plast Surg 2007;21(2):103–7.
3. Rutkauskas JS. The statistics (chapter 2). In: Shapiro FE, editor. Manual of office-based anesthesia procedures. Philadelphia: Lippincott, Williams and Wilkins; 2007. p. 6–10.
4. Kurrek MM, Twersky RS. Office-based anesthesia: how to start an office-based practice. Anesthesiol Clin 2010;28(2):353–67.
5. Rashewsky S, Parameswaran A, Sloane C, et al. Time and cost analysis: pediatric dental rehabilitation with general anesthesia in the office and the hospital settings. Anesth Prog 2012;59(4):147–53.
6. Prickett KK, Wise SK, DelGaudio JM. Cost analysis of office-based and operating room procedures in rhinology. Int Forum Allergy Rhinol 2012;2(3):207–11.
7. Byrd HS, Barton FE, Orenstein HH, et al. Safety and efficacy in an accredited outpatient plastic surgery facility: a review of 5316 consecutive cases. Plast Reconstr Surg 2003;112(2):636–41 [discussion: 42–6].
8. Vila H Jr, Soto R, Cantor AB, et al. Comparative outcomes analysis of procedures performed in physician offices and ambulatory surgery centers. Arch Surg 2003; 138(9):991–5.

9. Coldiron BM, Healy C, Bene NI. Office surgery incidents: what seven years of Florida data show us. Dermatol Surg 2008;34(3):285–91 [discussion: 91–2].

10. Keyes GR, Singer R, Iverson RE, et al. Analysis of outpatient surgery center safety using an internet-based quality improvement and peer review program. Plast Reconstr Surg 2004;113(6):1760–70.

11. Keyes GR, Singer R, Iverson RE, et al. Mortality in outpatient surgery. Plast Reconstr Surg 2008;122(1):245–50 [discussion: 51–3].

12. Soltani AM, Keyes GR, Singer R, et al. Outpatient surgery and sequelae: an analysis of the AAAASF Internet-based quality assurance and peer review database. Clin Plast Surg 2013;40(3):465–73.

13. Domino KB. Office-based anesthesia: lessons learned from the closed claims project. ASA Newsl 2001;65(6):9–11, 5.

14. Walsh MT, Kurrek MM, Desai M. Anesthesia outcomes in office based surgery. American Society of Anesthesiologists Annual Meeting, A798. San Diego, October 16–20, 2010.

15. Hoefflin SM, Bornstein JB, Gordon M. General anesthesia in an office-based plastic surgical facility: a report on more than 23,000 consecutive office-based procedures under general anesthesia with no significant anesthetic complications. Plast Reconstr Surg 2001;107(1):243–51 [discussion: 52–7].

16. Perrott DH, Yuen JP, Andresen RV, et al. Office-based ambulatory anesthesia: outcomes of clinical practice of oral and maxillofacial surgeons. J Oral Maxillofac Surg 2003;61(9):983–95 [discussion: 95–6].

17. Bitar G, Mullis W, Jacobs W, et al. Safety and efficacy of office-based surgery with monitored anesthesia care/sedation in 4778 consecutive plastic surgery procedures. Plast Reconstr Surg 2003;111(1):150–6 [discussion: 7–8].

18. Failey C, Aburto J, de la Portilla HG, et al. Office-based outpatient plastic surgery utilizing total intravenous anesthesia. Aesthet Surg J 2013;33(2):270–4.

19. Memtsoudis SG, Ma Y, Swamidoss CP, et al. Factors influencing unexpected disposition after orthopedic ambulatory surgery. J Clin Anesth 2012;24(2):89–95.

20. Qualifications of anesthesia providers in the office-based setting, statement on 2009. American Society of Anesthesiologists Web site. Available at: http://www.asahq.org/For-Healthcare-Professionals/Standards-Guidelines-and-Statements.aspx. Accessed September 7, 2013.

21. Urman RD, Punwani N, Shapiro FE. Office-based surgical and medical procedures: educational gaps. Ochsner J 2012;12(4):383–8.

22. Yates JA. American Society of Plastic Surgeons office-based surgery accreditation crosswalk. Plast Surg Nurs 2002;22(3):125–32.

23. Anesthesia machine obsolescence. American Society of Anesthesiologists web site. Available at: http://www.asahq.org/For-Healthcare-Professionals/Standards-Guidelines-and-Statements.aspx. Accessed September 7, 2013.

24. Standards for basic anesthetic monitoring. American Society of Anesthesiologists Web site. Available at: http://www.asahq.org/For-Healthcare-Professionals/Standards-Guidelines-and-Statements.aspx. Accessed September 7, 2013.

25. Difficult airway algorithm. American Society of Anesthesiologists. Available at: http://www.asahq.org/publicationsAndServices/Difficult%20Airway.pdf. Accessed September 7, 2013.

26. Kataria T, Cutter TW, Apfelbaum JL. Patient selection in outpatient surgery. Clin Plast Surg 2013;40(3):371–82.

27. Haeck PC, Swanson JA, Iverson RE, et al. Evidence-based patient safety advisory: patient selection and procedures in ambulatory surgery. Plast Reconstr Surg 2009;124(Suppl 4):6S–27S.

28. American Society of Anesthesiologists Task Force on Postanesthetic Care. Practice guidelines for postanesthetic care: a report by the American Society of Anesthesiologists Task Force on Postanesthetic Care. Anesthesiology 2002;96(3): 742–52.

29. Fortier J, Chung F, Su J. Unanticipated admission after ambulatory surgery–a prospective study. Can J Anaesth 1998;45(7):612–9.

30. American Society of Anesthesiologists. Statement on anesthesia care team. Last amended 2009. Available at: http://www.asahq.org/For-Members/Standards-Guidelines-and-Statements.aspx. Accessed January 5, 2014.

31. Owens WD, Felts JA, Spitznagel EL Jr. ASA physical status classifications: a study of consistency of ratings. Anesthesiology 1978;49(4):239–43.

32. Gaulton TG, Shapiro FE, Urman RD. Administrative issues to ensure safe anesthesia care in the office-based setting. Curr Opin Anaesthesiol 2013;26(6):692–7.

33. Ruskin KJ. Anesthesia information management systems for the office practitioner. Institute for Safety in Office Based Surgery. Available at: http://isobsurgery.org/?page_id=195. Accessed September 9, 2013.

Airway Management

Jennifer Anderson, MD*, P. Allan Klock Jr, MD

KEYWORDS

- Airway management • Difficult airway management • Videolaryngoscopy
- Supraglottic airway • Airway assessment • Difficult airway algorithm
- Airway equipment

KEY POINTS

- Large database studies have improved our understanding of airway management.
- New guidelines have been published to direct our management of the patient with a difficult airway.
- New airway devices have become commonly available and have improved outcomes but require modification of traditional techniques to maximize success and minimize complications.
- Airway assessment continues to be an imperfect science but should be performed to reduce the risk of patient harm.
- A strategy for airway management that preserves patient oxygenation and ventilation and avoids aspiration throughout the perioperative period should be used for every patient.

INTRODUCTION

The art and science of airway management have advanced considerably during the past 10 years. Airway management tools such as second-generation supraglottic airways (SGAs) and video-assisted devices have become commonly available in the ambulatory setting. These devices have improved patient care and safety, but they have required anesthesia providers to learn new skills and develop new airway strategies. The American Society of Anesthesiologists (ASA) practice guidelines for management of the difficult airway have been updated twice since 1993. The revised guidelines include new airway management techniques and devices and reflect an improved understanding of the science of airway management.[1] Concurrent with these improvements in our technology is the increasing prevalence of obesity and

Disclosures: Dr P.A. Klock is an unpaid member of the Scientific Advisory Board for Ambu Corporation. He does not have an equity position in this or any other medical device manufacturer. Dr J. Anderson has no conflict of Interest.
Department of Anesthesia and Critical Care, University of Chicago, 5841 South Maryland Avenue, MC-4028, Chicago, IL 60637, USA
* Corresponding author.
E-mail address: janderson@dacc.uchicago.edu

Anesthesiology Clin 32 (2014) 445–461
http://dx.doi.org/10.1016/j.anclin.2014.02.022
1932-2275/14/$ – see front matter © 2014 Elsevier Inc. All rights reserved.

anesthesiology.theclinics.com

obstructive sleep apnea (OSA), which have nearly doubled in the United States and substantially increased the number of patients at risk for difficult laryngoscopy, difficult ventilation, or aspiration of gastric contents. Ambulatory surgery patients are presenting with higher body mass indices (BMIs, calculated as weight in kilograms divided by the square of height in meters) and more comorbid conditions for increasingly complex surgical procedures. This constellation of events requires that anesthesia providers are fully capable of recognizing and managing patients with a hazardous airway.

Large database studies and review articles have been published that offer insight into the risk factors for a difficult airway, modes of injury, and clinicians' responses to challenging airway situations.[2–4] More high-risk patients receive care in ambulatory centers, in which providers may not have the luxury of extra personnel skilled in airway management and advanced airway equipment may be limited. Anesthesia providers in ambulatory centers must continue to stay current with airway management tools and techniques to continue to provide the best care for their patients.

To frame the conversation regarding airway management, it is helpful to review the prevalence of airway management difficulty. Relevant data are listed in **Box 1**.

LESSONS LEARNED FROM RECENT STUDIES

Adverse airway events are rare. As a result, it is difficult to conduct studies that have sufficient power to be meaningful. However, as electronic medical records and collaborative research increase, large database studies have been published. In the following section, the salient points of recent large-scale investigations are presented.

The Fourth National Audit Project of the United Kingdom

In 2011, the Royal College of Anesthetists of the United Kingdom and the Difficult Airway Society of the United Kingdom published the results of the Fourth National

---

Box 1
Prevalence of difficult airway management

- Difficult face mask ventilation occurs at a rate of 1% to 2%

- Impossible face mask ventilation occurs at a rate of 1 to 2 per 1000 anesthetics (0.1%–0.2%)

- The failure rate for the classic and flexible laryngeal mask airway (LMA) is 2%

- The failure rate for the intubating and Proseal LMA is 1%

- Difficult direct laryngoscopy occurs at a rate of 1% to 18% (but most of these patients are successfully intubated)

- Unsuccessful intubation with direct laryngoscopy occurs at a rate of 5 to 35 cases per 10,000 anesthetics

- For patients predicted to have a normal airway, the reported failure rate for videolaryngoscopy-assisted intubation ranges from 0.4% to 2.9%

- For patients predicted to have a difficult to manage airway the failure rate for intubation with videolaryngoscopy is 1.5% to 4.2%

- The cannot ventilate, cannot intubate scenario occurs at a rate of 0.01 to 2 per 10,000 anesthetics

- Difficult mask ventilation significantly increases the risk of difficult intubation by a factor of 4 and impossible intubation by a factor of 12

Data from Refs.[4–12]

Audit Project (NAP4).[2] The audit had 3 purposes: to determine what types of devices are used for airway management and their relative frequency of use, to determine the rate of major complications of airway management, and to perform an analysis of the events leading to these complications. All 309 National Health Service hospitals collected and returned data related to serious airway complications from September, 2008 to September, 2009. To determine the number of anesthetics delivered in a year, data were collected for all general anesthesia cases during a 2-week period. During this period, data were submitted for 114,904 general anesthetics, leading the investigators to estimate that approximately 2,900,000 anesthetics were delivered during the 12-month study period. There were 184 confirmed serious patient complications, with 133 complications occurring during anesthetic management; 36 occurred in the intensive care unit and 15 in the emergency department. The quality of care provided to patients who died or were seriously injured during anesthetic management was judged to be good in only 18% of the cases, mixed in 41%, and poor in 34% (7% of cases were not classified).[2] There is bad news and good news from this finding. The good news is that when good or appropriate care is delivered, the risk of a serious injury resulting from airway management is about 1 in 100,000, and the risk of death or brain damage is about 1 per million general anesthetics. The bad news is that most patients who were injured received suboptimal care. A conclusion that can be drawn from this study is that a significant opportunity exists to improve airway management across the United Kingdom; the same can likely be said for North America.

The major themes related to the adverse events captured in the NAP4 study are listed in **Box 2**.

There are 4 main lessons from this comprehensive observational study that relate to ambulatory anesthesia. First, anesthesia providers should plan for unanticipated airway difficulty and should have an airway strategy for every patient, which includes several viable plans that can be rapidly executed. Elements of a strategy might include face mask ventilation, direct laryngoscopy (DL) and videolaryngoscopy (VL), SGA use, and emergency surgical cricothyrotomy. If an airway management technique has failed, subsequent attempts of the same technique should be made only after conditions have been optimized. For example, with DL, proper head and neck position should be obtained, external laryngeal manipulation applied, and change of laryngoscope blade or operator considered between attempts. Because continued attempts with the same technique probably have decreasing usefulness and may lead to airway edema or bleeding, the number of attempts should be limited.

Providers should recognize that unlike emergency surgical airway techniques, percutaneous catheter cricothyrotomy has a high failure rate. Every ambulatory surgery facility should have the tools and appropriately skilled anesthesia providers to manage an unanticipated difficult airway situation.

The second main lesson from NAP4 is that anesthesia providers should recognize that not all patients are candidates for airway management using an SGA device. Patients at highest risk for an adverse event when an SGA is used include those with risk factors because of a recent meal, delayed gastric emptying, pregnancy or morbid obesity or those undergoing a procedure in which the operating table is rotated away from the anesthesia provider.[5] Third, if the patient is best managed with an awake intubation with a flexible bronchoscope, this technique should be used regardless of the practice setting. Patients should recover from their anesthetic in an appropriately monitored setting and should be discharged only when they are no longer at risk for airway obstruction.

Box 2
Lessons learned from the NAP4 study

- Poor airway assessment contributed to poor airway outcomes
- Poor planning contributed to poor airway outcomes
- Often, there was a failure to plan for failure, leading to an unstructured response to an unanticipated difficult airway situation
- The audit identified numerous cases in which awake intubation with a flexible bronchoscope was indicated but was not used
- Problems arose when patients were subjected to multiple attempts at tracheal intubation. The investigators state, "The airway problem regularly deteriorated to a 'can't intubate, can't ventilate' situation. It is well recognized (that) a change of approach is required rather than repeated use of a technique that has already failed"
- Inappropriate uses of SGA devices were reported; the most common themes were morbidly obese patients, patients with risk factors for aspiration of gastric contents, and the use of an SGA for a patient with a suspected difficult airway without a backup plan for SGA failure
- Complications related to anesthesia for head and neck surgery were disproportionately represented in the database; these cases require excellent teamwork and communication
- Obese and morbidly obese patients had more complications than would be expected based on their proportional representation of surgical cases; they had higher rates of aspiration, complications associated with SGA use, difficulty with tracheal intubation, and airway obstruction during emergence or recovery; airway rescue techniques were not as successful in obese patients as in the nonobese
- Emergency percutaneous small diameter catheter cricothyrotomy failed 60% of the time
- Emergency surgical airway techniques were almost universally successful
- Aspiration was the single most common cause of death in anesthesia events; many of these events were associated with poor assessment (not recognizing risk factors for aspiration) or poor judgment (eg, using an SGA when rapid sequence induction and tracheal intubation were indicated)
- One-third of adverse events occurred during emergence or recovery, and airway obstruction was the most common cause of harm in these events

Adapted from Cook TM, Woodall N, Frerk C. The NAP4 report: major complications of airway management in the UK. London: The Royal College of Anaesthetists; 2011.

2013 Update: ASA Difficult Airway Algorithm

The most recent version of the ASA guidelines for management of the difficult airway was published in 2013. Many of the changes in the guidelines seem subtle but have significant bearing on clinical practice.

First, in the, "assess likelihood and impact" section of the algorithm, "difficult supraglottic airway placement" was added. This factor is important to determine for all patients who may receive general anesthesia, because an SGA is likely the first strategy used if difficulty is encountered with face mask ventilation or intubation. Risk factors for SGA failure are discussed later. Second, in the same "assess likelihood and impact" section, "difficult laryngoscopy" has been added. The 2003 version of the guidelines listed only "difficult intubation" (DI).[6] The addition of difficult laryngoscopy to the algorithm recognizes the distinction between difficult laryngoscopy and DI. This distinction is particularly vexing when the operator is using a highly angulated videolaryngoscope and an excellent view of the laryngeal opening is obtained but it is difficult or impossible to pass the tube into the trachea.

The "consider the relative merits and feasibility of basic management choices" section now contains, "video-assisted laryngoscopy as an initial approach to intubation." This feature recognizes the usefulness of VL for routine and difficult airway management.

Throughout the guideline, LMA (laryngeal mask airway) has been changed to SGA or supraglottic airway. This change recognizes that all brands and types of supraglottic devices are candidates for use in the difficult airway algorithm. In the nonemergent pathway in which DL is unsuccessful but the patient can be ventilated by face mask, video-assisted laryngoscopy is now listed first under "alternative difficult intubation approaches." Again, this factor reflects the usefulness of VL when DL has failed.

One of the shortcomings of the algorithm is that "invasive airway access" appears twice in the algorithm: once as part of the nonemergency pathway and once as part of the emergency pathway. Retrograde intubation is listed in both sections, but this technique should not be considered as part of the emergency pathway. Although percutaneous airway techniques and jet ventilation remain in the algorithm, they are deemphasized because of the potential for technique failure with percutaneous catheter techniques and the risk for barotrauma and impaired venous return as a result of high intrathoracic pressure (pulmonary tamponade) caused by jet ventilation techniques. Although not explicitly stated in the 2013 difficult airway algorithm (**Fig. 1**), if VL has failed, providers should immediately consider DL, because there have been anecdotal reports of DL success after VL failure.[7]

The SGA: When Might It Fail?

In 2012, Ramachandran and colleagues[4] published results of a prospective database query of 15,795 anesthetics performed with the disposable LMA Unique (uLMA) (Teleflex, Research Triangle Park, NC, USA). The study was designed to glean information regarding characteristics and risk factors of uLMA failure in adults. Failure was defined as "any acute airway event occurring between insertion of uLMA and completion of surgical procedure that required uLMA removal and rescue endotracheal tube placement." Failures were associated with hypoxia (O_2 saturation <85%), hypercapnia, or airway obstruction. Obstruction occurred in more than 60% of the patients in whom the uLMA failed.

A 1.1% overall failure rate was found, which is consistent with other supraglottic devices. Univariate and multivariate analysis revealed that patients with the characteristics outlined in **Box 3** had a significantly increased frequency of uLMA failure.

Eighty-three percent of the LMA cases were ambulatory procedures. There was a lower frequency of uLMA failure in the ambulatory setting compared with inpatient (0.99% vs 1.48%). Of the 131 failed uLMA uses in the ambulatory setting, 14% required unplanned hospital admission.[4] Further evaluation of the ambulatory surgery subpopulation was not reported.

This study advances our understanding of the usefulness and failure of the uLMA. Although most SGAs have many features similar to the uLMA, caution is needed in extrapolating the results of this study to other devices.

Videolaryngoscopes: Glottic View Versus Successful Intubation

Traditional laryngoscopy depends on creating a line of sight from the viewer through the oropharynx to the glottis, which in some patients is difficult or impossible. Highly angulated videolaryngoscopes allow the user to view the glottis without requiring a line of sight. Many clinicians are frustrated when using these devices, because an excellent view of the glottis may be obtained, but intubation of the trachea can be technically difficult. It is important to appreciate the difference between laryngoscopy and intubation when using videolaryngoscopes.

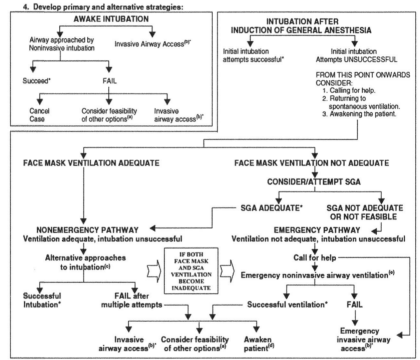

Fig. 1. The ASA difficult airway algorithm. (*From* Apfelbaum JL, Hagberg CA, Caplan RA, et al. Practice guidelines for management of the difficult airway: an updated report by the American Society of Anesthesiologists Task Force on Management of the Difficult Airway. Anesthesiology 2013;118(2):257; with permission.)

There are 3 major types of videolaryngoscopes. The first uses an integrated channel, through which the endotracheal tube (ETT) is threaded. The second uses a stylet over which the ETT is loaded and then slid down to intubate the trachea. The third is the most popular design, known as the rigid blade laryngoscope, with blades of

---

Box 3
Risk factors associated with uLMA failure

Univariate risk factors:

- Advanced age (>56 years)
- Increased BMI[a]
- Male sex
- Reduced thyromental distance (<6 cm)
- Thick neck (qualitatively analyzed by clinician)
- Poor dentition (includes missing some or all teeth)
- History of smoking (current smoker)
- Intraoperative surgical table rotation[b]

Multivariate risk factors:

- Intraoperative surgical table rotation[b]
- Male sex
- Poor dentition
- Increased BMI

[a] Mean BMI of patients in the LMA failure group was 29.3 kg/m^2, and 26.9 kg/m^2 in the successful LMA group.
[b] A 5-fold increased risk of failure was reported with table rotation.
Data from Ramachandran SK, Mathis MR, Tremper KK, et al. Predictors and clinical outcomes from failed Laryngeal Mask Airway Unique™: a study of 15,795 patients. Anesthesiology 2012; 116(6):1217–26.

---

varying curvature; ETT placement requires a separate stylet or guide to achieve intubation of the trachea.

Many studies indicate that videolaryngoscopes in each category[3,8] can provide a superior glottic view. However, successful intubation with these devices is not well documented. A recent systematic review of 77 studies[3] described the efficacy of 8 videolaryngoscopes in successful oral endotracheal intubation performed by trained operators. The following 8 devices were included: GlideScope (Verathon Inc, Bothell, WA, USA), V-MAC (including C-MAC and Storz Berci DCI) (KARL STORZ Endoscopy-America, Inc, El Segundo, CA, USA), Bullard (Olympus America Inc, Center Valley, PA, USA), McGrath (Aircraft Medical, Edinburgh, UK), Bonfils (KARL STORZ Endoscopy-America, Inc, El Segundo, CA, USA), Airtraq (Prodol Meditec S.A., Vizcaya, Spain), Pentax AWS (Ambu A/S, Ballerup, Denmark), and LMA CTrach (Teleflex, Research Triangle Park, NC, USA).

VL with these devices had an intubation success rate of 94% to 100% in unselected patients from the general population,[3] which is similar to the success rates for DL. The picture is not so clear for patients with suspected or known difficult DL. In patients assessed by Mallampati score to be at risk for difficult DL, Healy and colleagues[3] found good evidence for the overall success for use of Airtraq, CTrach, Glidescope, Pentax AWS, and V-MAC, but weak evidence of overall success with Bonfils and Bullard scopes. For patients with known difficult DL, there was weak evidence supporting the use of the Airtraq, Bonfils, Bullard, CTrach, Glidescope, and Pentax AWS, but this is because of low numbers of patients rather than a small clinical benefit (**Table 1**).

Table 1 Level of evidence for overall success for devices under study			
	Good Evidence (Level 1+)	Weak Evidence (Level 3)	No Evidence
Subjects at higher risk of difficulty during DL	Airtraq CTrach GlideScope Pentax AWS V-MAC	Bonfils Bullard	McGrath
Known difficult DL		Airtraq Bonfils Bullard CTrach GlideScope Pentax AWS	McGrath V-MAC
Failed DL		Airtraq Bonfils CTrach GlideScope McGrath Pentax AWS	Bullard V-MAC

From Healy DW, Maties O, Hovord D, et al. A systematic review of the role of videolaryngoscopy in successful orotracheal intubation. BMC Anesthesiol 2012;12(1):13.

Healy and colleagues[3] found that there are good data to show that some VLs are useful for anticipated DI. Because the predictive value of airway assessment tools is limited, we cannot confidently conclude that VLs are useful as rescue devices for patients with difficult airways when other devices have failed. Failed intubation and adverse airway events are rare, and it is difficult to prove the usefulness of VL for patients with known difficult or failed DL, but there may be some evidence that these devices can be useful for less experienced practitioners. In their meta-analysis of Glidescope use, Griesdale and colleagues[8] found that time to intubation and first time success were improved with Glidescope over DL for inexperienced providers.

The risks of using these devices must also be considered. According to Healy and colleagues,[3] there is no clear evidence that there is an increased risk of traumatic complications with VL compared with DL in the general population. However, adverse events with videolaryngoscopes have been reported, and mitigating these risks is important. Palatal perforation while using both the Glidescope and McGrath has been documented,[9,10] and 1 study of more than 2000 patients[7] found a 0.3% incidence of oropharyngeal injury using the Glidescope.

The 4-step process outlined in **Box 4** has been suggested by Walls to help avoid oropharyngeal injury with Glidescope intubation.[11]

Box 4 Four-step process for VL insertion and intubation
• First, look in the mouth to introduce the laryngoscope
• Second, look at the screen to obtain the best glottic view
• Third, look in the mouth to introduce the ETT, and watch as the tip of the tube goes behind the tongue, being careful to avoid the soft palate and tonsillar arches
• Fourth, look at the screen as the tube passes through the glottic opening

AIRWAY ASSESSMENT

The importance of patient airway assessment was highlighted by findings of NAP4.[2] Lack of proper airway assessment (one-quarter to one-third of patients with adverse airway events had no documented airway assessment) was associated with several poor outcomes. Poor planning was also associated with adverse events but was more the result of poor judgment than lack of knowledge.[2]

In recent literature, 3 main concerns stand out: aspiration, morbid obesity, and OSA. Aspiration was found to be the leading cause of anesthesia-related death in the NAP4. Clearly, attention must be paid to history and physical findings that suggest an increased risk of aspiration, including, but not limited to, history of gastroesophageal reflux disease, history of diabetes, opioid use, fasting status, and increased BMI. The NAP4 study showed that patients with aspiration, SGA failure, difficult mask ventilation, or DI had a higher BMI than the general population. Moreover, the risk of OSA causing postoperative complications is higher in obese patients. The confluence of these risks can make management of the obese patient difficult. Reliance on regional anesthesia or supraglottic devices without planning for backup techniques does not constitute an effective strategy, because no single approach is guaranteed. Along with patient characteristics, the type of procedure may alter the airway strategy. Considerations should include the need for table rotation, in which the patient's head is not near the anesthesia provider, and potential alteration of the airway by the surgery itself.[4]

Patient characteristics associated with difficult tracheal intubation and their predictive usefulness are listed in **Table 2**.

A review of multifactorial risk assessment for DI showed that scoring systems based on a practical bedside examination and analysis have sensitivities ranging from 60% to 95% and specificities of 65% to 92%.[17] When a test with 95% sensitivity and 91% specificity[18] is applied to an expected DI rate of 2%, the positive predictive value is 18% and the negative predictive value is more than 99%. In everyday practice, some anesthesia providers may not perform a complete assessment, and the analysis of the patient factors may be biased to minimize the risk of DI. Even if everything is carried out perfectly, some patients may have an impossible airway without any physical findings or history to suggest airway difficulty. One cause of this situation is lingual tonsil hypertrophy, which can lead to difficult or impossible ventilation with a face mask or SGA and difficult or impossible intubation.[19]

Performing and documenting a basic airway history and physical examination are recommended and prudent. The 2013 ASA difficult airway guidelines list characteristics to consider including in the examination (**Table 3**). If available, additional information from nasal endoscopy, imaging studies, or previous records should be reviewed.

Table 2 Sensitivity and specificity of patient factors associated with difficult intubation		
Examination	Sensitivity	Specificity
Interincisor gap	0.26–0.47	0.94–0.99
Thyromental distance	0.07–0.65	0.81–0.98
Chin protrusion (upper lip bite test)	0.16–0.29	0.85–0.95
Oropharyngeal grade (Mallampati)	0.14–0.67	0.66–0.96
Neck range of movement	0.15	0.98
History of difficult intubation	0.04–0.09	0.99

Data from Refs.[13–16]

Table 3
Components of the preoperative airway physical examination

Airway Examination Component	Nonreassuring Findings
Length of upper incisors	Relatively long
Relationship of maxillary and mandibular incisors during normal jaw closure	Prominent overbite (maxillary incisors anterior to mandibular incisors)
Relationship of maxillary and mandibular incisors during voluntary protrusion of mandible	Patient cannot bring mandibular incisors anterior to (in front of) maxillary incisors
Interincisor distance	<3 cm
Visibility of uvula	Not visible when tongue is protruded with patient in sitting position (eg., Mallampati class >2)
Shape of palate	Highly arched or very narrow
Compliance of mandibular space	Stiff, indurated, occupied by mass, or nonresilient
Thyromental distance	<3 ordinary finger breadths
Length of neck	Short
Thickness of neck	Thick
Range of motion of head and neck	Patient cannot touch tip of chin to chest or cannot extend neck

This table shows some findings of the airway physical examination that may suggest the presence of a difficult intubation. The decision to examine some or all of the airway components shown on this table is dependent on the clinical context and judgment of the practitioner. The table is not intended as a mandatory or exhaustive list of the components of an airway examination. The order or presentation in this table follows the line of sight that occurs during conventional oral laryngoscopy.

From Apfelbaum JL, Hagberg CA, Caplan RA, et al. Practice guidelines for management of the difficult airway: an updated report by the American Society of Anesthesiologists Task Force on Management of the Difficult Airway. Anesthesiology 2013;118(2):262; with permission.

Although performance of an airway assessment is the standard of care, a proper assessment only reduces and does not eliminate the incidence of an unexpected difficult to manage airway. For this reason, it is imperative to have an airway strategy that includes plans for unanticipated DI or ventilation.

Developing an Airway Strategy

With the information from the assessment, the anesthesia provider can create a strategy for airway management. Designing a strategy involves not only choosing a device but designing a plan for airway management that preserves patient oxygenation and ventilation and avoids aspiration throughout the perioperative period.[2] The strategy should include initial choices for airway management and backup plans if initial attempts fail.

Selection of techniques for any patient is outlined in section 3 of the ASA practice guidelines for management of the difficult airway, in which the practitioner is asked to "consider the relative merits and feasibility of basic management choices."[1]

- Awake intubation versus intubation after induction of general anesthesia
- Noninvasive technique versus invasive techniques for the initial approach to intubation
- Video-assisted laryngoscopy as an initial approach to intubation
- Preservation versus ablation of spontaneous ventilation

First, one should consider if awake intubation is necessary or feasible for the patient. NAP4 reported cases in which failure to secure the airway with the patient awake contributed to adverse events.[2] Although preferable, a flexible bronchoscope is not always required to secure the airway in a conscious patient. With proper topical anesthesia, the airway can be secured in a conscious or sedated patient with a conventional laryngoscope, a videolaryngoscope, or even an SGA. In some cases, an invasive technique (awake tracheostomy, cricothyrotomy, or retrograde intubation) may be the best choice for the patient, although these are rarely the primary plan in the ambulatory setting. The anesthesia provider must decide if tracheal intubation is required or an SGA may be used. If a patient has 1 or more risk factors for LMA failure as outlined by Ramachandran and colleagues,[4] intubation may be the preferred strategy. If an SGA is used, the decision to use a first-generation or second-generation device may depend on: (1) whether the plan calls for controlled ventilation or spontaneous ventilation, (2) the risk of aspiration, and (3) the benefit of suctioning the stomach. In some patients, such as those with limited neck mobility, VL may be the best first choice. An important decision is whether it is more advantageous to keep the patient breathing during airway management or if a neuromuscular blocker should be used to facilitate securing the airway. Regardless of the first choice, contingency planning must occur and assistance and equipment must be available.

SGA Tips for Success

Findings from large databases of patients[2,4] show that first-generation SGAs are safe, but certain patients and surgical case characteristics increase the risk of adverse outcomes with these devices. Second-generation supraglottic devices have certain modifications that may enhance their usefulness and safety, including an esophageal port designed to sit within the upper esophageal sphincter. The port provides a pathway for regurgitated gastric contents to drain without contaminating the airway and provides a conduit for orogastric tube placement and suctioning of stomach contents if desired.

The Proseal LMA (PLMA) (Teleflex, Research Triangle Park, NC, USA) is a second-generation SGA with a flexible reinforced tube with a cuff made of silicone. Because of its size and flexibility, the PLMA may be awkward to insert, and first time insertion success rates are lower with this device than with the classic LMA (Teleflex, Research Triangle Park, NC, USA).[20] There is a rigid curved introducer available that makes insertion easier, but anesthesia providers may not be aware of this device or it may be unavailable. Alternatively, styletting the drain tube of the PLMA with a fiber-optic scope, bougie, or 14-Fr gastric tube, directing the stylet into the esophagus with or without a laryngoscope, and then threading the PLMA into position over the chosen device have been described.[21] Using a gastric tube as the introducer and leaving it in place for gastric suctioning requires only a gastric tube, which is commonly available in the operating room. A 14-Fr orogastric tube is lubricated and inserted into the drain tube of the PLMA, with the tip protruding to 10 cm beyond the end, and this is then inserted into the oropharynx. Once placement has been confirmed by end-tidal CO_2, the gastric tube can be advanced into the stomach and used throughout the case.[22]

The LMA Supreme (Teleflex, Research Triangle Park, NC, USA) is a combination of the intubating LMA and the Proseal, with a similar sized esophageal port. It has a rigid curve and it is easy to insert, but sometimes, its rigidity impedes the ability of the operator to adjust it to create a satisfactory seal, because the fixed curvature may cause it to align incorrectly with the glottis and upper esophageal sphincter. If the device does not provide an adequate seal, another type of SGA (eg, uLMA or Proseal) should be considered. More information regarding supraglottic devices can be found in a comprehensive review article of the history of SGA development and tips for successful use by Klock and Hernandez.[5]

VL: Tips for Success

Although videolaryngoscopes have become popular, clinicians who are experienced with DL are often frustrated with their initial VL experiences because of some subtle differences between the techniques needed for the devices. Experienced users should continue to be vigilant to avoid VL-related airway injuries and consider using the following strategies. First, it is necessary to use a stylet when intubating with a highly curved VL such as a Glidescope. The curve of the stylet should be shaped to approximate the curve of the VL blade, which is significantly more angulated than the configuration for DL. Second, it is important to let the VL blade glide over the tongue rather than be closely opposed to the tongue as the blade is inserted. This strategy prevents the tongue from being pushed into the hypopharynx.

Third, it is important to avoid the common errors of inserting the blade more deeply than necessary or applying excessive lifting force. Although these maneuvers may provide a better view of the larynx, they hinder passage of the tube through the glottic opening. As with DL, if the esophagus or the posterior cricoid cartilage can be seen, the blade has been inserted too deeply. If it is difficult to introduce the ETT into the trachea, reducing the amount of lifting force and slightly withdrawing the blade to change the angle of the VL handle to a more horizontal position moves the larynx more posteriorly and brings the tracheal axis more in line with the ETT and stylet. These procedures are shown in **Fig. 2**. It is important to understand the interaction of the natural curve of the ETT, known as camber, with the curve of the stylet. Ordinarily, as the tube is advanced off the stylet, the tip of the tube curves to an increasingly anterior orientation, which can frustrate attempts to pass the tube into the trachea. This problem can be solved by loading the tube onto the stylet with reverse camber; the part of the tube that is normally concave is rotated so that it assumes a convex shape on the cephalad and posterior part of the stylet. This strategy allows the tip of the tube to be directed inferiorly toward the carina rather than anteriorly as it is advanced off the stylet. This procedure is shown in **Fig. 3**. If the tube is not preloaded with reverse camber, the operator may attempt a corkscrew maneuver; the tube is rotated along the axis of the stylet as gentle inward pressure is applied to advance the tube into the trachea.

ANESTHETIC EMERGENCE AND EXTUBATION

Anticipating and planning for intubation risks are mainstays of an anesthesiologist's practice, but attention should be paid to extubation as well. One-third of the adverse events from the NAP4 study occurred during emergence or recovery from general anesthesia. Evaluating extubation risk involves considering any previous anticipated or unanticipated DIs, possible side effects of the procedure (anatomic changes or edema), and whether or not access to the airway is an issue.[23] Anticipating extubation risk may be especially prudent for the anesthesia provider working in the ambulatory setting, who may have limited postoperative resources for airway management.

The Bailey Maneuver

The Bailey maneuver is useful for patients undergoing procedures where risk to the surgical sutures because of coughing and strain is undesirable but deep extubation is not optimal. It may also be helpful in patients with chronic obstructive pulmonary disease, severe asthma, or comorbidities, in whom increased sympathetic tone is

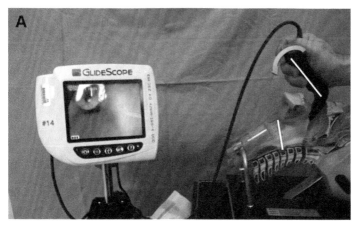

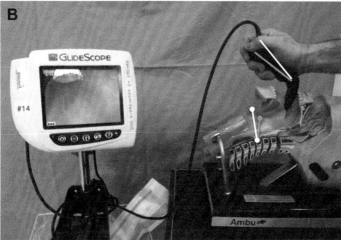

Fig. 2. (*A*) VL using excessive lifting force. The angle of the handle and the distance between a reference point on the posterior pharynx of the model and the vallecula are shown with white lines. Note that the laryngeal opening is well visualized. (*B*) VL using less lifting force and a more horizontal handle angle. The white lines show the angle of the laryngoscope and the relative position of the vallecula from (*A*). The green lines show the changes when the handle is slightly angled toward the patient's feet and less lifting force is applied. The larynx is not visualized so completely, but it has moved to a more posterior position, which makes intubation much easier.

undesirable. It entails placing a supraglottic device posterior to the ETT in a deeply anesthetized patient (**Fig. 4**). After proper placement of the SGA behind the ETT and assurance that the patient is at a depth of anesthesia sufficient to prevent laryngospasm, the ETT is removed and the patient is allowed to awaken without being stimulated until he or she rejects the supraglottic device. Placement of the SGA while the patient is intubated helps ensure that the airway is not lost after the ETT is removed, and the presence of the ETT prevents the SGA from pushing the epiglottis down over the glottic opening, which can cause obstruction. **Box 5** includes the sequence for this maneuver as described in the Difficult Airway Society extubation guidelines.[23]

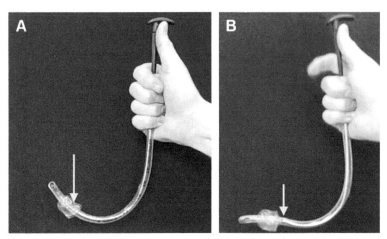

Fig. 3. (*A*) Endotracheal tube being deployed off rigid stylet with standard camber orientation. The arrow indicates the end of the stylet. Note that the tube is directed toward the location that would be the anterior wall of the trachea. (*B*) Endotracheal tube being deployed off rigid stylet with reverse camber orientation. The arrow indicates the end of the stylet. Note that the tube is directed parallel to the axis of the trachea.

EMERGENCY EQUIPMENT

The ability to manage the patient with a difficult airway requires appropriate equipment and experienced staff. Current assessment tools are not sensitive enough to always anticipate which patients may be difficult to mask ventilate or intubate, so equipment to deal with the unanticipated difficult airway must be readily available. The 2013 updated ASA practice guidelines suggest the contents of a portable difficult airway cart as listed in **Box 6**.[1]

The differences from the 2003 guidelines are the addition of a videolaryngoscope and the elimination of equipment for retrograde intubation.[6] This list should not be regarded as comprehensive but rather as suggestions for specific devices that meet the abilities of the least experienced staff and preferences of providers.[24] The cart should be well organized and labeled,[24,25] and a designated individual or a group should be in charge of maintenance of all airway equipment.[2,25] A system should be in place to restock the cart immediately after its use; premade sealed inserts with specific equipment may make this process more expeditious and reliable.[25]

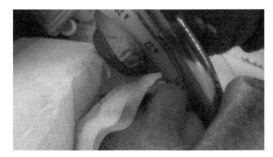

Fig. 4. The Bailey maneuver. The SGA is inserted cephalad and posterior to the endotracheal tube.

Box 5
Sequence for LMA exchange in at-risk extubation

1. Administer 100% oxygen

2. Avoid airway stimulation: either deep anesthesia (1 MAC) or neuromuscular blockade is essential

3. Perform laryngoscopy and suction under direct vision

4. Insert deflated SGA behind the tracheal tube

5. Ensure SGA placement with the tip in its correct position

6. Inflate cuff of SGA

7. Deflate tracheal tube cuff and remove tube while maintaining positive pressure

8. Continue oxygen delivery via SGA

9. Insert a bite block

10. Sit the patient upright

11. Allow undisturbed emergence from anesthesia

Adapted from Mitchell V, Dravid R, Patel A, et al. Difficult Airway Society Guidelines for the management of tracheal extubation. Anaesthesia 2012;67(3):327; with permission.

Flexible bronchoscopes are expensive, and their limited role in managing the cannot intubate, cannot ventilate patient may not support having them immediately available at every airway cart location. If laryngoscopy and mask ventilation are impossible, there is no role for the use of the flexible bronchoscope in the 2013 guidelines.

Box 6
Suggested contents of the portable storage unit for difficult airway management

Rigid laryngoscope blades of alternative design and size to those routinely used; this may include a rigid fiber-optic laryngoscope

Videolaryngoscope

Tracheal tubes of assorted sizes

Tracheal tube guides; examples include (but are not limited to) semirigid stylets, ventilating tube-changer, light wands, and forceps designed to manipulate the distal portion of the tracheal tube

SGAs (eg, LMA or intubating LMA of assorted sizes for noninvasive airway ventilation/ intubation)

Flexible fiber-optic intubation equipment

Equipment suitable for emergency invasive airway access

An exhaled carbon dioxide detector

The items listed in this table represent suggestions. The contents of the portable storage unit should be customized to meet the specific needs, preferences, and skills of the practitioner and health care facility.

From Apfelbaum JL, Hagberg CA, Caplan RA, et al. Practice guidelines for management of the difficult airway: an updated report by the American Society of Anesthesiologists Task Force on Management of the Difficult Airway. Anesthesiology 2013;118(2):262; with permission.

However, if ventilation is adequate with a face mask or SGA, there is time to obtain a flexible bronchoscope. Therefore, one recommendation is to have a fiber-optic scope within 5 minutes of any anesthetizing location.[26] Greenland[24] questioned the need for fiber-optic intubation equipment, because practitioners may lose skills with the device if continuing practice does not occur. To maintain operator skills, flexible broncho-scopes can be used regularly in nondifficult situations or in ongoing training sessions. The investigators of the NAP4 study state, "Anesthetic departments should provide a service where the skills and the equipment are available to deliver awake fiber-optic intubation whenever it is indicated."[2]

SUMMARY

The tools and techniques that are available to anesthesia providers in the ambulatory setting have improved considerably during the past 10 years. To fully use these gains, clinicians must understand the risks and benefits and appropriate clinical settings for each technique and device. Patients are presenting for ambulatory procedures with increasing comorbidities and risk factors for difficult airway management. To mitigate this risk, it is important to develop an airway strategy that includes addressing difficult mask ventilation, intubation, and SGA use. In doing so, the specialty of anesthesiology can improve on its strong record of providing excellent patient safety and care.

REFERENCES

1. Apfelbaum JL, Hagberg CA, Caplan RA, et al. Practice guidelines for management of the difficult airway: an updated report by the American Society of Anesthesiologists Task Force on Management of the Difficult Airway. Anesthesiology 2013;118(2):251–70.
2. Cook TM, Woodall N, Frerk C. The NAP4 report: major complications of airway management in the UK. London: The Royal College of Anaesthetists; 2011.
3. Healy DW, Maties O, Hovord D, et al. A systematic review of the role of videolaryngoscopy in successful orotracheal intubation. BMC Anesthesiol 2012;12(1):32.
4. Ramachandran SK, Mathis MR, Tremper KK, et al. Predictors and clinical outcomes from failed Laryngeal Mask Airway Unique™: a study of 15,795 patients. Anesthesiology 2012;116(6):1217–26.
5. Hernandez MR, Klock PA, Ovassapian A. Evolution of the extraglottic airway: a review of its history, applications, and practical tips for success. Anesth Analg 2012;114(2):349–68.
6. Caplan RA, Benumof JL, Berry FA, et al. American Society of Anesthesiologists Task Force on Management of the Difficult Airway. Practice guidelines for management of the difficult airway. An updated report by the American Society of Anesthesiologists Task Force on Management of the Difficult Airway. Anesthesiology 2003; 98(5):1269–77.
7. Aziz MF, Healy D, Kheterpal S, et al. Routine clinical practice effectiveness of the Glidescope® in difficult airway management: an analysis of 2,004 Glidescope® intubations, complications, and failures from two institutions. Anesthesiology 2011;114(1):34–41.
8. Griesdale DE, Liu D, McKinney J, et al. Glidescope® video-laryngoscopy versus direct laryngoscopy for endotracheal intubation: a systematic review and meta-analysis. Can J Anaesth 2012;59(1):41–52.
9. Vincent RD Jr, Wimberly MP, Brockwell RC, et al. Soft palate perforation during orotracheal intubation facilitated by the GlideScope® videolaryngoscope. J Clin Anesth 2007;19(8):619–21.

10. Williams D, Ball DR. Palatal perforation associated with McGrath® videolaryngo-scope. Anaesthesia 2009;64(10):1144–5.
11. Walls RM. Essential techniques for using the GlideScope video laryngoscope. In: A clinician's guide to video laryngoscopy: tips and techniques. New York: McMahon Publishing and Verathon, Inc; 2009. p. 16–8. Available at: http://www.anesthesiologynews.com/download/PG093_finalwebWM.pdf. Accessed October 8, 2013.
12. Cormack RS, Lehane J. Difficult tracheal intubation in obstetrics. Anaesthesia 1984;39:1105–11.
13. el-Ganzouri AR, McCarthy RJ, Tuman KJ, et al. Preoperative airway assessment: predictive value of a multivariate risk index. Anesth Analg 1996;82:1197–204.
14. Oates JD, Macleod AD, Oates PD, et al. Comparison of two methods for predicting difficult intubation. Br J Anaesth 1991;66(3):305–9.
15. Yamamoto K, Tsubokawa T, Shibata K, et al. Predicting difficult intubation with indirect laryngoscopy. Anesthesiology 1997;86(2):316–21.
16. Savva D. Prediction of difficult tracheal intubation. Br J Anaesth 1994;73(2):149–53.
17. Karkouti K, Rose DK, Wigglesworth D, et al. Predicting difficult intubation: a multivariate analysis. Can J Anaesth 2000;47(8):730–9.
18. Naguib M, Malabarey T, AlSatli RA, et al. Predictive models for difficult laryngoscopy and intubation. A clinical, radiologic and three-dimensional computer imaging study. Can J Anaesth 1999;46(8):748–59.
19. Ovassapian A, Glassenberg R, Randel GI, et al. The unexpected difficult airway and lingual tonsil hyperplasia: a case series and a review of the literature. Anesthesiology 2002;97(1):124–32.
20. Brimacombe J, Keller C. The ProSeal™ laryngeal mask airway: a randomized, crossover study with the standard laryngeal mask airway in paralyzed, anesthetized patients. Anesthesiology 2000;93(1):104–9.
21. Brimacombe J, Keller C, Judd DV. Gum elastic bougie-guided insertion of the ProSeal™ laryngeal mask airway is superior to the digital and introducer tool techniques. Anesthesiology 2004;100(1):25–9.
22. Nagata T, Kishi Y, Tanigami H, et al. Oral gastric tube-guided insertion of the ProSeal™ laryngeal mask is an easy and noninvasive method for less experienced users. J Anesth 2012;26(4):531–5.
23. Mitchell V, Dravid R, Patel A, et al. Difficult Airway Society guidelines for the management of tracheal extubation. Anaesthesia 2012;67(3):318–40.
24. Greenland KB. Difficult airway management in an ambulatory surgical center? Curr Opin Anaesthesiol 2012;25(6):659–64.
25. Berkow LC, Greenberg RS, Kan KH, et al. Need for emergency surgical airway reduced by a comprehensive difficult airway program. Anesth Analg 2009;109(6):1860–9, 28.
26. Australian and New Zealand College of Anaesthetists (ANZCA) guidelines on equipment to manage a difficult airway during anaesthesia. Available at: http://www.anzca.edu.au/resources/professional-documents/documents/professional-standards/pdf-files/PS56-guidelines-on-equipment-to-manage-a-difficult-airway-during-anaesthesia.pdf. Accessed October 8, 2013.

New Medications and Techniques in Ambulatory Anesthesia

M. Stephen Melton, MD, Karen C. Nielsen, MD,
Marcy Tucker, MD, PhD, Stephen M. Klein, MD,
Tong J. Gan, MD, MHS, FRCA, MB, FFARCSI*

KEYWORDS

- Medications • Techniques • Ambulatory anesthesia • Analgesia

KEY POINTS

- There are several new anesthetic and analgesic medications, including novel sedative-hypnotics, neuromuscular blocking and reversal agents, and analgesics.
- Novel propofol formulations and etomidate derivatives show improved side effect profiles.
- Remimazolam is an ultra–short-acting benzodiazepine derivative showing more rapid recovery compared with midazolam.
- Suggamadex provides rapid reversal of profound steroid neuromuscular blockade.
- Peripherally selective kappa-opioid agonists improve visceral pain and reduce centrally mediated mu-opioid–related side effects.
- Liposomal bupivacaine provides an extended analgesia duration of 72 to 96 hours, with decreased opioid consumption and opioid-related side effects.
- Inhaled fentanyl has shown a similar pharmacokinetic profile to intravenous fentanyl.

INTRODUCTION

Advancing anesthetic care reflects the continued development of novel anesthetic drugs and drug delivery systems. This development has matched the need of a growing outpatient surgical population for efficient same-day surgery with minimal side effects and maximum pain control. From 1996 to 2006, the number of outpatient surgery visits in the United States increased from 20.8 million to 34.7 million, accounting for approximately half of all surgery visits in 1996 and two-thirds of all surgery visits in 2006.[1] Advancements in surgical technique and technology resulting in less invasive surgery, and advancements in anesthesia care and postoperative pain management, are allowing patients and surgeries once requiring inpatient care and resources to be scheduled in the outpatient setting. These advancements have resulted in reduced

Disclosures: T.J. Gan has received research grant support and honoraria from Acacia, Baxter, GSK, Helsinn and Merck.
Department of Anesthesiology, Duke University Medical Center, Box 3094, Durham, NC 27710, USA
* Corresponding author.
E-mail address: tjgan@duke.edu

Anesthesiology Clin 32 (2014) 463–485
http://dx.doi.org/10.1016/j.anclin.2014.02.003
1932-2275/14/$ – see front matter © 2014 Elsevier Inc. All rights reserved.

expenses in a competitive, cost-conscious health care environment with improved patient satisfaction.[2] In this article, novel sedative-hypnotic, analgesic, neuromuscular blocking, and reversal agents, as well as drug delivery systems currently under investigation, are reviewed, providing the anesthesia practitioner with insights into an encouraging area of activity.

NOVEL SEDATIVE-HYPNOTICS DRUGS AND DELIVERY SYSTEMS

Strategies used by the pharmaceutical industry to improve hypnotic/sedative drugs include (1) reformulations of existing drugs to improve the formulation vehicle, (2) development of prodrugs of existing agents to circumvent issues such as poor water solubility, and (3) synthesis of novel active compounds that are broken down rapidly in the body to inactive metabolites (so-called soft-drugs).[3]

Propofol Formulations

Propofol (2,6-diisopropylphenol) is a commonly used intravenous anesthetic and sedative. Propofol is the most commonly used induction agent in daily practice. In addition, propofol is used as a continuous infusion for anesthetic maintenance or sedation, including prolonged sedation in the intensive care unit (ICU). The ability to formulate propofol in a biocompatible vehicle having minimal side effects and an appropriate pharmacokinetic/pharmacodynamic profile is critical to the use of propofol as an intravenous agent.[4] Although a rapid onset of action and redistribution phase makes it an attractive sedative-hypnotic agent, it has limitations.

Propofol is a challenging compound to formulate in stable aqueous vehicles suitable for routine clinical use. Because propofol is water insoluble, current formulations of propofol use a soybean oil emulsion that is composed of long-chain triglycerides (LCTs). Approved propofol formulations in the United States include Diprivan Injectable Emulsion 1% (AstraZeneca Pharmaceuticals LP, Wilmington, DE) and Propofol Injectable Emulsion 1% (Baxter Healthcare Corporation, Deerfield, IL). Drawbacks associated with current formulations include emulsion instability,[5] bacterial growth and the addition of antimicrobial agents,[6–9] hyperlipidemia,[10,11] pain on injection,[12] and propofol infusion syndrome.[13] In addition, propofol has a long context-sensitive half-time.

Alternate Propofol Emulsion Formulations

Alternate propofol emulsion formulations are being investigated in an effort to overcome these limitations. Formulation modifications have included (1) increasing propofol concentrations in the emulsion, (2) creating emulsions containing less than 10% oil, (3) creating emulsions having oils with different fatty acid contents, and (4) modifying emulsion droplets with protein.[4] Formulations include Ampofol, Insoluble Delivery-MicroDroplet (IDD-D) Propofol 2%, AM149, Propofol-Lipuro 1% and 2%, and albumin-stabilized emulsions.

Ampofol

Ampofol (Amphastar Pharmaceuticals, Inc, Rancho Cucamonga, CA) 1% propofol emulsion containing 5% soybean oil has shown similar pharmacokinetics to Diprivan 1% propofol in a 10% soybean oil emulsion. Although benefits include a reduction in both triglyceride dose and possibly microbe growth, Ampofol was associated with more pain on injection.[14–16]

IDD-D Propofol 2%

IDD-D Propofol 2% (SkyePharma Inc, New York, NY) is an oil-in-water emulsion composed of medium-chain triglycerides (MCTs) and showing similar pharmacokinetics to the 1% propofol in 10% soybean oil emulsions composed of LCTs.[17,18] Using a reduced oil vehicle content (4% vs 10%) and a lipid emulsion consisting of MCT, IDD-D Propofol lessens the risk of hypertriglyceridemia during prolonged infusion. In addition, IDD-D Propofol has inherent antimicrobial properties and thus does not contain preservative additives (**Table 1**).[17] However, IDD-D Propofol showed increased pain on injection compared with a 1% propofol in 10% soybean oil emulsion.[17] Although the administration of MCTs at sufficient concentrations has resulted in the production of both ketone bodies and octanoate, an MCT metabolite associated with neurotoxic effects including somnolence and coma, neither has been shown in humans. Their safety requires further investigation in a larger population of patients and after prolonged periods of infusion.[17]

AM149

AM149, another medium-chain triglyceride formulation of 1% propofol (AM149; AMRAD Operations Pty Ltd, Richmond, Victoria, Australia) is under investigation.[19] The MCT formulation of 1% propofol was associated with a significantly higher incidence of pain on injection (80%) and thrombophlebitis (93.3%) compared with the standard formulation (20% and 6.6%, respectively).[4]

Propofol-Lipuro 1% and 2%

Propofol-Lipuro 1% and 2% (B. Braun, Melsungen, Germany), which are available outside the United States, are formulated in a 10% fat emulsion (Lipofundin@ MCT; B. Braun, Melsungen, Germany) composed of LCTs and MCTs. These formulations showed similar pharmacokinetics, less pain on injection, and more rapid triglyceride elimination compared with propofol 1% soybean emulsion.[20–22]

Table 1	
Patented propofol emulsion excipients	
Excipient	**Patent**
Disodium ethylenediaminetetraacetate	Jones CB, Platt JH. Propofol composition containing edetate. Zeneca Ltd. US patent 5,714,520. February 3, 1998
Sodium metabisulfite	Mirejovsky D, Tanudarma L, Ashtekar DR. Propofol composition containing sulfite. Gensia Sicor. US patent 6,147,122. November 14, 2000
Tromethamine	George MM, Yuen P-H, Joyce MA. Propofol formulation containing TRIS. American Home Products Corporation (Madison, NJ). US patent 6,177,477. January 23, 2001
Pentetate	George MM. Propofol composition comprising pentetate. American Home Products Corporation (Madison, NJ). US patent 6,028,108. February 22, 2000
Benzyl alcohol	Carpenter JR. Propofol-based anesthetic and method of making same. Phoenix Scientific (St Joseph, MO). US patent 6,534,547. March 18, 2003
Benzethonium chloride and sodium benzoate	May T, Hofstetter J, Olson KL, Menon SK, Mikrut BA, Ovenshire CS, Rhodes LJ, Speicher ER, Waterson JR. Propofol composition. Abbott Laboratories (Abbott Park, IL). US patent 6,140,374. October 31, 2000

From Baker MT, Naguib M. Propofol: the challenges of formulation. Anesthesiology 2005;103:867; with permission.

Albumin emulsions

Several formulations of propofol using a novel Protosphere technology are under investigation. This technology uses proteins such as human albumin to form nanoparticles of water-insoluble drugs such as propofol.[4] Protosphere formulations of propofol prepared in albumin and either 0% or 3% soybean oil showed similar anesthetic activity in preclinical trials to propofol in a 10% soybean oil emulsion (Diprivan),[4] eliminating the hyperlipidemia seen with current formulations.

Nonemulsion Formulations

Propofol cyclodextrin formulation

Cyclodextrins form inclusion complexes with lipophilic drugs, providing an attractive alternative to emulsion formulations (**Fig. 1**). These complexes can initiate different physical, chemical, and biological attributes from those of either the parent drug or cyclodextrin alone, such as increasing solubility and dissolution rate, decreasing volatility, altering release rates, modifying local irritation, and/or increasing the stability.[23] Structural features and a complex interplay of intermolecular forces confer aqueous solubility on the cyclodextrin molecule, but allow it to transport water-insoluble compounds such as propofol.[4]

Pharmacodynamic studies of propofol cyclodextrin formulations showed reduced induction times and longer duration of action in rats compared with propofol in emulsion.[24] A propofol sulfobutylether β-cyclodextrin formulation (Captisol; CyDex Inc,

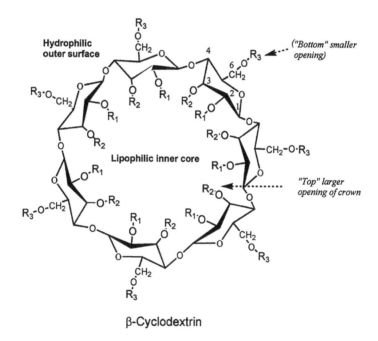

β-Cyclodextrin

Hydroxypropyl-β-cyclodextrin   Sulfobutylether-β-cyclodextrin
R_1, R_2, R_3 = $CH_2CHOHCH_3$ or H R_1, R_2, R_3 = $(CH_2)_4SO_3Na$ or H

Fig. 1. Basic structure of β-cyclodextrin and the hydroxyl-propyl and sulfobutylether forms used to form propofol inclusion complexes. (*From* Baker MT, Naguib M. Propofol: the challenges of formulation. Anesthesiology 2005;103:872; with permission.)

Lenexa, KS) showed similar pharmacodynamic and pharmacokinetic effects to Diprivan in a porcine model during a 3-hour infusion.[25] Concerns with the administration of propofol cyclodextrin formulations include potential renal toxicity,[26] hemolysis,[27] severe bradycardia and hypotension in association with injection,[28] and potential binding of coadministered lipophilic drugs such as rocuronium, substantially shortening its duration of action.[4,29]

Micelle formulations

Micelles made from poloxamers have been considered for formulating propofol.[4] Poloxamers consist of nonionic surfactants containing chains of polyethylene oxide (PEO), which form the outer shell of the micelle, and chains of polypropylethylene oxide (PPO), which form the inner hydrophobic core (**Fig. 2**). In vivo data from the administration of propofol in polymeric micelles has yet to be reported. Advantageous characteristics of polymeric micelles include inherent stability compared with emulsion formulations, spontaneous micelle formation, and sterilization by filtration.[4]

Propofol Prodrugs (Fospropofol, HX0969w)

The primary objective of synthesizing propofol prodrugs is to fulfill a need that exists for a water-soluble, stable, nontoxic pharmaceutical composition that is readily converted to propofol in vivo without the need for additives, solubilizers, or emulsifiers.

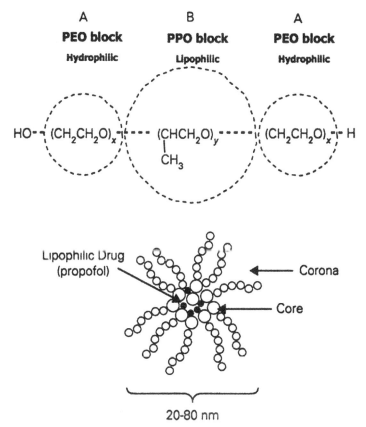

Fig. 2. Structural features of poloxamers for micelle formulation. (*From* Baker MT, Naguib M. Propofol: the challenges of formulation. Anesthesiology 2005;103:873; with permission.)

More specifically, they have the potential to circumvent the complications of emulsion instability, lipid infusion, and the need for antimicrobial additives in the formulation.[2]

Novel potential prodrugs include propofol esters such as propofol hemisuccinate, propofol hemiglutarate, propofol hemiadipate, monopropofol phosphate, and dipropofol phosphate.[4] In addition, several cyclic amino acid esters of propofol have been proposed.[30] Fospropofol disodium (Lusedra) is the only water-soluble propofol prodrug approved by the Food and Drug Administration (FDA) in the United States. Fospropofol seems to be a promising new agent, but further studies are necessary to better assess its pharmacokinetic and pharmacodynamic properties. Retraction of 6 such studies, because of possible errors in propofol assays, has disrupted the clinical characterization of fospropofol. New pharmacokinetic studies are awaited. Studies to date have shown safety and efficacy for monitored anesthesia care sedation in colonoscopies[31] and bronchoscopies,[32] short-term induction and maintenance of sedation in mechanically ventilated ICU patients using an infusion/bolus or infusion-only regimen,[33] and total intravenous anesthesia for coronary artery bypass surgery.[34] There are no published clinical trials investigating the use of fospropofol for ambulatory surgery. Although its metabolite, formaldehyde, is an endogenous compound, it has not shown accumulation in the body after administration (**Fig. 3**). Similar to fospropofol, HX0969w is an effective, water-soluble prodrug that is capable of inducing a sedative-hypnotic effect in animal models; however, it releases gamma-hydroxybutyrate instead of formaldehyde. Further studies regarding the efficacy and safety of HX0969w are necessary.[35]

SEDASYS System

Several propofol infusion platforms have been devised to address the inherent safety problems associated with propofol administration. Patient-controlled and target-controlled infusion systems have been described in the literature.[36] The SEDASYS System, approved by the FDA in May 2013, is a computer-assisted personalized sedation system integrating propofol delivery with patient monitoring to enable endoscopist/nurse teams to safely administer propofol.[37] In a nonblinded comparison with a standard benzodiazepine/opioid combination sedation protocol, the SEDASYS System showed significantly less oxygen desaturation, greater patient and clinician satisfaction, and faster recovery (**Fig. 4**).[37] However, the SEDASYS Computer-Assisted Personalized Sedation System is not intended for the sedation of high-risk patients.[38] No matter what the infusion platform, there are important safety concerns that should be addressed whenever propofol is administered by nonanesthesiologists.[36] These

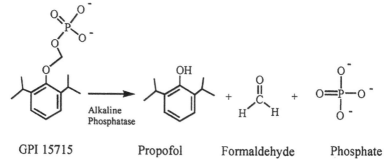

GPI 15715   Propofol   Formaldehyde   Phosphate

Fig. 3. Metabolism of fospropofol. (*From* Baker MT, Naguib M. Propofol: the challenges of formulation. Anesthesiology 2005;103:873; with permission.)

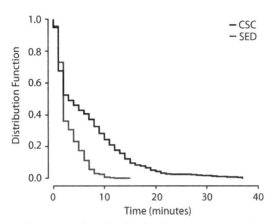

Fig. 4. Log-rank test of recovery time distribution between groups, showing statistical significance (P<.001). CSC, current standard of care (benzodiazepine/opioid combination); SED, SEDASYS System. (*From* Pambianco DJ, Vargo JJ, Pruitt RE, et al. Computer-assisted personalized sedation for upper endoscopy and colonoscopy: a comparative, multicenter randomized study. Gastrointest Endosc 2011;73:770; with permission.)

concerns are addressed in the American Society of Anesthesiologists' Practice Guidelines for Sedation and Analgesia by Non-Anesthesiologists.[39] Continued development of such systems may one day provide robotic anesthesia and teleanesthesia.[40]

Benzodiazepine Receptor Agonists

PF0713
PF0713 is a propofol analogue, gamma-aminobutyric acid A (GABA$_A$) agonist, developed to improve on propofol for intravenous induction and maintenance of general anesthesia and sedation.[41] A phase I clinical trial showed rapid induction of general anesthesia without injection pain, dose-related depth and duration of anesthetic effect, hemodynamic stability, and no serious adverse events.[42] Further data have not become available, and there are no additional registered clinical trials.

Remimazolam (CNS 7056)
Remimazolam, or CNS 7056, is a novel, ultra–short-acting benzodiazepine derivative that is highly selective for the GABA$_A$ receptor at the alpha-1–containing subtype, which is thought to mediate the sedative effects of benzodiazepines.[43] In phase I clinical trials,[44,45] remimazolam showed a rapid onset with dose-dependent sedation, and more rapid recovery compared with midazolam, with a 10-minute median time for return to fully alert, compared with 40 minutes for midazolam. The context-sensitive half-time of remimazolam seems to be insensitive to infusion duration, reaching its maximum of 7 to 8 minutes after a 2-hour infusion (**Fig. 5**). Remimazolam showed dose-dependent cardiorespiratory depression similar to propofol and midazolam.[44–46]

AZD 3043 (previously named TD-4756)
AZD3043, previously named TD-4756, is a novel sedative-hypnotic with rapid onset, showing direct GABA$_A$ receptor agonist activity in humans.[47,48] It is a close structural analogue of propanidid, a nonbarbiturate hypnotic; however, molecular modifications have increased its hydrophobicity and hypnotic potency.[49] As a result, it is formulated as an emulsion. Metabolism by ester hydrolysis to an inactive metabolite provides rapid emergence that is primarily unaffected by infusion duration, in contrast with

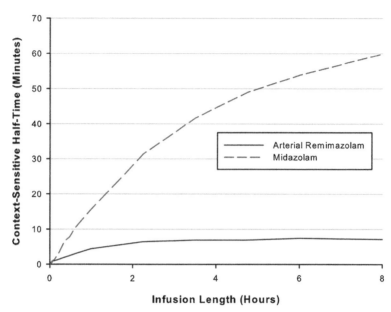

Fig. 5. Comparison of context-sensitive half-times for remimazolam and midazolam. Midazolam dosages, 0.075 mg/kg/h; remimazolam dosages, 50 mg/h. (*From* Wiltshire HR, Kilpatrick GJ, Tilbrook GS, et al. A placebo- and midazolam-controlled phase I single ascending-dose study evaluating the safety, pharmacokinetics, and pharmacodynamics of remimazolam (CNS 7056). Anesth Analg 2012;115:293; with permission.)

redistribution kinetics associated with propofol.[48] Three phase I clinical trials have been completed (a fourth was withdrawn), but data have not been published (Clinicaltrials.gov).

JM-1232 (-) (MR04A3)

JM-1232 (2) is a novel isoindoline-1-one derivative, benzodiazepine receptor agonist that is fully reversible by flumazenil.[50] JM-1232 (-) was synthesized in effort to develop an alternative to emulsion-based formulations of propofol. Kanamitsu and colleagues[50] and Maruishi Pharmaceutical Company sought to discover an easy-to-formulate water-soluble anesthetic and sedative drug with reduced respiratory depression. Using a nonbenzodiazepine, isoindolin-1-one skeleton compound with selective pharmacologic sedative and anxiolytic actions, approximately 170 compounds were synthesized and their hypnotic effects evaluated in mice after intravenous administration. JM-1232 (-) was selected for further investigation. In a phase I clinical trial, JM-1232 (-) produced dose-dependent sedation with rapid onset and resolution, and a satisfactory hemodynamic and safety profile.[51]

Etomidate Derivatives

Etomidate is a widely used, short-acting intravenous induction agent that provides rapid onset with minimal cardiovascular depression.[52] It is metabolized by ester hydrolysis. However, it is associated with postoperative nausea and vomiting, pain on injection, myoclonus, and adrenocortical suppression through 11β-hydroxylase inhibition.[52] Although the clinical impact of adrenocortical suppression after a single induction dose of etomidate in non–critically ill patients is uncertain, increased mortality related to its use in critically ill patients with sepsis[53,54] has decreased its use overall. These limitations have driven drug discovery toward etomidate analogues (**Fig. 6**).

Methoxycarbonyl etomidate

Methoxycarbonyl (MOC) etomidate is an ultra–rapid-acting etomidate analogue. Animal data show rapid recovery from both hypnosis and adrenal suppression after single induction doses and short-duration infusions.[55] However, hypnotic recovery depends heavily on infusion duration.[55] The ultrarapid metabolism and recovery of MOC-etomidate necessitates administration of large volumes of drug for prolonged infusions, resulting in the accumulation of its metabolite, MOC-etomidate carboxylic acid (MOC-ECA), which has 350-fold less hypnotic potency.[55] As a result of MOC-ECA accumulation, prolonged infusions ($\geq$30 minutes) are associated with delayed recovery time. Further study will define recovery profiles and the influence of metabolite production in humans. In an effort to reduce metabolite accumulation, etomidate analogue development was directed toward agents with higher potency and increased duration of action.[55] These analogues, termed spacer-linked etomidate esters, contain molecular modifications between the susceptible ester moiety and the etomidate backbone. These modifications sterically hinder ester hydrolysis, tailoring metabolic stability and pharmacokinetics.[56]

Cyclopropyl MOC etomidate

Cyclopropyl MOC etomidate (CPMM) shows the most promise of 13 new spacer-linked etomidate esters.[56] Developed in effort to reduce metabolite accumulation, compared with MOC-etomidate, CPMM showed a higher potency, and duration of action intermediate to those of MOC etomidate and etomidate. Its recovery time was independent of infusion duration, suggesting minimal metabolite accumulation.[57] Investigation in humans will define its clinical usefulness.

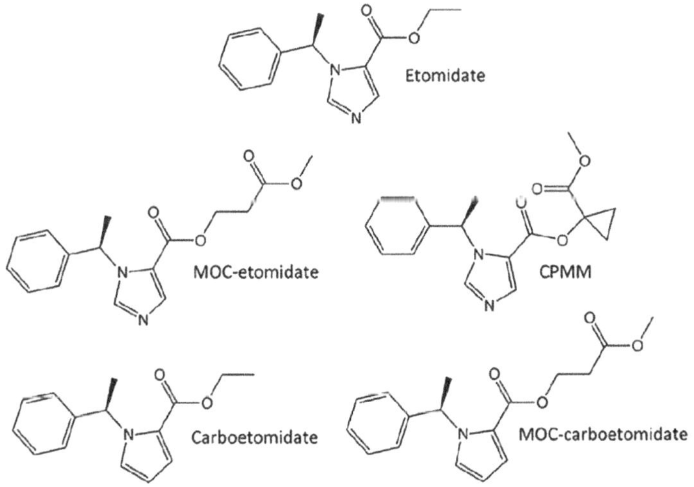

Fig. 6. Etomidate derivatives: methoxycarbonyl (MOC) etomidate, cyclopropyl MOC-etomidate (CPMM), carboetomidate, and MOC-carboetomidate. (*From* Chitilian H, Eckenhoff R, Raines D. Anesthetic drug development: novel drugs and new approaches. Surg Neurol Int 2013;4:2; with permission.)

MOC-carboetomidate

MOC-carboetomidate combined the unique structural features of MOC-etomidate and carboetomidate.[55,58,59] It showed potent hypnotic activity with intermediate metabolism and clearance, and maintained hemodynamic stability and adrenocortical function.[55] However, water insolubility limits onset time and ease of formulation.[55] Future development will be directed toward water-soluble MOC-carboetomidate analogues, providing faster onset times and non–emulsion-based formulations.[55]

Other Class

Melatonin

Melatonin (*N*-acetyl-5-methoxytryptamine) is a secretory product of the pineal gland. It possesses sedative, hypnotic, analgesic, antiinflammatory, antioxidative, and chronobiotic properties making it an attractive preoperative medication.[60–63] Although melatonin is not an FDA-approved medication, randomized clinical trials have shown no significant adverse events, showing fewer side effects than midazolam, including excessive sedation, disorientation, impaired psychomotor performance, and amnesia.[60,64] A systematic review of eligible clinical trials in the current literature suggests that melatonin possesses a significant anxiolytic effect and thus may be useful as an anxiolytic in patients undergoing surgery.[60] The mechanism by which melatonin exerts its hypnotic activity is still under investigation. It is proposed that endogenous melatonin participates in the regulation of the sleep-wake cycle, leading to a cascade of events that may activate somnogenic structures or that melatonin metabolites possess a hypnotic effect.[65] The effects of melatonin may be minimized with the application of the benzodiazepine antagonist, flumazenil.[63] The evidence regarding its potential analgesic effect in the perioperative setting is inconsistent and limited.[60] Additional clinical investigation will determine whether preoperative melatonin with its anxiolytic and possible analgesic effects may serve as the ideal alternative for premedication, potentially leading to better patient care and less opioid-related morbidity.[60]

NOVEL NEUROMUSCULAR BLOCKING/REVERSAL AGENTS

Development of a novel muscle relaxant with a rapid onset to facilitate tracheal intubation and an ultrashort duration to afford intraoperative variability is the current focus of drug discovery in this category. The ideal agent would posses a clinical profile similar to succinylcholine without the adverse effects of depolarization. At present, rocuronium, a nondepolarizing alternative to succinylcholine, shows rapid onset only at high doses. This rapid onset comes at the expense of increased duration of action, which may require reversal, increasing the risk for residual neuromuscular blockade. The lack of availability of a compound with these characteristics has led to the development of a new series of fumarate compounds, olefinic (double-bonded) isoquinolinium diesters, as neuromuscular blockers.[66] These include gantacurium (GW280430A) and CW 002.

The ability to safely and rapidly reverse varying levels of neuromuscular blockade, both weak and profound, has been the focus of investigation. A novel aspect of fumarate neuromuscular blocking agents is the rapid reversal by L-cysteine. Intravenous administration of L-cysteine antagonizes block from these drugs within 2 to 3 minutes (immediate chemical reversal) when given 1 minute after 4 to 5 times their effective dose to achieve a 95% neuromuscular blockade (ED95).[67]

Selective relaxant binding agents (SRBAs) are a class of drugs that selectively encapsulate and bind steroid neuromuscular blocking agents (NMBAs) via a chelating mechanism of action that effectively terminates the ability of an NMBA to bind to acetylcholine receptors at the neuromuscular junction.[68,69] Development of an SRBA using a cyclodextrin (discussed earlier) molecule has provided a novel neuromuscular blocking reversal agent.

Gantacurium (GW280430A)

Gantacurium, an asymmetric alpha-chlorofumarate, is under investigation as a promising nondepolarizing neuromuscular relaxant. Gantacurium administration at 2 to 3 times the ED95 dose showed an onset time of 60 to 90 seconds, 10-minute duration of action, and complete recovery (train of four (TOF) of 90% or greater) within 15 minutes, in the absence of side effects, making it an attractive alternative to succinylcholine (1 mg/kg).[70] Gantacurium is currently undergoing phase III clinical development.[71]

CW 002

CW 002 is a fumarate compound synthesized to undergo slower L-cysteine antagonism to yield an intermediate duration of action.[67] It is further characterized by a rapid onset of action and a higher potency compared with gantacurium.[67] Maximal block (100%) occurred 1 minute after administration of 3 times the ED95 dose in monkeys, with complete spontaneous recovery in 30 minutes.[67,72] A volunteer trial of the pharmacokinetics and pharmacodynamics of CW 002 has recently begun.[71]

Sugammadex

Sugammadex was the first modified cyclodextrin to be used as a therapeutic agent (**Fig. 7**). As such, suggamadex selectively inhibits steroidal NMBAs by encapsulating them and thereby rendering them inactive (**Fig. 8**).[69] A review by Akha and colleagues[69] details the pharmacology, clinical usefulness, and FDA concerns associated with this agent. In summary, clinical trials have effectively shown safe and rapid (0.9–4 minutes) dose-dependent (0.5–16 mg/kg) reversal of varying levels of neuromuscular blockade, including profound blockade (reversal administered 5 minutes after high-dose rocuronium 1.2 mg/kg for intubation), with the use of sugammadex in healthy volunteers and surgical subjects.[73–81] Recovery times were significantly shorter than the respective times to spontaneous recovery from succinylcholine-induced block (**Fig. 9**).[69,80] However, in 2008, an FDA nonapproval letter for the use of sugammadex in the United States cited concern about its potential effects on bone and tooth modeling, safety in pediatric and parturient populations, and the potential risk of hypersensitivity reactions and bleeding as reasons for its disapproval. It is hoped that expanded approval for its clinical use in Europe and ongoing US clinical investigation will provide data to meet FDA criteria for eventual approval in the United States (clinical trials.gov; sugammadex).

NOVEL ANALGESICS AND ANALGESIC DELIVERY SYSTEMS

Multimodal analgesia, or balanced analgesia, is the cornerstone of current analgesic practice. Compared with unimodal therapy, the concept of multimodal analgesia involves the use of different classes of analgesics and different sites of analgesic administration to provide optimal pain relief with reduced analgesic-related side effects.[82] Peripherally acting analgesics are a key aspect to this balanced analgesic approach.[83–85] Development of novel peripherally selective intravenous opioid agonist and peripherally administered local anesthetics, through wound infiltration or perineural administration with peripheral nerve blockade (PNB), are under investigation. In addition, the development of nonintravenous formulations of fentanyl may expand its use beyond the operating or recovery room.[86] Whether such reformulations could

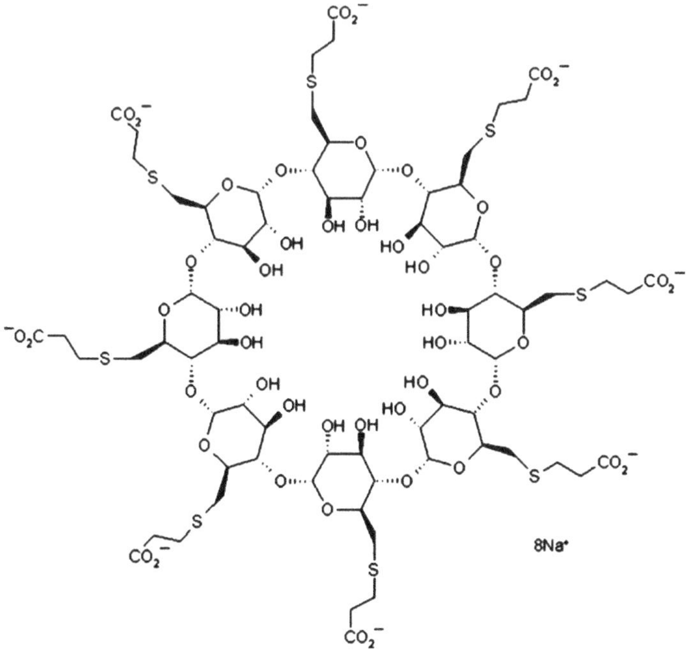

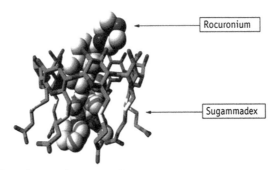

Fig. 7. Chemical structure of sugammadex, a modified cyclodextrin. (*From* Groudine SB, Soto R, Lien C, et al. A randomized, dose-finding, phase II study of the selective relaxant binding drug, sugammadex, capable of safely reversing profound rocuronium-induced neuromuscular block. Anesth Analg 2007;104:556; with permission.)

safely be applied to an outpatient population to improve postoperative pain control and reduce unanticipated admissions and readmissions secondary to pain has not been evaluated.

Kappa-Opioid Agonists

Centrally acting mu-opioid receptor agonists are a mainstay of traditional postoperative pain management. However, inadequate analgesia and/or excessive centrally

Fig. 8. Complex formulation of sugammadex and rocuronium. (*From* Sorgenfrei IF, Norrild K, Larsen PB, et al. Reversal of rocuronium-induced neuromuscular block by the selective relaxant binding agent sugammadex: a dose-finding and safety study. Anesthesiology 2006;104:668; with permission.)

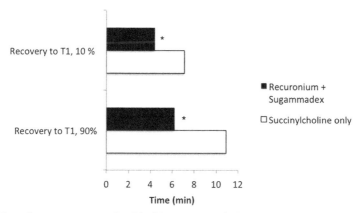

Fig. 9. Time from neuromuscular blocking agent administration to T_1 10% and 90%. * $P<.001$ between treatment groups. (*Data from* Lee C, Jahr JS, Candiotti KA, et al. Reversal of profound neuromuscular block by sugammadex administered three minutes after rocuronium. Anesthesiology 2009;110:1020–5.)

mediated adverse effects including euphoria, sedation, respiratory depression, and nausea limit their usage.[87] Drug development targeting peripherally selective kappa-opioid receptors was explored because of the proposed absence of centrally mediated affects. As such, peripherally selective kappa-opioid agonists were developed to provide a well-tolerated opioid addition and/or alternative to reduce classic mu-opioid agonist action. Kappa-opioid receptors are located both centrally and peripherally, and activation results in antinociception. Activation of supraspinal kappa-opioid receptors is associated with unwanted side effects. Novel kappa-agonists are under investigation to selectively target peripheral kappa-opioid receptors in an effort to improve visceral pain analgesia, which is often resistant to conventional mu-opioid receptor activation, and to limit centrally mediated adverse effects.[88–90]

CR665 (JNJ-38488502)
CR665 (JNJ-38488502) is a novel peripherally selective kappa-opioid receptor agonist that has shown efficacious visceral pain management.[90,91] FE200041 (an earlier analogue of CR665) and CR665 have been developed in an effort to reduce centrally mediated adverse effects.[90,92] Evaluation of CR665 showed peripheral kappa-opioid selectivity and antinociceptive activity in a wide range of preclinical visceral pain models.[90,92] However, central nervous system effect was shown in the form of paresthesias, which were reported as an adverse event in 61.1% of healthy volunteers receiving CR665. As such, it cannot be excluded that CR665 also exerted analgesic effects in the central nervous system.[93]

CR845
CR845 is an additional peripherally selective kappa-opioid receptor with potential analgesic and morphine-sparing effects. In a phase 2 clinical investigation, CR845 was safe, well tolerated, and showed robust analgesic activity for postoperative pain in female patients undergoing laparoscopy, with a significant reduction in postoperative morphine consumption and opioid-related side effects. In this study, CR845 administered both before and after surgery provided greater benefit compared with single-dose administration. These data establish the viability of developing CR845 as a novel analgesic for the treatment of acute pain.[94]

Local Anesthetics

Surgical site infiltration of local anesthetic is one aspect of multimodal postsurgical analgesia. However, postsurgical analgesia after local anesthetic infiltration with traditional long-acting local anesthetics such as bupivacaine is limited to local anesthetic duration of action, usually lasting 12 hours or less. Extending the analgesic duration of local wound infiltration with continuous catheter techniques produces complications.[95]

Perineural local anesthetic administration with PNB is another multimodal postoperative analgesic approach. The use of PNBs has shown improved postoperative analgesia, with significant reductions in opioid consumption and opioid-related side effects.[96,97] PNBs with long-acting local anesthetics provide site-specific surgical anesthesia and prolonged postoperative analgesia. Nevertheless, like surgical wound infiltration, PNBs are limited by local anesthetic duration of action. The duration of analgesia can be extended further with the placement of perineural catheters and subsequent continuous local anesthetic infusion in the hospital and/or at home (continuous PNBs [CPNBs]).[96] However, CPNBs transition from dense anesthetic blocks, achieved with an initial PNB bolus injection of high concentration (0.5%) local anesthetic, to analgesic blocks achieved with continuous infusion at a lower concentration (0.2%). This transition is associated with diminished sensory blockade leading to pain, frequently requiring opioids.

Development of longer-acting local anesthetics may prolong analgesia with surgical wound infiltration and initial PNB injection, eliminating the need for continuous infusions.

EXPAREL (bupivacaine liposome injectable suspension 1.3%)

In October 2011, the FDA-approved bupivacaine liposome injectable suspension 1.3% (EXPAREL, Pacira Pharmaceuticals Inc, San Diego, CA) for single-dose surgical site infiltration for postsurgical analgesia. Bupivacaine liposome injectable suspension is an innovative formulation that delivers bupivacaine HCl in a novel drug delivery system called DepoFoam. This system involves a preservative-free aqueous suspension of multivesicular liposomes containing a 1.33% bupivacaine concentration with 3% of this concentration existing in free nonencapsulated form. Although local anesthetic absorption is multifactorial,[98] liposomal bupivacaine offers time-to-onset characteristics similar to traditional bupivacaine HCl.[99] A review of pharmacokinetic parameters based on data compiled from 4 randomized, active-controlled and placebo-controlled trials in patients undergoing inguinal herniorrhaphy, total knee arthroplasty, hemorrhoidectomy, or bunionectomy was completed.[100] Patients in this review receiving liposomal bupivacaine surgical infiltration doses of 106, 266, 399, and 532 mg compared with bupivacaine HCl 100-mg or 150-mg doses, collectively showed concentration versus time profiles that were quantitatively similar across these 4 doses. The results showed an initial peak occurring within 1 hour after administration followed by a second peak about 12 to 36 hours later.[100] The initial peak reflects free, unencapsulated drug present in the aqueous phase, and the second reflects slow release from the DepoFoam delivery system (**Fig. 10**).

Lower peak plasma concentrations associated with EXPAREL pharmacokinetics, compared with the same dose of bupivacaine HCl, may confer potential safety advantages with liposomal formulation. The overall incidence of adverse events was lower in the group given liposome bupivacaine at less than 266 mg than in the groups given greater than 266 mg liposome bupivacaine and bupivacaine HCl.[100] The prescribing information (package insert) emphasizes that the maximum dose of EXPAREL is not to exceed 266 mg (chemically equivalent to 300 mg bupivacaine HCl), and, like all local

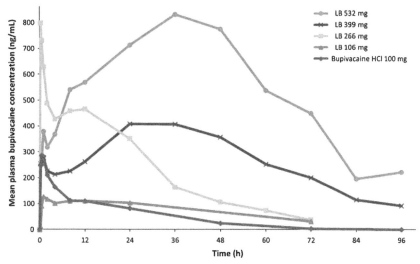

Fig. 10. Plasma bupivacaine concentration versus time for liposome bupivacaine 106, 266, 399, and 532 mg, and bupivacaine HCl 100 mg. LB, liposome bupivacaine. (*From* Hu D, Onel E, Singla N, et al. Pharmacokinetic profile of liposome bupivacaine injection following a single administration at the surgical site. Clin Drug Investig 2012;33:113; with permission.)

anesthetics undergoing metabolism by the liver, it should be used cautiously in patients with hepatic impairment. In addition, bupivacaine HCl, when injected immediately before EXPAREL, may affect the pharmacokinetic and/or physiochemical properties of each drug when the milligram dose of bupivacaine HCl solution exceeds 50% of the EXPAREL dose.

Liposomal bupivacaine was well tolerated across the 4 studies and varied surgical models, and showed bimodal kinetics with rapid uptake observed during the first few hours and prolonged release up to 96 hours after administration.[100] Compared with bupivacaine HCl with and without epinephrine, liposomal bupivacaine showed improved postsurgical pain from 72 to 96 hours, with reduced time to first opioid rescue, total opioid consumption, opioid-related side effects, and adverse events, including serious adverse events.[100] Electrocardiogram changes and cardiac adverse events were similar compared with bupivacaine HCl.[101] Three patients had excessive plasma concentrations, thought to be caused by unintentional intravascular injection of 150-mg doses of liposomal bupivacaine in 2 patients and a 450-mg dose in 1 patient, with resultant mean plasma concentrations of 255 and 520 ng/mL, respectively.[101] In these 3 patients, there were no clinically relevant changes from baseline to indicate cardiac repolarization abnormalities.[101]

In addition, in patients undergoing ileostomy reversal[102,103] and colectomy,[104] multimodal analgesia with liposomal bupivacaine infiltration showed reduced opioid consumption, postsurgical hospital stay, and associated hospitalization costs compared with standard opioid-based analgesia. However, alternative multimodal strategies including PNB with paravertebral blocks and traditional long-acting, nonliposomal local anesthetics may further reduce the use of hospital resources and economic costs without compromising patient care. A study by Kalady and colleagues[105] showed that select patients undergoing loop ileostomy closure using this multimodal approach showed safe discharge after overnight observation without increased complications or hospital readmissions.

Liposomal bupivacaine is currently under clinical investigation for perineural use with PNB. Single-dose toxicology studies (up to 30 mg/kg) investigating the use of EXPAREL for brachial plexus interscalene block in animal models did not show histologic evidence of increased bupivacaine toxicity. From a toxicology standpoint, slower uptake into the systemic circulation as a result of bimodal kinetics associated with EXPAREL may avoid high plasma concentrations. A small study investigating perineural administration of liposomal bupivacaine for femoral nerve blockade in healthy volunteers showed significant block magnitude variability, with an inverse relationship between dose and response magnitude and no relationship between dose and motor block duration.[106] As noted by the investigators, limitations of this study make interpretation and extrapolation of these results to clinical practice difficult. Further investigation will determine the safety and pharmacokinetic profile of perineural liposomal bupivacaine injection and the clinical usefulness of this route of administration compared with surgical infiltration.

SABER-Bupivacaine
SABER-Bupivacaine, an extended-release bupivacaine HCl formulation, is being developed by DURECT Corporation (Cupertino, CA). SABER-Bupivacaine is a semi-viscous solution of sucrose acetate isobutyrate (SAIB), a well-known food additive, containing the active ingredient bupivacaine 12%. The controlled-release delivery system is a matrix formulation containing SAIB and solvent. On administration, the solvent subsequently quickly diffuses away allowing the SAIB/bupivacaine mixture to form an in situ depot, providing drug delivery for 72 hours. Surgical infiltration of SABER-Bupivacaine showed safe and effective, prolonged postsurgical pain management in patients undergoing elective, open inguinal herniorrhaphy, with a reduction in opioid requirements and opioid-related side effects.[107]

Nonintravenous formulations of fentanyl
Nonintravenous fentanyl administration includes transmucosal, transdermal, and inhaled routes. Transmucosal routes provide fast delivery (time to reach maximum fentanyl plasma concentrations, 20 minutes [range, 20–180 minutes] and 12 minutes [range, 12–21 minutes], respectively) and are suitable for rapid onset of analgesia in acute pain conditions, with time to onset of analgesia of 5 or 2 minutes, respectively.[86] Passive transdermal patches and iontophoretic transdermal systems release fentanyl at a constant zero-order rate for 2 to 3 days, making them suitable for chronic pain management.[86]

Staccato Fentanyl for Inhalation (Alexza Pharmaceuticals Inc, Mountain View, CA) is a novel combination drug-device delivery system for rapid, systemic delivery of aerosolized fentanyl via the lung through a single metered inspiration (**Fig. 11**).[108] A study by Macleod and colleagues[108] showed that single-breath delivery of fentanyl using the Staccato system results in a pharmacokinetic profile identical to intravenous administration of a similar dose of fentanyl in terms of onset, extent, and reliability of absorption. Furthermore, the administration of repeated doses resulted in predictable, dose-dependent serum concentrations. The side effect profile of inhaled fentanyl is consistent with the known opioid side effects, namely nausea and vomiting. The most frequent side effect reported was nausea, seen at the higher dose ranges. Serial spirometry was unaltered, and none of the subjects reported any symptoms of bronchoconstriction, a known potential side effect resulting from direct airway irritation.[108] Future studies will determine whether

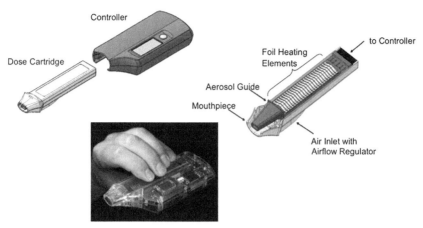

Fig. 11. Staccato fentanyl controller and dose cartridge. (*From* Macleod DB, Habib AS, Ikeda K, et al. Inhaled fentanyl aerosol in healthy volunteers: pharmacokinetics and pharmacodynamics. Anesth Analg 2012;115:1071–7; with permission.)

pharmacokinetic and safety profiles are suitable for trials in outpatient surgical populations.

SUMMARY

The drug development process explores novel drug formulations and delivery systems to improve anesthetic care and patient recovery. The pharmacokinetic and analgesic profiles of these agents meet growing health care expectations for provision of rapid and efficacious anesthesia and analgesia care to an expanding outpatient surgical population. This development has been pursued to address and overcome current pharmaceutical limitations. Although many of these agents are in early stages of development, preliminary evidence is encouraging.

REFERENCES

1. Cullen KA, Hall MJ, Golosinskiy A. Ambulatory surgery in the United States, 2006. Natl Health Stat Report 2009;11:1–25.
2. White PF. Ambulatory anesthesia advances into the new millennium. Anesth Analg 2000;90:1234–5.
3. Kilpatrick GJ, Tilbrook GS. Drug development in anaesthesia: industrial perspective. Curr Opin Anaesthesiol 2006;19:385–9.
4. Baker MT, Naguib M. Propofol: the challenges of formulation. Anesthesiology 2005;103:860–76.
5. Park JW, Park E-S, Chi S-C, et al. The effect of lidocaine on the globule size distribution of propofol emulsions. Anesth & Analg 2003;97:769–71.
6. Bennett SN, McNeil MM, Bland LA, et al. Postoperative infections traced to contamination of an intravenous anesthetic, propofol. N Engl J Med 1995;333:147–54.
7. Langevin PB, Gravenstein N, Doyle TJ, et al. Growth of Staphylococcus aureus in Diprivan and Intralipid: implications on the pathogenesis of infections. Anesthesiology 1999;91:1394–400.

8. Rieschke P, LaFleur BJ, Janicki PK. Effects of EDTA- and sulfite-containing formulations of propofol on respiratory system resistance after tracheal intubation in smokers. Anesthesiology 2003;98:323–8.

9. Barr J, Zaloga GP, Haupt MT, et al. Cation metabolism during propofol sedation with and without EDTA in patients with impaired renal function. Intensive Care Med 2000;26(Suppl 4):S433–42.

10. Wolf A, Weir P, Segar P, et al. Impaired fatty acid oxidation in propofol infusion syndrome. Lancet 2001;357:606–7.

11. McKeage K, Perry CM. Propofol: a review of its use in intensive care sedation of adults. CNS Drugs 2003;17:235–72.

12. Tan CH, Onsiong MK. Pain on injection of propofol. Anaesthesia 1998;53: 468–76.

13. Kam PCA, Cardone D. Propofol infusion syndrome. Anaesthesia 2007;62: 690–701.

14. Song D, Hamza M, White PF, et al. The pharmacodynamic effects of a lower-lipid emulsion of propofol: a comparison with the standard propofol emulsion. Anesth Analg 2004;98:687–91 [table of contents].

15. Song D, Hamza MA, White PF, et al. Comparison of a lower-lipid propofol emulsion with the standard emulsion for sedation during monitored anesthesia care. Anesthesiology 2004;100:1072–5.

16. Zhang Y, Lou Z, Ding J, et al. Comparison of Microbial Growth Retardation of Propofol Formulations: Ampofol™ vs Diprivan™ with and without EDTA Anesthesiology 2003;99:A57.

17. Ward SD, Norton JR, Guivarc'h PH, et al. Pharmacodynamics and pharmacokinetics of Propofole in a Medium-Chain Triglyceride Emulsion. Anesthesiology 2002;97:1401–8.

18. Cox EH, Knibbe CA, Koster VS, et al. Influence of different fat emulsion-based intravenous formulations on the pharmacokinetics and pharmacodynamics of propofol. Pharm Res 1998;15:442–8.

19. Paul M, Dueck M, Kampe S, et al. Pharmacological characteristics and side effects of a new galenic formulation of propofol without soyabean oil. Anaesthesia 2003;58:1056–62.

20. Doenicke AW, Roizen MF, Rau J, et al. Pharmacokinetics and pharmacodynamics of propofol in a new solvent. Anesth Analg 1997;85:1399–403.

21. Rau J, Roizen MF, Doenicke AW, et al. Propofol in an emulsion of long- and medium-chain triglycerides: the effect on pain. Anesth Analg 2001;93:382–4, 3rd contents page.

22. Theilen HJ, Adam S, Albrecht MD, et al. Propofol in a medium- and long-chain triglyceride emulsion: pharmacological characteristics and potential beneficial effects. Anesth Analg 2002;95:923–9 [table of contents].

23. Irie T, Uekama K. Pharmaceutical applications of cyclodextrins. III. Toxicological issues and safety evaluation. J Pharm Sci 1997;86:147–62.

24. Trapani G, Latrofa A, Franco M, et al. Inclusion complexation of propofol with 2-hydroxypropyl-beta-cyclodextrin. Physicochemical, nuclear magnetic resonance spectroscopic studies, and anesthetic properties in rat. J Pharm Sci 1998;87:514–8.

25. Egan TD, Kern SE, Johnson KB, et al. The pharmacokinetics and pharmacodynamics of propofol in a modified cyclodextrin formulation (Captisol) versus propofol in a lipid formulation (Diprivan): an electroencephalographic and hemodynamic study in a porcine model. Anesth Analg 2003;97:72–9 [table of contents].

26. Frank DW, Gray JE, Weaver RN. Cyclodextrin nephrosis in the rat. Am J Pathol 1976;83(2):367–82.

27. Bost M, Laine V, Pilard F, et al. The hemolytic properties of chemically modified cyclodextrins. J Inclus Phenom Mol 1997;29:57–63.

28. Bielen SJ, Lysko GS, Gough WB. The effect of a cyclodextrin vehicle on the cardiovascular profile of propofol in rats. Anesth Analg 1996;82:920–4.

29. Adam JM, Bennett DJ, Bom A, et al. Cyclodextrin-derived host molecules as reversal agents for the neuromuscular blocker rocuronium bromide: synthesis and structure-activity relationships. J Med Chem 2002;45:1806–16.

30. Altomare C, Trapani G, Latrofa A, et al. Highly water-soluble derivatives of the anesthetic agent propofol: in vitro and in vivo evaluation of cyclic amino acid esters. Eur J Pharm Sci 2003;20:17–26.

31. Bergese SD, Dalal P, Vandse R, et al. A double-blind, randomized, multicenter, dose-ranging study to evaluate the safety and efficacy of fospropofol disodium as an intravenous sedative for colonoscopy in high-risk populations. Am J Ther 2013;20:163–71.

32. Silvestri GA, Vincent BD, Wahidi MM. Fospropofol Disodium for Sedation in Elderly Patients Undergoing Flexible Bronchoscopy. J Bronchology Interv Pulmonol 2011;18:15–22.

33. Candiotti KA, Gan TJ, Young C, et al. A randomized, open-label study of the safety and tolerability of fospropofol for patients requiring intubation and mechanical ventilation in the intensive care unit. Anesth & Analg 2011;113:550–6.

34. Fechner J, Ihmsen H, Schüttler J, et al. A randomized open-label phase I pilot study of the safety and efficacy of total intravenous anesthesia with fospropofol for coronary artery bypass graft surgery. J Cardiothorac Vasc Anesth 2013;27: 908–15.

35. Zhou Y, Yang J, Liu J, et al. Efficacy comparison of the novel water-soluble propofol prodrug HX0969w and fospropofol in mice and rats. Br J Anaesth 2013; 111(5):825–32.

36. Maurer WG, Philip BK. Propofol infusion platforms: opportunities and challenges. Digestion 2010;82:127–9.

37. Pambianco DJ, Vargo JJ, Pruitt RE, et al. Computer-assisted personalized sedation for upper endoscopy and colonoscopy: a comparative, multicenter randomized study. Gastrointest Endosc 2011;73:765–72.

38. Martin JF, Bridenbaugh P, Gustafson M. The SEDASYS System is not intended for the sedation of high-risk patients. Gastrointest Endosc 2011;74:723.

39. American Society of Anesthesiologists Task Force on Sedation and Analgesia by Non-Anesthesiologists. Practice guidelines for sedation and analgesia by non-anesthesiologists. Anesthesiology 2002;96:1004–17.

40. Hemmerlingg TM, Terrasini N. Robotic anesthesia: not the realm of science fiction any more. Curr Opin Anaesthesiol 2012;25:736–42.

41. Siegel LC, JW. Initial studies of the mechanism of action of PF0713, an investigational anesthetic agent. asaabstractscom. 2008. Available at: http://www.asaabstracts.com/strands/asaabstracts/abstract.htm;jsessionid=07BA0389432C8F9E37BC34BC59D83D4B?year=2008&index=2&absnum=1019. Accessed October 16, 2008.

42. Siegel LC, Konstantatos A. PF0713 produced rapid induction of general anesthesia without injection pain in a phase 1 study. Anesthesiology 2009. Available at: http://www.asaabstracts.com/strands/asaabstracts/abstract.htm;jsessionid=CB6A81BF5CC6EB138F94DF701B4F93BD?year=2009&index=7&absnum=841. Accessed September 16, 2013.

43. Kilpatrick GJ, McIntyre MS, Cox RF, et al. CNS 7056: a novel ultra-short-acting benzodiazepine. Anesthesiology 2007;107:60–6.

44. Antonik LJ, Goldwater DR, Kilpatrick GJ, et al. A placebo- and midazolam-controlled phase I single ascending-dose study evaluating the safety, pharmacokinetics, and pharmacodynamics of remimazolam (CNS 7056): Part I. Safety, efficacy, and basic pharmacokinetics. Anesth Analg 2012;115:274–83.

45. Wiltshire HR, Kilpatrick GJ, Tilbrook GS, et al. A placebo- and midazolam-controlled phase I single ascending-dose study evaluating the safety, pharmacokinetics, and pharmacodynamics of remimazolam (CNS 7056): Part II. Population pharmacokinetic and pharmacodynamic modeling and simulation. Anesth Analg 2012;115:284–96.

46. Upton RN, Martinez AM, Grant C. Comparison of the sedative properties of CNS 7056, midazolam, and propofol in sheep. Br J Anaesth 2009;103:848–57.

47. Jonsson Fagerlund M, Sjödin J, Dabrowski MA, et al. Reduced efficacy of the intravenous anesthetic agent AZD3043 at GABA(A) receptors with β2 (N289M) and β3 (N290M) point-mutations. Eur J Pharmacol 2012;694:13–9.

48. Egan TD, Obara S, Jenkins TE, et al. AZD-3043: a novel, metabolically labile sedative-hypnotic agent with rapid and predictable emergence from hypnosis. Anesthesiology 2012;116:1267–77.

49. Chitilian H, Eckenhoff R, Raines D. Anesthetic drug development: novel drugs and new approaches. Surg Neurol Int 2013;4:2.

50. Kanamitsu N, Osaki T, Itsuji Y, et al. Novel water-soluble sedative-hypnotic agents: isoindolin-1-one derivatives. Chem Pharm Bull 2007;55:1682–8.

51. Sneyd JR, Rigby-Jones AE, Cross M, et al. First human administration of MR04A3: a novel water-soluble nonbenzodiazepine sedative. Anesthesiology 2012;116:385–95.

52. Forman SA. Clinical and molecular pharmacology of etomidate. Anesthesiology 2011;114:695–707.

53. Chan CM, Mitchell AL, Shorr AF. Etomidate is associated with mortality and adrenal insufficiency in sepsis. Crit Care Med 2012;40:2945–53.

54. Jabre P, Combes X, Lapostolle F, et al, KETASED Collaborative Study Group. Etomidate versus ketamine for rapid sequence intubation in acutely ill patients: a multicentre randomised controlled trial. Lancet 2009;374:293–300.

55. Pejo E, Ge R, Banacos N, et al. Electroencephalographic recovery, hypnotic emergence, and the effects of metabolite after continuous infusions of a rapidly metabolized etomidate analog in rats. Anesthesiology 2012;116:1057–65.

56. Husain SS, Pejo E, Ge R, et al. Modifying methoxycarbonyl etomidate inter-ester spacer optimizes in vitro metabolic stability and in vivo hypnotic potency and duration of action. Anesthesiology 2012;117:1027–36.

57. Ge R, Pejo E, Husain SS, et al. Electroencephalographic and hypnotic recoveries after brief and prolonged infusions of etomidate and optimized soft etomidate analogs. Anesthesiology 2012;117:1037–43.

58. Cotten JF, Forman SA, Laha JK, et al. Carboetomidate. Anesthesiology 2010;112:637–44.

59. Cotten JF, Le Ge R, Banacos N, et al. Closed-loop continuous infusions of etomidate and etomidate analogs in rats: a comparative study of dosing and the impact on adrenocortical function. Anesthesiology 2011;115:764–73.

60. Yousaf F, Seet E, Venkatraghavan L, et al. Efficacy and safety of melatonin as an anxiolytic and analgesic in the perioperative period. Anesthesiology 2010;113:968–76.

61. Ambriz-Tututi M, Rocha-González HI, Cruz SL, et al. Melatonin: a hormone that modulates pain. Life Sci 2009;84:489–98.
62. Ebadi M, Govitrapong P, Phansuwan-Pujito P, et al. Pineal opioid receptors and analgesic action of melatonin. J Pineal Res 1998;24:193–200.
63. Golombek DA, Martini M, Cardinali DP. Melatonin as an anxiolytic in rats: time dependence and interaction with the central GABAergic system. Eur J Pharmacol 1993;237:231–6.
64. Seabra ML, Bignotto M, Pinto LR, et al. Randomized, double-blind clinical trial, controlled with placebo, of the toxicology of chronic melatonin treatment. J Pineal Res 2000;29:193–200.
65. Tzischinsky O, Lavie P. Melatonin possesses time-dependent hypnotic effects. Sleep 1994;17:638–45.
66. Van Toi V, Toan NB, Khoa TQ, et al. 4th International Conference on Biomedical Engineering in Vietnam. Springer, January 10-12, 2012.
67. Savarese JJ, McGilvra JD, Sunaga H, et al. Rapid chemical antagonism of neuromuscular blockade by L-cysteine adduction to and inactivation of the olefinic (double-bonded) isoquinolinium diester compounds gantacurium (AV430A), CW 002, and CW 011. Anesthesiology 2010;113:58–73.
68. Ren WH, Jahr JS. Reversal of neuromuscular block with a selective relaxant-binding agent: sugammadex. Am J Ther 2009;16:295–9.
69. Akha AS, Rosa J, Jahr JS, et al. Sugammadex: cyclodextrins, development of selective binding agents, pharmacology, clinical development, and future directions. Anesthesiol Clin 2010;28:691–708.
70. Belmont MR, Lien CA, Tjan J, et al. Clinical pharmacology of GW280430A in humans. Anesthesiology 2004;100:768–73.
71. Lien CA. Development and potential clinical impairment of ultra-short-acting neuromuscular blocking agents. Br J Anaesth 2011;107(Suppl 1):i60–71.
72. Lien CA, Savard P, Belmont M, et al. Fumarates: unique nondepolarizing neuromuscular blocking agents that are antagonized by cysteine. J Crit Care 2009; 24:50–7.
73. Sorgenfrei IF, Norrild K, Larsen PB, et al. Reversal of rocuronium-induced neuromuscular block by the selective relaxant binding agent sugammadex: a dose-finding and safety study. Anesthesiology 2006;104:667.
74. Bom A, Bradley M, Cameron K, et al. A novel concept of reversing neuromuscular block: chemical encapsulation of rocuronium bromide by a cyclodextrin-based synthetic host. Angew Chem Int Ed Engl 2002;114:275–80.
75. Suy K, Morias K, Cammu G, et al. Effective reversal of moderate rocuronium- or vecuronium-induced neuromuscular block with sugammadex, a selective relaxant binding agent. Anesthesiology 2007;106:283–8.
76. Vanacker BF, Vermeyen KM, Struys MM, et al. Reversal of rocuronium-induced neuromuscular block with the novel drug sugammadex is equally effective under maintenance anesthesia with propofol or sevoflurane. Anesth Analg 2007; 104:563–8.
77. Groudine SB, Soto R, Lien C, et al. A randomized, dose-finding, phase II study of the selective relaxant binding drug, sugammadex, capable of safely reversing profound rocuronium-induced neuromuscular block. Anesth Analg 2007;104:555–62.
78. Duvaldestin P, Kuizenga K, Saldien V, et al. A randomized, dose-response study of sugammadex given for the reversal of deep rocuronium- or vecuronium-induced neuromuscular blockade under sevoflurane anesthesia. Anesth Analg 2010;110:74–82.

79. Pühringer FK, Rex C, Sielenkämper AW, et al. Reversal of profound, high-dose rocuronium-induced neuromuscular blockade by sugammadex at two different time points. Anesthesiology 2008;109:188–97.

80. Lee C, Jahr JS, Candiotti KA, et al. Reversal of profound neuromuscular block by sugammadex administered three minutes after rocuronium. Anesthesiology 2009;110:1020–5.

81. Rex C, Wagner S, Spies C, et al. Reversal of neuromuscular blockade by sugammadex after continuous infusion of rocuronium in patients randomized to sevoflurane or propofol maintenance anesthesia. Anesthesiology 2009;111:30–5.

82. Dalury DF, Lieberman JR, MacDonald SJ. Current and innovative pain management techniques in total knee arthroplasty. J Bone Joint Surg Am 2011;93:1938–43.

83. Kehlet H. Balanced analgesia: a prerequisite for optimal recovery. Br J Surg 1998;85:3–4.

84. Kehlet H, Werner M, Perkins F. Balanced analgesia: what is it and what are its advantages in postoperative pain? Drugs 1999;58:793–7.

85. Kehlet H, Dahl JB. The value of "multimodal" or "balanced analgesia" in postoperative pain treatment. Anesth Analg 1993;77:1048–56.

86. Lötsch J, Walter C, Parnham MJ, et al. pharmacokinetics of non-intravenous formulations of fentanyl. Clin Pharm 2012;52:23–36.

87. Oderda GM, Gan TJ, Johnson BH, et al. Effect of opioid-related adverse events on outcomes in selected surgical patients. J Pain Palliat Care Pharmacother 2013;27:62–70.

88. Rivière P. Peripheral kappa-opioid agonists for visceral pain. Br J Pharmacol 2004;141(8):1331–4. Rivière - 2009-British Journal of Pharmacology - Wiley Online Library.

89. Stein C, Schäfer M, Machelska H. Attacking pain at its source: new perspectives on opioids. Nat Med 2003;9:1003–8.

90. Vanderah TW, Largent-Milnes T, Lai J, et al. Novel D-amino acid tetrapeptides produce potent antinociception by selectively acting at peripheral kappa-opioid receptors. Eur J Pharmacol 2008;583:62–72.

91. Arendt-Nielsen L, Olesen AE, Staahl C, et al. Analgesic efficacy of peripheral kappa-opioid receptor agonist CR665 compared to oxycodone in a multimodal, multi-tissue experimental human pain model: selective effect on visceral pain. Anesthesiology 2009;111:616–24.

92. Binder W, Machelska H, Mousa S, et al. Analgesic and antiinflammatory effects of two novel kappa-opioid peptides. Anesthesiology 2001;94:1034–44.

93. Olesen AE, Kristensen K, Staahl C, et al. A population pharmacokinetic and pharmacodynamic study of a peripheral κ-opioid receptor agonist CR665 and oxycodone. Clin Pharm 2013;52:125–37.

94. Gan TJ, Jones JB, Schuller R, et al. Analgesic and morphine-sparing effects of the peripherally-restricted kappa opioid agonist CR845 after intravenous administration in women undergoing a laparoscopic hysterectomy. Anesth & Analg 2012;114.

95. Liu SS, Richman JM, Thirlby RC, et al. Efficacy of continuous wound catheters delivering local anesthetic for postoperative analgesia: a quantitative and qualitative systematic review of randomized controlled trials. J Am Coll Surg 2006;203:914–32.

96. Klein SM, Grant SA, Greengrass RA, et al. Interscalene brachial plexus block with a continuous catheter insertion system and a disposable infusion pump. Anesth Analg 2000;91:1473–8.

97. Macfarlane AJ, Prasad GA, Chan VW, et al. Does regional anaesthesia improve outcome after total hip arthroplasty? A systematic review. Br J Anaesth 2009; 103:335–45.

98. Rosenberg P, Veering B, Urmey W. Maximum recommended doses of local anesthetics: a multifactorial concept. Reg Anesth Pain Med 2004;29:564–75.

99. Apseloff G, Onel E, Patou G. Time to onset of analgesia following local infiltration of liposome bupivacaine in healthy volunteers: a randomized, single-blind, sequential cohort, crossover study. Int J Clin Pharmacol Ther 2013;51:367–73.

100. Hu D, Onel E, Singla N, et al. Pharmacokinetic profile of liposome bupivacaine injection following a single administration at the surgical site. Clin Drug Investig 2012;33:109–15.

101. Bergese SD, Onel E, Morren M, et al. Bupivacaine extended-release liposome injection exhibits a favorable cardiac safety profile. Reg Anesth Pain Med 2012;37:145–51.

102. Salerno S, Vogel J. Liposome bupivacaine (EXPAREL) for extended pain relief in patients undergoing ileostomy reversal at a single institution with a fast-track discharge protocol: an IMPROVE phase IV health economics trial. J Pain Res 2013;6:605–10.

103. Marcet J, Nfonsam L. An extended pain relief trial utilizing the infiltration of a long-acting Multivesicular liPosome foRmulation Of bupiVacaine, EXPAREL (IMPROVE): a phase IV health economic trial in adult patients undergoing ileostomy reversal. J Pain Res 2013;6:549–55.

104. Cohen S. Extended pain relief trial utilizing infiltration of Exparel, a long-acting multivesicular liposome formulation of bupivacaine: a phase IV health economic trial in adult patients undergoing open colectomy. J Pain Res 2012;5:567–72.

105. Kalady MF, Fields RC, Klein S, et al. Loop ileostomy closure at an ambulatory surgery facility: a safe and cost-effective alternative to routine hospitalization. Dis Colon Rectum 2003;46:486–90.

106. Ilfeld BM, Malhotra N, Furnish TJ, et al. Liposomal bupivacaine as a single-injection peripheral nerve block. Anesth Analg 2013;117:1248–56.

107. Hadj A, Hadj A, Hadj A, et al. Safety and efficacy of extended-release bupivacaine local anaesthetic in open hernia repair: a randomized controlled trial. ANZ J Surg 2012;82:251–7.

108. Macleod DB, Habib AS, Ikeda K, et al. Inhaled fentanyl aerosol in healthy volunteers: pharmacokinetics and pharmacodynamics. Anesth Analg 2012;115: 1071–7.

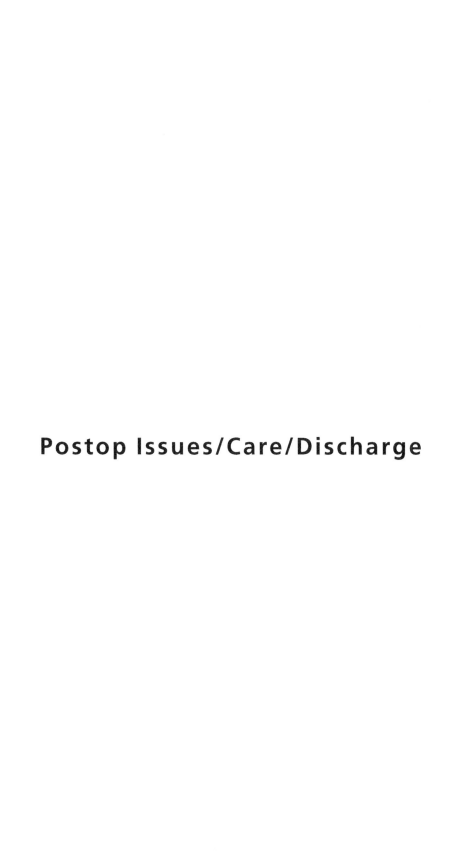

Postop Issues/Care/Discharge

Postoperative Issues
Discharge Criteria

Hairil Rizal Abdullah, MBBS, MMed[a], Frances Chung, MBBS, FRCPC[b],*

KEYWORDS

- Ambulatory surgery • Discharge criteria • Fast-track • Discharge scoring

KEY POINTS

- Use of discharge criteria provides a safe and reliable mechanism for postanesthetic recovery assessment in the ambulatory surgery setting.
- Fast-tracking (bypassing the postanesthesia care unit) is an acceptable and safe pathway, provided careful patient selection and assessment are performed.
- Having an adult escort to accompany the patient after discharge is a prerequisite.
- Recovery continues even after hospital discharge, with current evidence of cognitive impairment for up to 3 days after general anesthesia.

POSTANESTHETIC RECOVERY

With the continuous increase in the numbers and complexity of cases being done as ambulatory procedures, striking a balance between operational efficiency, patient safety, and patient satisfaction has become increasingly difficult. This article summarizes the latest evidence and consensus with regard to discharging an ambulatory patient home, the use of patient recovery scoring systems for protocol-based decision making, the concept of fast-track recovery, and requirements for patient escort.

Recovery has been defined as an ongoing process that begins from the end of intraoperative care until the patient returns to his or her preoperative state. It may be simplified into 3 phases: early recovery (Phase 1), which starts from the moment anesthetic agents are discontinued until the recovery of protective reflexes and motor function; intermediate recovery (Phase 2), when the patient has recovered enough to allow discharge to home; and late recovery (Phase 3), when the patient returns to his or her preoperative physiologic state.[1] Traditionally, Phase 1 occurs in the postanesthetic care unit (PACU) and Phase 2 in the ambulatory surgical unit (ASU) (or similar stepdown units). With modern drugs and anesthetic techniques, Phase 1 may be complete

[a] Department of Anesthesiology, Singapore General Hospital, Outram Road, 169608, Singapore;
[b] Department of Anesthesiology, Toronto Western Hospital, University Health Network, University of Toronto, Room 405, 2McL, 399 Bathurst Street, Toronto, Ontario M5T2S8, Canada
* Corresponding author.
E-mail address: Frances.chung@uhn.ca

Anesthesiology Clin 32 (2014) 487–493
http://dx.doi.org/10.1016/j.anclin.2014.02.013
1932-2275/14/$ – see front matter © 2014 Elsevier Inc. All rights reserved.

by the time the patient leaves the operating room, which allows for fast-tracking such patients directly to the ASU and bypassing the PACU (Phase 1) completely. This approach is increasingly being taken in many ambulatory surgical centers.[2]

DISCHARGE SCORING SYSTEM

Although the decision to discharge a patient is ultimately a physician's responsibility, it may be delegated to the nursing staff using standardized discharge criteria and procedures.[3] The use of discharge criteria is associated with reduced length of stay in the PACU in comparison with traditional time-based criteria.[4]

The modified Aldrete score has been used extensively as an objective assessment tool during Phase 1 recovery to guide discharge from the PACU to a ward (**Table 1**).[5,6] Though not originally designed for ambulatory patients, it has been applied in the ambulatory setting with success. The system assigns a score of 0, 1, or 2 for activity, respiration, circulation, consciousness, and oxygen saturation, giving a maximum score of 10. A score of 9 denotes a patient who is ready to be discharged to an ambulatory surgical ward.

Fast-Tracking

As stated earlier, fast-tracking in ambulatory anesthesia is the process of bypassing the PACU and directly transferring a patient from the operating room to the

Table 1 The modified Aldrete scoring system for determining when patients are ready for discharge from the postanesthesia care unit	
Discharge Criteria from Postanesthesia Care Unit	**Score**
Activity: able to move voluntarily or on command	
Four extremities	2
Two extremities	1
Zero extremities	0
Respiration	
Able to breathe deeply and cough freely	2
Dyspnea, shallow or limited breathing	1
Apneic	0
Circulation	
Blood pressure ±20 mm of preanesthesia level	2
Blood pressure ±20–50 mm preanesthesia level	1
Blood pressure ±50 mm of preanesthesia level	0
Consciousness	
Fully awake	2
Arousable on calling	1
Not responding	0
O_2 saturation	
Able to maintain O_2 saturation >92% on room air	2
Needs O_2 inhalation to maintain O_2 saturation >90%	1
O_2 saturation <90% even with O_2 supplementation	0

A score ≥9 was required for discharge.
From Aldrete JA. The post-anesthetic recovery score revisited. J Clin Anesth 1995;7:89–91; with permission.

step-down unit or ASU. It has become an acceptable postoperative pathway to improve efficiency without compromising safety and patient satisfaction.[7] Use of short-acting and ultrashort-acting anesthetic agents, nonsedating analgesics, and monitoring technologies such as bispectral index monitoring may facilitate the process. Fast-tracking has also been successful in the pediatric and geriatric age groups.[2,8–10]

The fast-track concept has been developed and driven by its perceived benefit of reducing nursing workload and hospital costs. Song and colleagues[11] found that reduction of nursing workload may not be straightforward, reporting that the total numbers of nursing interventions and nursing hours between fast-tracked patients and conventional PACU discharge were not significant. In turn, this did not result in cost savings as there was merely a shift in the workload from PACU to ASU. Moreover, subgroups of patients undergoing different types of surgeries required different patient-care hours, suggesting that rather than fast-tracking all patients, careful selection based on type of surgery may be more appropriate. This finding is supported by Williams and colleagues,[12] who showed 12% hospital cost reduction from PACU bypass in patients who underwent anterior cruciate ligament reconstruction with the routine use of peripheral nerve-block analgesia/anesthesia. Hadzic and colleagues[13] showed more successful PACU bypass in patients who underwent rotator cuff surgery under interscalene brachial plexus block. A study by Twersky and colleagues[7] preliminarily suggests factors that can be identified preoperatively to predict the success of fast-tracking. Patients younger than 60 years, of American Society of Anesthesiologists grade III, and undergoing general surgery rather than ophthalmology and orthopedics were more likely to be ineligible for fast-tracking. More studies on predictors of failure or success should undoubtedly be encouraged to optimize the flow of ASUs.

Serious complications in the immediate postoperative period are not increased by fast-tracking, most likely because well-defined criteria, adopted from the PACU discharge criteria, are used.[14] Whereas the Aldrete score only considers stable vital signs and alertness, the White criteria also include pain and nausea/vomiting, and have been adopted for fast-track pathways (**Table 2**).[15]

Discharge from Ambulatory Surgical Unit

Discharging the patient home from the ASU (Phase 2) requires guidelines based on validated criteria and should not be done in a hurried manner. The decision must also incorporate common sense, clinical judgment, and a shared responsibility between the health care staff and the patient. A recent review by Metzner and Kent[16] showed that adverse events occurring after discharge following ambulatory anesthesia are at increased risk for legal action. Several scoring systems have been developed,[17] one of the more widely used being the Postanesthesia Discharge Scoring System, introduced by Chung and colleagues in 1995 (**Table 3**).

Discharge After Regional Anesthesia

For patients recovering from a spinal anesthetic, certain conditions should be met before discharge, including return of sensation in S4-S5, plantar flexion at preoperative levels, proprioception of the big toe, and minimal sedation or hypovolemia.[1,17] Patients undergoing peripheral nerve block may be discharged home before full regression of motor and sensory block, but should be given verbal and written advice on how to take care of the insensate limb, including the use of crutches or walker, and the need to take analgesic medications early.[1,18] If possible, these instructions should be given in the presence of the person who will be escorting and caring for the patient postoperatively.[18]

Table 2
Scoring system to determine whether outpatients can be transferred directly from the operating room to the step-down (phase II) unit

Level of consciousness	
Awake and oriented	2
Arousable with minimal stimulation	1
Responsive only to tactile stimulation	0
Physical activity	
Able to move all extremities on command	2
Some weakness in movement of extremities	1
Unable to voluntarily move extremities	0
Hemodynamic stability	
Blood pressure <15% of baseline MAP value	2
Blood pressure 15%–30% of baseline MAP value	1
Blood pressure >30% below baseline MAP value	0
Respiratory stability	
Able to breathe deeply	2
Tachypnea with good cough	1
Dyspneic with weak cough	0
Oxygen saturation status	
Maintains value >90% on room air	2
Requires supplemental oxygen (nasal prongs)	1
Saturation <90% with supplemental oxygen	0
Postoperative pain assessment	
None, or mild discomfort	2
Moderate to severe pain controlled with intravenous analgesics	1
Persistent severe pain	0
Postoperative emetic symptoms	
None, or mild nausea with no active vomiting	2
Transient vomiting or retching	1
Persistent moderate to severe nausea and vomiting	0
Total possible score	14

A minimal score of 12 (with no score <1 in any individual category) would be required for a patient to be fast-tracked (ie, bypass the postanesthesia care unit) after general anesthesia.
Abbreviation: MAP, mean arterial pressure.
From White PF, Song D. New criteria for fast tracking after outpatient anesthesia: a comparison with the modified Aldrete's scoring system. Anesth Analg 1999;88:1069–72; with permission.

Requiring patients to void before discharge is not a standard of care, and this is reflected in practice guidelines.[18,19] It may be necessary to identify patients with a high risk of urinary retention, such as those undergoing anorectal surgeries and lower limb joint arthroplasty, those with benign prostatic hyperplasia, or those who have received neuraxial anesthesia with opioids and intraoperative fluids of more than 1000 mL with possible bladder distension. Ultrasonographic assessment of the bladder may help in the management of these patients.[20,21] Mandatory oral intake is also not necessary, and may provoke nausea and vomiting and delay discharge unnecessarily.[1,18,19]

Table 3	
Revised postanesthetic discharge scoring system (PADS)	
Vital signs	
Within 20% of preoperative baseline	2
20%–40% of preoperative baseline	1
40% of preoperative baseline	0
Activity level	
Steady gait, no dizziness, consistent with preoperative level	2
Requires assistance	1
Unable to ambulate/assess	0
Nausea and vomiting	
Minimal: mild, no treatment needed	2
Moderate: treatment effective	1
Severe: treatment not effective	0
Pain	
VAS = 0–3: the patient has minimal or no pain before discharge	2
VAS = 4–6: the patient has moderate pain	1
VAS = 7–10: the patient has severe pain	0
Surgical bleeding	
Minimal: does not require dressing change	2
Moderate: required up to 2 dressing changes with no further bleeding	1
Severe: required 3 or more dressing changes and continues to bleed	0

Maximum score = 10; patients scoring ≥9 are fit for discharge.
  Abbreviation: VAS, visual analog scale.
  From Chung F. Recovery pattern and home-readiness after ambulatory surgery. Anesth Analg 1995;80(5):896–902; with permission.

Postdischarge Instructions

Patients should be advised to not drink alcohol, operate machinery, or drive for 24 hours after a general anesthetic or sedation.[22] Those who have had regional anesthesia should also refrain from driving if they have an insensate limb. Patients should also be advised to not drive until the pain or immobility from their operation and anesthetic diminishes enough for them to control their car safely and perform an emergency stop.[18] In a 10-year review of litigations in ambulatory surgery in Canada by Chung and Assmann,[23] there were 3 malpractice cases of car accidents after ambulatory surgery in patients without an escort, which included a patient who was sedated with intravenous midazolam 2 mg, fentanyl 50 μg, and propofol 50 mg, and who appeared completely alert before discharge. The patient was subsequently involved in a single vehicle accident and became quadriplegic. Sedation with as little as 1 mg lorazepam as a premedication could result in a clinician being deemed negligent for allowing the patient to drive home.[24,25]

Patients should thus be aware of the importance of having a responsible adult escort them home and stay with them overnight. Ideally this conversation should take place at the time when the decision for surgery is made.[25] A responsible adult may be defined as a person who has the physical and mental ability to assist the patient, recognize when help is needed, and summon help should the patient be unable to do so. The minimum age of this individual ranges from 16 to 18 years.[25,26] For children, the Academy of Pediatrics/American Academy of Pediatric Dentistry guideline suggests that a child transported in a car safety seat should be accompanied by at least 2 adults on discharge, so that transportation to and from a treatment facility is provided by one of the adults while the other one takes care of the child.[27]

Major life and financial decisions should also be discouraged, as it has been shown that cognitive function may be impaired up to 3 days after general anesthesia.[24,28] Attempts to assess full functional recovery include the Postoperative Quality Recovery Scale, which tests across the 6 domains of physiologic, nociceptive, cognitive, emotive, overall patient perspective, and activities of daily living at various time points.[28] Wong and colleagues[29] have produced and validated a 14-item questionnaire grouped across 3 factors (pain and social activity, lower limb activity, general physical activity) called the Functional Recovery Index, which may be used for postdischarge assessment.

SUMMARY

The incorporation of formal discharge criteria to assess patients postoperatively after ambulatory surgery provides a safe and reliable mechanism that could help in improving efficiency, workflow processes, and costs of an ambulatory surgical center. These criteria should be backed up by sound clinical judgment and evidence-based decisions to ensure patient safety, especially in circumstances where an anesthesiologist's liability extends to the postdischarge period.

REFERENCES

1. Awad IT, Chung F. Factors affecting recovery and discharge following ambulatory surgery. Can J Anaesth 2006;53:858–72.
2. White PF, Kehlet H, Neal JM, et al. The role of the anesthesiologist in fast-track surgery: from multimodal analgesia to perioperative medical care. Anesth Analg 2007;104:1380–96.
3. Whitaker DK, Booth H, Clyburn P, et al. Guidelines: immediate post anaesthesia recovery 2013. Anaesthesia 2013;68:288–97.
4. Truong L, Moran JL, Blum P. Post anaesthesia care unit discharge: a clinical scoring system versus traditional time based criteria. Anaesth Intensive Care 2004;1:33–42.
5. Aldrete JA. The post-anesthetic recovery score revisited. J Clin Anesth 1995;7: 89–91.
6. Ead H. From Aldrete to PADSS: reviewing discharge criteria after ambulatory surgery. J Perianesth Nurs 2006;21:259–67.
7. Twersky RS, Sapozhnikova S, Toure B. Risk factors associated with Fast Track ineligibility after monitored anesthesia care in ambulatory surgery patients. Anesth Analg 2008;106:1421–6.
8. Ornek D, Metin S, Deren S, et al. The influence of various techniques on postoperative recovery and discharge criteria among geriatric patients. Clinics (Sao Paulo) 2010;65:941–6.
9. White PF, Tang J, Wender RH, et al. Desflurane versus sevoflurane for maintenance of outpatient anesthesia: the effect on early versus late recovery and perioperative coughing. Anesth Analg 2009;109:387–93.
10. White PF, Eng M. Fast-track anesthetic techniques for ambulatory surgery. Curr Opin Anaesthesiol 2007;20:545–57.
11. Song D, Chung F, Ronayne M, et al. Fast tracking (bypassing the PACU) does not reduce nursing workload after ambulatory surgery. Br J Anaesth 2004;93:768–74.

12. Williams BA, Kentor ML, Vogt MT, et al. The economics of nerve block pain management after anterior cruciate ligament reconstruction: significant hospital cost savings via associated PACU bypass and same day discharge. Anesthesiology 2004;100:697–706.
13. Hadzic A, Williams BA, Karaca PE, et al. For outpatient rotator cuff surgery, nerve block anesthesia provides superior same day recovery over general anesthesia. Anesthesiology 2005;102:1001–7.
14. Millar J. Fast tracking in day surgery. Is your journey to the recovery room really necessary? [editorial]. Br J Anaesth 2004;93:756–8.
15. White PF, Song D. New criteria for fast tracking after outpatient anesthesia: a comparison with the modified Aldrete's scoring system. Anesth Analg 1999;88: 1069–72.
16. Metzner J, Kent CD. Ambulatory surgery: is the liability risk lower? Curr Opin Anaesthesiol 2012;25:654–8.
17. Rastogi S, Vickers AP. Postoperative analgesia and discharge criteria for day surgery. Anaesth Intensive Care Med 2010;11:153–6.
18. Verma R, Alladi R, Jackson I, et al. Guidelines: day case and short stay surgery: 2. Association of Anaesthetists of Great Britain and Ireland, British Association of Day Surgery. Anaesthesia 2011;66:417–34.
19. Apfelbaum J, Silverstein J, Chung F, et al. Practice guidelines for postanesthetic care: an updated report by the American Society of Anesthesiologists task force on postanesthetic care. Anesthesiology 2013;118:291–307.
20. Choi S, Awad I. Maintaining micturition in the perioperative period: strategies to avoid urinary retention. Curr Opin Anaesthesiol 2013;26:361–7.
21. Baldini G, Bagry H, Aprikian A, et al. Postoperative urinary retention: anesthetic and perioperative considerations. Anesthesiology 2009;110:1139–57.
22. Chung F, Kayumov L, Sinclair DR, et al. What is the driving performance of ambulatory surgical patients after general anesthesia? Anesthesiology 2005;103: 951–6.
23. Chung F, Assmann N. Car accidents after ambulatory surgery in patients without an escort. Anesth Analg 2008;106:817–20.
24. Ward B, Imarengiaye C, Peirovy J, et al. Cognitive function is minimally impaired after ambulatory surgery. Can J Anaesth 2005;52:1017–21.
25. Ip HY, Chung F. Escort accompanying discharge after ambulatory surgery: a necessity or a luxury? Curr Opin Anaesthesiol 2009;22:748–54.
26. Springman SR, Hines R, editors. Ambulatory anesthesia: the requisites in anesthesiology. Philadelphia: Mosby Elsevier; 2006.
27. Cote CJ, Wilson S. Guidolincs for monitoring and management of pediatric patients during and after sedation for diagnostic and therapeutic procedures: an update. Pediatrics 2006;118:2587–602.
28. Royse CF, Newman S, Chung F, et al. Development and feasibility of a scale to assess postoperative recovery: the post-operative quality recovery scale. Anesthesiology 2010;113:892–905.
29. Wong J, Tong D, Silva Y, et al. Development of the functional recovery index for ambulatory surgery and anesthesia. Anesthesiology 2009;110:596–602.

Acute Pain Management

David M. Dickerson, MD

KEYWORDS

- Acute pain management • Multimodal analgesia • Multimodal pain management
- Ambulatory surgery • Outpatient surgery

KEY POINTS

- The cost to the patient and society of uncontrolled postoperative pain and chronic post-surgical pain requires a focus on prevention and effective multimodal intervention.
- The ambulatory anesthesiologist should be skilled at regional anesthesia and the application of continuous peripheral nerve catheters.
- The ambulatory surgical setting should make these techniques and their implementation possible.
- Effective communication in the perioperative period among the patient, nursing staff, and providers is necessary for rapid assessment and treatment of a patient's pain.
- The cost of maintaining a formulary with multiple analgesic drug classes and supplies and equipment for regional anesthesia may be offset by revenue in an outcomes-based reimbursement model.

INTRODUCTION

Acute postsurgical pain poses treatment challenges for the anesthesiologist, challenges augmented by the ambulatory surgical setting. The "fifth vital sign," pain, has become a focal point and continues to be a primary determinant of delayed discharge, unanticipated admission, and quality of recovery.[1–5] Although the prevalence of uncontrolled postoperative pain, frequently moderate to severe, has been characterized, the continued cost of uncontrolled pain has led to publication of practice guidelines for its control.[6] Most recently, the American Society of Anesthesiologists practice guidelines for acute pain management establish a paradigm for the more frequent and specific use of multimodal analgesia (MMA) (**Table 1**).[7]

This article updates acute pain management in ambulatory surgery and proposes a practical three-step approach, the "three I's" (**Box 1**), for reducing the impact and incidence of uncontrolled surgical pain. By identifying at-risk patients, implementing MMA, and intervening promptly with rescue therapies, the anesthesiologist may

Disclosure: No conflicts or relationships to disclose.
Department of Anesthesia and Critical Care, University of Chicago Medicine, 5841 South Maryland Avenue MC4028, Office O-416, Chicago, IL 60637, USA
E-mail address: ddickerson@dacc.uchicago.edu

Anesthesiology Clin 32 (2014) 495–504
http://dx.doi.org/10.1016/j.anclin.2014.02.010   anesthesiology.theclinics.com
1932-2275/14/$ – see front matter © 2014 Elsevier Inc. All rights reserved.

Table 1
American Society of Anesthesiologists practice guidelines for acute pain management in the perioperative setting

	Recommendations

Institutional policies	• Anesthesiologists should provide ongoing, up-to-date education and training on the safe and effective use of available treatment options within the institution. Including:
	  ○ Basic bedside pain assessment
	  ○ Nonpharmacologic techniques
	  ○ Sophisticated pain management techniques (eg, regional anesthesia)
	• Providers should use standardized, validated instruments for the regular evaluation and documentation of pain intensity, therapeutic response, and side effects.
	• Anesthesiologists responsible for perioperative analgesia should be available at all times to assist in the evaluation and treatment of perioperative pain.
	• Standardized, institutional policies and procedures should be developed and an integrated approach used for pain management by an anesthesiologist-led acute pain service.

Preoperative preparation of the patient	• A directed pain history, directed physical examination, and pain control plan should be included in the anesthetic preoperative evaluation.
Perioperative techniques	• Anesthesiologists who manage perioperative pain should use therapeutic options, such as central regional opioids, systemic opioid PCA, or peripheral regional techniques after an analysis of the risk/benefit ratio for the individual patient. • The therapy implemented should reflect the individual anesthesiologist's expertise and a respect for the capacity for safe application of the modality in the specific practice setting. This includes the ability to recognize and treat adverse effects from the therapy.
Multimodal techniques for pain management	• Whenever possible, anesthesiologists should use multimodal pain management therapy, regional block should be considered. • Unless contraindicated, patients should receive an around-the-clock regimen of COXIBs, NSAIDS, or acetaminophen. • Dosing regimens should optimize efficacy and minimize adverse events. • Specific medication, dose, route, and duration of therapy should be individualized.

Abbreviations: COXIB, cyclooxygenase-2 inhibitor; NSAID, nonsteroidal anti-inflammatory drugs; PCA, Patient-Controlled Analgesia.

Adapted from American Society of Anesthesiologists Task Force on Acute Pain Management. Practice guidelines for acute pain management in the perioperative setting. Anesthesiology 2012;116:255–6; with permission.

Box 1
Planning for pain: the three "I's"

Identify patients at risk for uncontrolled postoperative pain

Implement effective preventative multimodal analgesia

Intervene with rescue regional analgesia, additional opioids, or nonopioid agents improve outcomes, reduce cost, and optimize the patient's experience and quality of recovery.

IDENTIFY: RISK STRATIFICATION, PREPROCEDURAL PLANNING

The preanesthetic assessment identifies a history of uncontrolled postsurgical pain, intolerance or contraindications to analgesics, contraindications to regional anesthesia, and presence of preoperative pain or anxiety.[7] Several patient and surgical characteristics predispose to moderate or severe postoperative pain (**Box 2**).[8–12] Identifying a high-risk cohort preoperatively warrants prompt initiation of MMA. Comprehensive MMA may impact the patient's quality of recovery, prevent discharge delay or unanticipated admission, and reduce the risk of chronic postsurgical pain (**Box 3**).[13–22]

Katz[23] suggested controlling pain throughout all phases of the perioperative period and not just the period of surgical intervention.[24] Uncontrolled postdischarge pain can lead to unanticipated admission, defined as readmission within 24 hours of surgery, and greater risk for chronic postsurgical pain. For these reasons, the anesthesiologist should assist the surgical team in planning postdischarge multimodal analgesic regimens for the most immediate and intense period of surgical pain. Appreciation of the multitude of neural pathways involved in nociceptive afferent neurotransmission is the foundation for a targeted, comprehensive multimodal approach (**Table 2**). Preoperative blocking of the afferent injury barrage during and after surgery prevents the induction of central sensitization, lowering postoperative pain and analgesic requirements.

IMPLEMENT: MMA, REGIONAL ANESTHESIA

Multiple days of effective analgesia minimizing adverse effects can be accomplished with continuous peripheral neural blockade (cPNB). A single-shot PNB reduces opioid exposure, improves patient comfort and circulation to the anesthetized extremity, reduces time in recovery, increases patient satisfaction, and lowers rates of adverse events.[25] Catheter-based continuous techniques have similar benefit.[4,26] Compared with single-shot PNBs, cPNBs are associated with better pain control and the need for decreased opioid analgesics, resulting in less nausea. Chronic pain after surgery

---

Box 2
Preoperative predictors of moderate-to-severe postoperative pain

- Increased preoperative pain
- Increased preoperative anxiety
- Younger patients
- Female gender
- Surgery type
  - Appendectomy
  - Cholecystectomy
  - Hemorrhoidectomy
  - Tonsillectomy
- Duration of surgery

Box 3
Preoperative predictors of the development of chronic postsurgical pain

- Increased preoperative pain
- Increased preoperative anxiety
- Increased postoperative pain
- Female gender
- Surgical type

---

also is decreased and patient satisfaction is augmented.[27,28] cPNBs can be safely placed at multiple sites with proved analgesic efficacy for a multitude of ambulatory surgeries (**Table 3**).[29] The cost and risks of these techniques must be weighed in the context of the benefit to the patient during the first postoperative days. Some

Table 2
Pathway approach to multimodal analgesia

	Peripheral vs Central Nervous Site of Action	Analgesic Agent	Receptor Target
Peripheral afferent blockade, inhibition of central hyperexcitability	Peripheral +/− central	Local anesthetic (wound infiltration)	Sodium channel (free nerve endings of peripheral)
		Local anesthetic (peripheral nerve block)	Sodium channel (peripheral afferent neuron)
		Local anesthetic systemic infusion	Sodium channel (central and peripheral)
Inflammation reduction (reduction in proinflammatory mediators, decreased afferent neurotransmission)	Peripheral and central	Acetaminophen, paracetamol	Cox-II, cannabinoid
		NSAIDs	Cox-I, Cox-II
		Dexamethasone	Cox-II
Afferent slowing	Peripheral and central	Gabapentanoids (Lyrica, gabapentin)	Calcium-channel
Spinal and supraspinal modulation	Central	Opioids	Opioid receptors
Antinociceptive interneuron activation	Membrane stabilization	Benzodiazepines SNRI/TCA (chronic use)	GABAa Norepinephrine reuptake, serotonin reuptake
Pronociceptive interneuron blockade	Central (dorsal horn of spinal cord)	Ketamine, dextromethorphan, levorphanol, methadone	NMDA receptor
Descending inhibition	Central	Tizanidine, clonidine, dexmedetomidine	Alpha-2 in locus ceruleus

Abbreviations: Cox, cyclooxygenase; GABA, γ-aminobutyric acid; NMDA, N-methyl-D-aspartate; NSAID, nonsteroidal anti-inflammatory drugs; SNRI, selective norepinephrine reuptake inhibitor; TCA, tricyclic antidepressant.

Table 3
Indications for continuous nerve blocks in orthopedic procedures and trauma

Surgical Procedure or Site of Injury	Continuous Block	Doses for Initial Bolus Followed by Continuous Infusion
Total shoulder arthroplasty, shoulder hemiarthroplasty, rotator cuff repair, shoulder arthrodesis, "frozen" shoulder physical therapy, biceps surgery, proximal humerus fractures	Interscalene	20 mL ropivacaine 0.5% 5–10 mL·h^{-1} ropivacaine 0.2%
Distal humerus fractures, elbow arthroplasty, elbow arthrodesis, radius fractures and surgery, ulna fractures and surgery, wrist arthrodesis, reimplantation surgery	Supraclavicular, infraclavicular, axillary	20 mL ropivacaine 0.5% 5–10 mL·h^{-1} ropivacaine 0.2%
Breast surgery	Thoracic paravertebral (T4-5)	15 mL ropivacaine 0.5% via catheter 5–10 mL·h^{-1} ropivacaine 0.2% via catheter
Total knee arthroplasty, anterior cruciate ligament reconstruction, patella repair, knee active and passive physical therapy	Femoral nerve	20 mL ropivacaine 0.5% 5–10 mL·h^{-1} ropivacaine 0.2%
Total knee arthroplasty, posterior cruciate ligament reconstruction	Femoral + sciatic	6–12 mL ropivacaine 0.2%–0.5% 3–8 mL·h^{-1} ropivacaine 0.1%–0.2%
Tibia fracture and repair, fibular fracture and repair, ankle fusion, subtalar fusion, total knee arthroplasty, hallux valgus repair	Sciatic or popliteal	5–10 mL ropivacaine 0.2%–0.5% 3–8 mL·h^{-1} ropivacaine 0.1%–0.2%
Ankle fusion, total ankle arthroplasty	Femoral or saphenous + sciatic	20 mL ropivacaine 0.2% 5–10 mL·h^{-1} ropivacaine 0.1%

Adapted from Chelly JE, Ghisi D, Fanelli A. Continuous peripheral nerve blocks in acute pain management. Br J Anaesth 2010;105(Suppl 1):i88; with permission.

procedures and patients, however, are not suitable for regional anesthesia because of contraindication or surgical site. These patients should still receive local anesthetic infiltration at incision sites.

IMPLEMENT: MMA, PHARMACOTHERAPY

Much emphasis has been placed on MMA to improve the quality of recovery, decrease length of postanesthesia care unit stay, and potentially reduce the opioid requirement.[1–3,30–33] Opioid-sparing methods help to reduce delayed discharge, prevent unanticipated admission, and potentially alter the rates of cancer recurrence or metastasis.[34–36] The American Society of Anesthesiologists practice guidelines provide a framework for incorporating nonopioid medications perioperatively.[7] The selection of the type and number of specific nonopioid agents should be evidence-based and directed toward minimizing risk and maximizing benefit.

Several studies support preoperative initiation of nonsteroidal anti-inflammatory drugs (NSAIDs), yet the necessary dose, route, frequency, and duration are unclear. The potent inhibition of prostaglandin synthesis by NSAID therapy may have analgesic benefits that must be weighed against the potential renal, cardiovascular, gastrointestinal, and bleeding risks.[37–39] Whether or not NSAIDs impair bone healing is controversial.[40]

Among its potent antiemetic effects, dexamethasone also may contribute to postoperative pain relief and reduce opioid consumption.[41,42] α_2-Agonists, ketamine, β-blockers, local anesthetics, and acetaminophen can improve postoperative pain management (see **Table 1**).[43–50] When acetaminophen and an NSAID were combined, the benefit was synergistic. When not contraindicated, these agents should be administered concurrently for maximal benefit.[51]

The efficacy of preoperative gabapentinoids in reducing postoperative pain has been evaluated in randomized controlled trials and meta-analyses. Most studies demonstrated a reduction in postoperative pain scores, but there was discrepancy in the reduction of opioid consumption; postoperative nausea and vomiting; and other adverse effects, such as sedation, dizziness, or visual disturbances.[52–55]

Because preoperative anxiety correlates with severe postoperative pain, anxiolysis may be another target for intervention. A 1200-mg dose of gabapentin significantly reduced preoperative anxiety and pain catastrophization in highly anxious patients compared with placebo.[56] In a recent, randomized, double-blind study, preoperative coadministration of midazolam and diclofenac resulted in significant reduction of pain scores and postoperative nausea and vomiting compared with diclofenac alone for hernia repair surgery performed with general anesthesia.[57]

IMPLEMENT: NONPHARMACOLOGIC TECHNIQUES

Nonpharmacologic techniques may influence patient stress, anxiety, and pain. Intraoperative music has been shown to reduce opioid consumption and increase patient comfort after gynecologic surgery.[58] Transcutaneous electrical nerve stimulation and other complementary therapies offer additional patient comfort.[59]

INTERVENE: RECOVERY ROOM RESCUE

If preoperative and intraoperative interventions fail to produce patient comfort, the anesthesiologist must first rule out superimposed medical issues in a timely fashion (eg, anginal chest pain, pneumoperitoneum-related shoulder or abdominal pain). Assuming surgical pain, the anesthesiologist must implement a treatment algorithm to promptly intervene in hopes of improving the patient's comfort and preventing potential discharge delay or admission. Application of other classes or doses of nonopioid analgesics and additional opioids should be initiated while the possible need for a neuraxial block is evaluated.

SUMMARY

The cost to the patient and society of uncontrolled postoperative pain and chronic postsurgical pain requires a focus on prevention and effective intervention. The ambulatory anesthesiologist should be skilled at regional anesthesia and the application of continuous peripheral nerve catheters.

The ambulatory surgical setting should make these techniques and their implementation possible. For rapid assessment and treatment of a patient's pain, communication in the perioperative period among the patient, nursing staff, and providers is necessary. The cost of maintaining a formulary with multiple analgesic drug classes and supplies and equipment for regional anesthesia may be offset by revenue in an outcomes-based reimbursement model.

REFERENCES

1. Pavlin DJ. Pain as a factor complicating recovery and discharge after ambulatory surgery. Anesth Analg 2002;95:627–34.
2. Pavlin DJ. A survey of pain and other symptoms that affect recovery process after discharge from an ambulatory surgical unit. J Clin Anesth 2004;16:200–6.
3. Pavlin DJ. Factors affecting discharge time in adult outpatients. Anesth Analg 1998;89:1352–9.
4. Coley KC, Williams BA, DaPos SV, et al. Retrospective evaluation of unanticipated admissions and readmissions after same day surgery and associated costs. J Clin Anesth 2002;14(5):349–53.
5. Mezei G, Chung F. Return hospital visits and hospital readmissions after ambulatory surgery. Ann Surg 1999;230:721–7.
6. Apfelbaum JL, Chen C, Mehta SS, et al. Postoperative pain experience results: results from a national survey suggest postoperative pain continues to be undermanaged. Anesth Analg 2003;97:534–40.
7. American Society of Anesthesiologists Task Force on Acute Pain Management. Practice guidelines for acute pain management in the perioperative setting. Anesthesiology 2012;116:248–73.
8. Ip HY, Abrishami A, Peng PW, et al. Predictors of postoperative pain and analgesic consumption: a qualitative systematic review. Anesthesiology 2009;111: 657–77.
9. Herbershagen HJ, Aduckathil A, Van Wijck AJ, et al. Pain intensity on the first day after surgery. Anesthesiology 2013;118:934–44.
10. Kalkman CJ, Visser K, Moen J, et al. Preoperative prediction of severe postoperative pain. Pain 2004;105:415–23.
11. Caumo W, Schmidt AP, Schneider CN, et al. Preoperative predictors of moderate to intense acute postoperative pain in patients undergoing abdominal surgery. Acta Anaesthesiol Scand 2002;46:1265–71.
12. Singh JA, Gabriel S, Lewallen D. The impact of gender, age, and preoperative pain severity on pain after TKA. Clin Orthop Relat Res 2008;466(11):2717–23.
13. Kehlet H, Jensen TS, Woolf CJ. Persistent postsurgical pain risk factors and prevention. Lancet 2006;267(9522):1618–25.
14. Macrae WA, Davies HT. Chronic postsurgical pain. In: Crombie IK, editor. Epidemiology of pain. Seattle (WA): IASP Press; 1999. p. 125–42.
15. Macrae WA, Bruce J. Chronic pain after surgery. In: Wilson PR, Watson PJ, Haythornthwaite JA, et al, editors. Clinical pain management: chronic pain. London: Hodder Arnold; 2008. p. 405–14,
16. Singh JA, Lewallen D. Predictors of pain and use of pain medications following primary total hip arthroplasty (THA): 5,707 THAs at 2-years and 3,289 THAs at 5-years. BMC Muscloskelet Disord 2010;11:90.
17. Perkins FM, Kehlet H. Chronic pain as an outcome of surgery: a review of predictive factors. Anesthesiology 2000;93(4):1123–33.
18. Forsythe MD, Dunbar MJ, Hennigar AW, et al. Prospective relation between catastrophizing and residual pain following knee arthroplasty: two year follow-up. Pain Res Manag 2008;13:335–41.
19. Katz J, Seltzer Z. Transition from acute to chronic postsurgical pain: risk factors and protective factors. Expert Rev Neurother 2009;9(5):723–44.
20. Jung BF, Ahrendt GM, Oaklander AL, et al. Neuropathic pain following breast cancer surgery: proposed classification and research update. Pain 2003; 204(102):1–13.

21. Granot M, Ferber SG. The roles of catastrophising and anxiety in the prediction of postoperative pain intensity: a prospective study. Clin J Pain 2005;21: 429–45.
22. Katz J, Poleshuck EL, Andrus CH, et al. Risk factors for acute pain and its persistence following breast cancer surgery. Pain 2005;119(1–3):16–25.
23. Katz J, Clark H, Seltzer Z. Preventive analgesia: quo vadimus? Anesth Analg 2011;24:545–50.
24. Diatchenko L, Slade GD, Nackley AG, et al. Genetic basis for individual variations in pain perception and the development of a chronic pain condition. Hum Mol Genet 2005;14(1):135–43.
25. Carli F, Kehlet H, Baldini G, et al. Evidence basis for regional anesthesia in multidisciplinary fast-track surgical care pathways. Reg Anesth Pain Med 2011;36: 63–72.
26. Lenart MJ, Wong K, Gupta RK, et al. The impact of peripheral nerve techniques on hospital stay following major orthopedic surgery. Pain Med 2012;13(6): 828–34.
27. Borghi B, D'Addabbo M, White PF, et al. The use of prolonged peripheral neural blockade after lower extremity amputation: the effect on symptoms associated with phantom limb syndrome. Anesth Analg 2010;111:1308–15.
28. Ilfeld BM. Continuous peripheral nerve blocks: a review of the published evidence. Anesth Analg 2011;113(4):904–25.
29. Chelly JE, Ghisi D, Fanelli A. Continuous peripheral nerve blocks in acute pain management. Br J Anaesth 2010;105(Suppl 1):i86–96.
30. White PF, Kehlet H. Improving postoperative pain management: what are the unresolved issues? Anesthesiology 2010;112:220–5.
31. Elvir-Lazo O, White PF. The role of multimodal analgesia in pain management after ambulatory surgery. Curr Opin Anesthesiol 2010;23:697–703.
32. Joshi GP. Multimodal analgesia techniques for ambulatory surgery. Int Anesthsiol Clin 2005;43:197–204.
33. Bisgaard T. Analgesic treatment after laparoscopic cholecystectomy: a critical assessment of the evidence. Anesthesiology 2006;104:835–46.
34. Exadaktylos AK, Buggy DJ, Moriary DC, et al. Can anesthetic technique for primary breast cancer surgery affect recurrence or metastasis? Anesthesiology 2006;105(4):660–4.
35. Singleton PA, Moreno-Vinaco L, Sammani S, et al. Attenuation of vascular permeability by methylnaltrexone: role of mOP-R and S1P3 transactivation. Am J Respir Cell Mol Biol 2007;37(2):222–31.
36. De Oliveira GS, Ahmad S, Schink JC, et al. Intraoperative neuraxial anesthesia but not postoperative neuraxial analgesia is associated with increased relapse-free survival in ovarian cancer patients after primary cytoreductive surgery. Reg Anesth Pain Med 2011;36(3):271–7.
37. White PF, Sacan O, Tufanogullari B, et al. Effect of short-term postoperative celecoxib administration on patient outcome after outpatient laparoscopic surgery. Can J Anaesth 2007;54:342–8.
38. Gan TJ, Joshi GP, Viscusi E, et al. Preoperative parenteral paracoxib and follow-up oral valdecoxib reduce length of stay and improve quality of patient recovery after laparoscopic cholecystectomy surgery. Anesth Analg 2004;98: 1665–73.
39. De Oliviera GS, Agarwal D, Benzon HT. Perioperative single dose ketorolac to prevent postoperative pain: a meta-analysis of randomized trials. Anesth Analg 2012;114:424–33.

40. Pountos I, Georgouli T, Calori GM, et al. Do nonsteroidal anti-inflammatory drugs affect bone healing? A critical analysis. Scientific World Journal 2012;2012: 606404.
41. Mattila K, Kontinen VK, Kalso E, et al. Dexamethasone decreases oxycodone consumption following osteotomy of the first metatarsal bone: a randomized controlled trial in day surgery. Acta Anaesthesiol Scand 2010;54:268–76.
42. De Oliviera GS, Almeida MD, Benzon HT, et al. Perioperative single dose systemic dexamethasone for postoperative pain. Anesthesiology 2011;115: 575–88.
43. Salman N, Uzun S, Coskun F, et al. Dexmedetomidine as a substitute for remi-fentanil in ambulatory gynecologic laparoscopic surgery. Saudi Med J 2009; 102:117–22.
44. Viscomi CM, Friend A, Parker C, et al. Ketamine as an adjuvant in lidocaine intravenous regional anesthesia: a randomized, double-blind, systematic control trial. Reg Anesth Pain Med 2009;34:130–3.
45. Suzuki M. Role of *N*-methyl-D-aspartate receptor antagonists in postoperative pain management. Curr Opin Anesthesiol 2009;22:618–22.
46. Laskowski K, Stirling A, McKay WP, et al. A systematic review of intravenous ketamine for postoperative analgesia. Can J Anesth 2011;58:911–23.
47. Collard V, Mistraletti G, Taq A, et al. Intraoperative esmolol infusion in the absence of opioids spares postoperative fentanyl in patients undergoing ambulatory laparoscopic cholecystectomy. Anesth Analg 2007;105:1255–62.
48. McCarthy GC, Megalla SA, Habib AS. Impact of intravenous lidocaine infusion on postoperative analgesia and recovery from surgery: a systematic review of randomized controlled trials. Drugs 2010;70:1149–63.
49. Wininger SJ, Miller H, Minkowitz HS, et al. A randomized, double-blind, placebo-controlled, multicenter, repeat-dose study of two intravenous acetaminophen dosing regimens for the treatment of pain after abdominal laparoscopic surgery. Clin Ther 2010;32(14):2348–69.
50. Api O, Unal O, Ugurel V, et al. Analgesic efficacy of intravenous paracetamol for outpatient fractional curettage: a randomized controlled trial. Int J Clin Pract 2009;63(1):105–11.
51. Ong CK, Seymour RA, Lirk P, et al. Combining paracetamol (acetaminophen) with nonsteroidal anti-inflammatory drugs: a qualitative systematic review of analgesic efficacy for acute postoperative pan. Anesth Analg 2010;110:1170–9.
52. Moore A, Costello J, Wieczorek P, et al. Gabapentin improves postcesarean delivery pain management: a randomized, placebo-controlled trial. Anesth Analg 2011,112.167–73.
53. McQuay HJ, Poon KH, Derry S, et al. Acute pain: combination treatments and how we measure their efficacy. Br J Anaesth 2008;101:69–76.
54. Kim SY, Song JW, Park B, et al. Pregabalin reduces postoperative pain after mastectomy: a double blind, randomized, placebo-controlled study. Acta Anaesthesiol Scand 2011;55:290–6.
55. Engleman E, Cateloy F. Efficacy and safety of perioperative pregabalin for postoperative pain: a meta-analysis of randomized-controlled trials. Acta Anaesthesiol Scand 2011;55:290–6.
56. Clarke H, Kirkham KR, Orser BA, et al. Gabapentin reduces preoperative anxiety and pain catastrophizing in highly anxious patients prior to major surgery: a blinded randomized placebo-controlled trial. Can J Anesth 2013;60:432–43.
57. Hasani A, Maloku H, Sallahu F, et al. Preemptive analgesia with midazolam and diclofenac for hernia repair pain. Hernia 2011;15:267–72.

58. Angioli R, Cicco Nardone CD, Plotti F, et al. The use of music to reduce anxiety during office hysteroscopy: a prospective randomized trial. J Minim Invasiv Gynecol 2013. http://dx.doi.org/10.1016/j.jmig.2013.07.020.
59. Chen L, Tang J, White PF, et al. The effect of location of transcutaneous electrical nerve stimulation on postoperative opioid analgesic requirement: acupoint versus nonacupoint stimulation. Anesth Analg 1998;87:1129–34.

Long-Acting Serotonin Antagonist (Palonosetron) and the NK-1 Receptor Antagonists
Does Extended Duration of Action Improve Efficacy?

M. Stephen Melton, MD, Karen C. Nielsen, MD,
Marcy Tucker, MD, PhD, Stephen M. Klein, MD,
Tong J. Gan, MD, MHS, FRCA, MB, FFARCSI*

KEYWORDS

- Postoperative • Postdischarge • Nausea • Vomiting • Palonosetron • Aprepitant
- Casopitant • Rolapitant

KEY POINTS

- In a growing outpatient surgical population, postdischarge nausea and vomiting (PDNV) is unfortunately a common and costly anesthetic complication.
- Specific risk factors for PDNV through 7 days have been identified and validated.
- Palonosetron and aprepitant, with extended durations of action, are attractive pharmacologic interventions for PDNV.
- Although neurokinin-1 antagonists demonstrate improved antiemesis, nausea outcomes are comparable with more traditional and less-expensive options.
- Further investigation is necessary to strengthen current PONV and PDNV predictive models, and to determine the success of these models in directing prophylactic regimens before and after ambulatory patient discharge.

INTRODUCTION

Postoperative nausea and vomiting (PONV) is a common anesthetic complication that occurs in approximately 20% to 30% of the surgical population, and as many as 30% to 55% of patients discharged after same-day surgery (**Fig. 1**).[1–11] Approximately half of those affected by postdischarge nausea and vomiting (PDNV) will not have

Disclosures: Dr T.J. Gan has received research grant support and honoraria from Acacia, Baxter, GSK, Helsinn, and Merck.
Department of Anesthesiology, Duke University Medical Center, Durham, NC 27710, USA
* Corresponding author. Duke University Medical Center, Box 3094, Durham, NC 27710.
E-mail address: tjgan@duke.edu

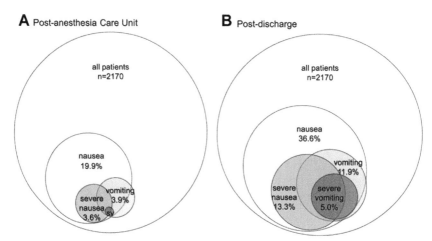

Fig. 1. Percentage of patients who experienced nausea and/or vomiting (*A*) in the PACU and (*B*) postdischarge. The incidence of severe vomiting (SV) in the postanesthesia care unit was 0.2%. (*From* Apfel CC, Philip BK, Cakmakkaya OS, et al. Who is at risk for postdischarge nausea and vomiting after ambulatory surgery? Anesthesiology 2012;117:479; with permission.)

experienced PONV before discharge.[3] Although intravenous pharmacologic treatments are easily administered within the health care facility, duration of action limits their effectiveness on PDNV.[4] This article discusses 2 of the latest pharmacologic interventions with extended durations of action providing efficacy for both PONV and PDNV prevention and management.

RISK FACTOR IDENTIFICATION

Risk factor identification is the hallmark of efficacious, evidence-based, cost-effective PONV and PDNV prevention and management. In patients undergoing general anesthesia, Apfel and colleagues[12] demonstrated a simple, validated predictive criteria score for early PONV. However, independent predictors for early PONV may not correlate to late PONV, or PDNV.[13] Recently, however, Apfel and colleagues[4] developed and validated a prediction model for PDNV up to 48 hours after ambulatory surgery (**Fig. 2, Table 1**). Additional risk factors after patient discharge may impact PDNV, such as postoperative pain and resultant opioid use, premature ambulation, drug interactions, and lack of patient education.[14] Odom-Forren and colleagues[2] subsequently demonstrated Apfel and colleagues[4] PDNV predictive criteria for PDNV up to 7 days, and verified which risk factors were applicable in the 3-day to 7-day period (**Fig. 3**, see **Table 1**).

PHARMACOLOGIC INTERVENTION

Pharmacologic intervention for PONV and PDNV should consist of combination therapy targeting different mechanisms of action,[5,13] including long-acting antiemetics and/or postdischarge oral regimens for prophylactic and therapeutic treatment at home in those patients at risk for PDNV. Specifically, this article discusses the 5-hydroxytryptamine3 (5-HT3) receptor antagonist palonosetron, and the neurokinin-1 (NK-1) receptor antagonists, aprepitant, casopitant, and rolapitant, all of which provide extended efficacy for PDNV, whether used alone or in combination with traditional PONV prophylactic regimens. The corticosteroid dexamethasone and anticholinergic transdermal scopolamine, which additionally provide extended efficacy for PDNV, are discussed

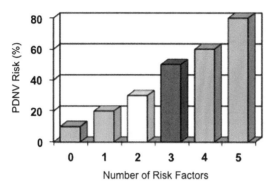

Risk Factors	Points
Female sex	1
History of PONV	1
Age <50 years	1
Use of opioids in the PACU	1
Nausea in the PACU	1
Sum	**0...5**

Fig. 2. Risk factors for PDNV and associated incidences. (*Adapted from* Odom-Forren J, Jalota L, Moser DK, et al. Incidence and predictors of postdischarge nausea and vomiting in a 7-day population. J Clin Anesth 2013;25(7):551–9, with permission; and Apfel CC, Philip BK, Cakmakkaya OS, et al. Who is at risk for postdischarge nausea and vomiting after ambulatory surgery? Anesthesiology 2012;117:484, with permission.)

only in context with a review of the literature when combined or compared to palonosetron or neurokinin-1 (NK-1) receptor antagonists. Postdischarge regimens with oral ondansetron disintegrating tablets and granisetron, or promethazine, which has also proven beneficial for PDNV, are not discussed.[15–18] Current literature specifically investigating palonosetron and the NK-1 receptor antagonists are reviewed. **Table 2** summarizes the pharmacology of the 2 antiemetics.

Table 1
PONV and PDNV risk factors

PONV Risk Factors	PDNV Risk Factors (48 h)	PDNV Risk Factors (Postoperative Day 3–7)
Female gender	Female gender	Operating room time
History of motion sickness or PONV	PONV history	PONV history
Nonsmoking status	Age <50 y	Use of ondansetron
Postoperative opioid status	Opioids administered in PACU Nausea in PACU	Pain during days 3–7
If 0, 1, 2, 3, or 4 of these risk factors were present, the incidence of PONV was 10%, 21%, 39%, 61%, and 79%, respectively	If 0, 1, 2, 3, 4, or 5 of these risk factors were present, the associated PDNV incidences were 40.0%, 19.4%, 39.7%, 65.0%, 88.4%, and 93.8%	

Abbreviations: PACU, postanesthesia care unit; PDNV, postdischarge nausea and vomiting; PONV, postoperative nausea and vomiting.

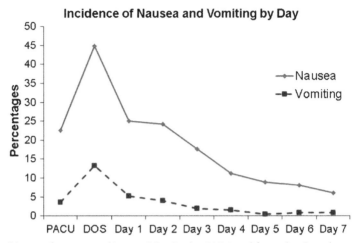

Fig. 3. Incidence of nausea and/or vomiting in the PACU and from the day of surgery (DOS) to postoperative day 7. Solid line = nausea; dotted line = vomiting. (*From* Odom-Forren J, Jalota L, Moser DK, et al. Incidence and predictors of postdischarge nausea and vomiting in a 7-day population. J Clin Anesth 2013;25(7):554; with permission.)

Palonesetron

Palonosetron is a 5-HT3 receptor antagonist (**Fig. 4**). Activation of the serotonin system through 5-HT3 receptors in the central chemoreceptor trigger zone or vagal gastrointestinal afferents plays a role in PONV pathogenesis.[19,20] Additionally, genetic variations in 5-HT3 genes may modulate susceptibility to nausea or vomiting.[21] Receptor binding is thought to be the most important factor influencing the duration of action of 5-HT3 antagonists.[22] Palonosetron, with a binding affinity 100 times that of ondansetron and a 40-hour half-life, makes it an attractive antiemetic for PDNV.[22] Palonosetron at a dose of 0.075 mg is approved for PONV prophylaxis by the Food and Drug Administration (FDA).[23,24]

Aprepritant, Casopitant, Rolapitant

Aprepritant, casopitant, and rolapitant are Substance P/NK-1 receptor antagonists. Neurokinin receptors are largely expressed in the nucleus of the solitary tract (NST), where they are involved in the central regulation of visceral function.[25] NK-1 receptor antagonists are believed to provide antiemetic activity by suppressing activity at the NST, where vagal afferents from the gastrointestinal tract converge with inputs from

Table 2
Pharmacology of palonosetron and aprepritant

Agent	Class	Dose (mg)	Route	$T_{1/2}$ (h)	Efficacy	Side Effects
Palonosetron	5-HT3 receptor antagonist	0.075	IV	40	Nausea and vomiting 0–72 h	Headache, constipation, QT prolongation
Aprepitant	Substance P/NK-1 receptor antagonist	40	PO	9–14	Vomiting and nausea 0–48 h	Pruritus, nausea, hypotension, constipation

Abbreviations: IV, intravenous; NK-1, neurokinin-1; PO, by mouth; 5-HT3, 5-hydroxytryptamine3.

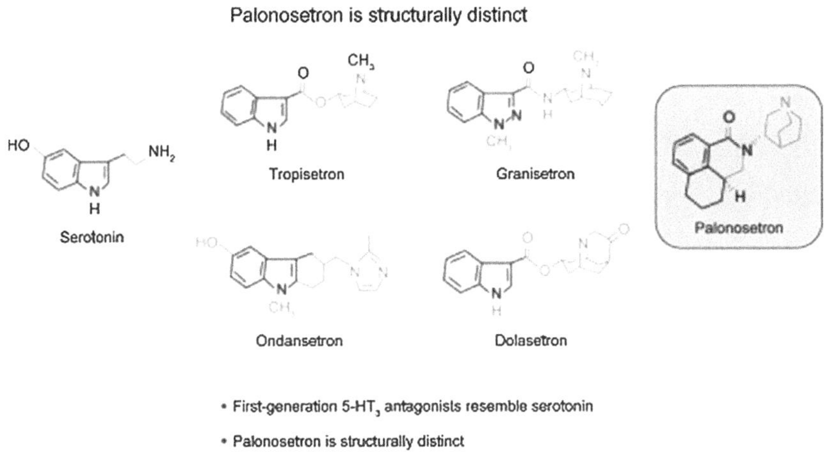

Palonosetron is structurally distinct

Serotonin

Tropisetron

Granisetron

Ondansetron

Dolasetron

Palonosetron

• First-generation 5-HT₃ antagonists resemble serotonin

• Palonosetron is structurally distinct

Fig. 4. Structures of palonosetron and other 5-HT3 antagonists. (*From* Rojas C, Grunberg S, Rosti G. Creating real benefit for patients at risk of nausea and vomiting: palonosetron— from bench to bedside. Clin Adv Hematol Oncol 2007;5(12 Suppl 19):14; with permission.)

the area postrema and other regions of the brain believed to be important in the control and initiation of emesis.[26] Aprepitant, a highly selective, brain-penetrating NK-1 antagonist with a long half-life (9–14 hours), is FDA approved for PONV management (**Fig. 5**).[27] Casopitant is another highly selective NK-1 antagonist with a long half-life that is under investigation (**Fig. 6**). The pharmacologic effects of casopitant again are related to brain penetration and subsequent receptor occupancy, important factors that influence its onset and duration.[26] Substantial brain concentrations of casopitant, in excess of their median inhibition concentration (concentration that reduces the effect by 50%) for protracted periods, may explain its prolonged duration of action.[26] Rolapitant is yet another NK-1 receptor antagonist that is characterized by rapid absorption after oral administration and a remarkably long half-life of 180 hours (**Fig. 7**).

CLINICAL EVIDENCE OF EFFICACIES
Palonosetron

Palonosetron has demonstrated inconsistent results when compared with other 5-HT3 receptor antagonists. Palonosetron 0.075 mg compared with ondansetron

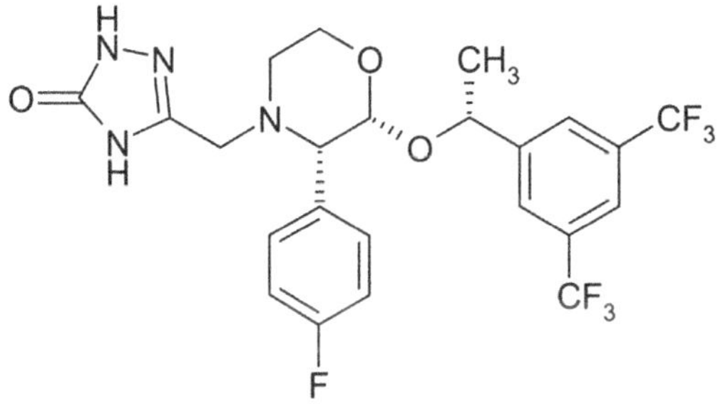

Fig. 5. Structure of aprepitant.

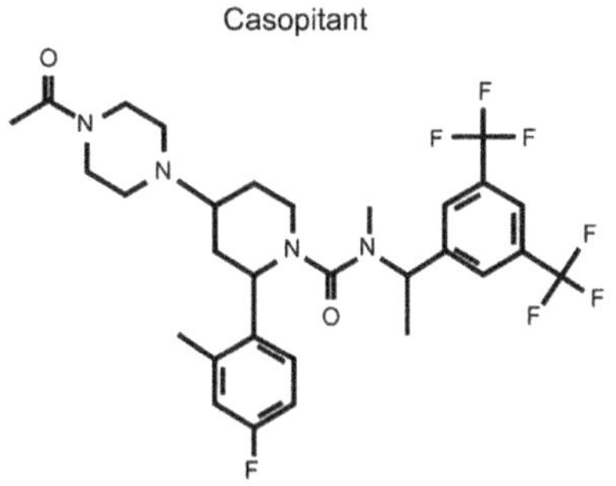

Fig. 6. Structure of casopitant.

4 mg demonstrated significantly reduced incidence of nausea and vomiting and the need for rescue antiemetic therapy at all time periods up to 48 hours in a high-risk patient population undergoing laparoscopic surgery.[28] In a lower-risk population undergoing laparoscopic surgery, palonosetron demonstrated similar efficacy to that of ondansetron 4 mg for up to 24 hours.[29] Studies comparing palonosetron 0.075 mg with ondansetron 8 mg demonstrated reduced PONV and rescue antiemetics at 2 to 24 hours in a high-risk group with postoperative opioid patient controlled analgesia (**Fig. 8**),[30] reduced overall PONV at 24 hours after surgery due to a reduction in nausea,[31] and reduced PONV up to 72 hours.[32] In the later study, the incidence of rescue antiemetic intervention and postoperative headache was significantly lower in the palonosetron group.[32] Although Kim and colleagues[28] demonstrated decreased vomiting at up to 72 hours, there was no difference in rescue antiemetics. Comparing palonosetron 0.075 mg with granisetron 2.5 mg, palonosetron demonstrated a significant reduction in the incidence of complete response, nausea, and vomiting for up to 48 hours.[33] Palonosetron 0.075 mg compared with ramosetron 0.3 mg, significantly reduced the incidence of nausea and vomiting and the need for rescue antiemetic therapy for up to 48 hours in high-risk patients undergoing laparoscopic surgery.[34] In a lower-risk population undergoing laparoscopic surgery, palonosetron was associated with significantly less vomiting for up to 48 hours.[35] Ironically, this reduction was due to early, not late, antiemetic efficacy.

Combination therapy of palonosetron 0.075 mg with dexamethasone 4 mg[36] or dexamethasone 8 mg[37] did not reduce the incidence of PONV or PDNV when compared with palonosetron alone over 24 hours and 72 hours, respectively. Both groups had a low incidence of vomiting in the postanesthesia care unit (PACU) at

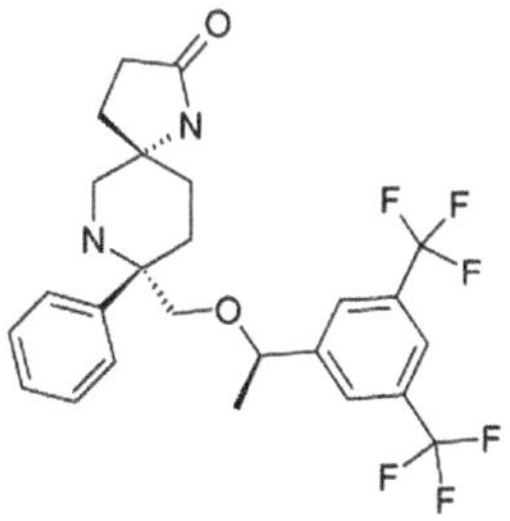

Fig. 7. Structure of rolapitant.

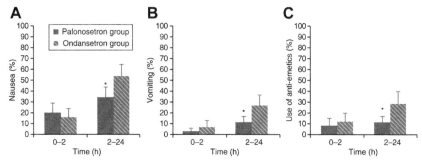

Fig. 8. Incidence of (*A*) nausea and (*B*) vomiting, and (*C*) the use of antiemetics in palonosetron and ondansetron groups during the 24-hour postoperative period. For each group, the error bar indicates the value of the upper limit of the 95% confidence interval for the percentage of patients achieving the end point. * *P* = .05 compared with the ondansetron group. (*From* Moon YE, Joo J, Kim JE, et al. Anti-emetic effect of ondansetron and palonosetron in thyroidectomy: a prospective, randomized, double-blind study. Br J Anaesth 2012;108:420; with permission.)

24 and 72 hours. There was no difference in complete response, defined as no vomiting and no rescue medication.

Neurokinin Receptor Antagonist

Preoperative oral aprepitant 40 mg compared with intravenous ondansetron 4 mg demonstrated significantly reduced vomiting up to 24,[38] 48,[27] and 72 hours,[39] with a delayed time to first vomiting. Aprepitant 40 mg in combination with ondansetron 4 mg reduced vomiting up to 48 hours[40] as compared with ondansetron alone (**Fig. 9**).[27,38,40] There were no differences in complete response and rescue treatments. Although aprepitant was not associated with a reduced incidence of

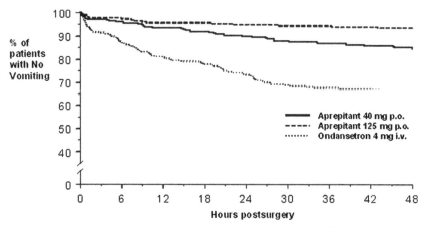

Fig. 9. Kaplan-Meier curves for the time to first vomiting during the 48 hours after surgery. The time to first vomiting was delayed by aprepitant; *P* = .001 based on the log-rank test. IV, intravenous; PO, by mouth. (*From* Gan TJ, Apfel CC, Kovac A, et al. A randomized, double-blind comparison of the NK1 antagonist, aprepitant, versus ondansetron for the prevention of postoperative nausea and vomiting. Anesth Analg 2007;104:1087; with permission.)

nausea, it reduced nausea severity (**Fig. 10**).[27,40] In a small study of patients undergoing total knee arthroplasty under spinal anesthesia with extended-release epidural morphine, aprepitant 40 mg demonstrated a significant reduction in PONV through 48 hours.[41]

The combination of aprepitant 40 mg and dexamethasone 10 mg was significantly more effective than ondansetron 4 mg in combination with dexamethasone 10 mg for prophylaxis against postoperative vomiting in adult patients undergoing craniotomy.[42] There was, however, no difference in the incidence or severity of nausea.[42] In patients undergoing gynecologic surgery, aprepitant plus ramosetron was more effective than ramosetron alone in decreasing PONV, use of rescue antiemetics, and nausea severity for up to 24 hours.[43] Last, there was no significant difference in clinical efficacy between aprepitant alone and aprepitant with scopolamine.[44,45]

Casopitant in combination with ondansetron 4 mg compared with ondansetron alone demonstrated a significantly higher complete response rate (no vomiting, retching, or the use of rescue) for up to 120 hours, but no difference in nausea. A subsequent trial comparing casopitant 50 mg in combination with ondansetron 4 mg with ondansetron alone demonstrated no significant difference in complete response and nausea severity during the first 24 hours after surgery.[46]

In a dose-ranging study[47] comparing rolapitant 5 mg, 20 mg, 70 mg, or 200 mg with placebo and ondansetron 4 mg control groups, rolapitant (70 and 200 mg) had a higher complete response (no emesis or rescue) rate at 72, 96, and 120 hours and rolapitant 200 mg alone at 48 hours after surgery in comparison with placebo only. Ondansetron showed no difference in comparison with placebo at these time points. The rolapitant 200-mg group showed a significantly higher incidence of no emetic episodes at 72 and 96 hours compared with ondansetron.[47] Ondansetron was administered before induction in this study, as recommended in the package insert, as opposed to a more clinically effective time of administration at the end of surgery, which may have diminished the effects of ondansetron.[48,49]

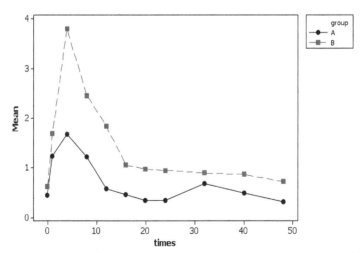

Fig. 10. Mean nausea verbal rating scale scores over time. Group A, aprepitant plus ondansetron; group B, ondansetron only. (*From* Vallejo MC, Phelps AL, Ibinson JW, et al. Aprepitant plus ondansetron compared with ondansetron alone in reducing postoperative nausea and vomiting in ambulatory patients undergoing plastic surgery. Plast Reconstr Surg 2012;129:524; with permission.)

SUMMARY

Palonosetron and the NK-1 receptor antagonists are attractive pharmacologic interventions for PDNV. Palonosetron demonstrates clinical efficacy equal to or greater than ondansetron. Although NK-1 antagonists have promising profiles and demonstrate improved antiemesis, nausea outcomes are comparable with more traditional and less-expensive options. Further studies are needed to better define the clinical utility of these drugs in ambulatory settings.

REFERENCES

1. Gupta A, Wu CL, Elkassabany N, et al. Does the routine prophylactic use of antiemetics affect the incidence of postdischarge nausea and vomiting following ambulatory surgery? A systematic review of randomized controlled trials. Anesthesiology 2003;99:488–95.
2. Odom-Forren J, Jalota L, Moser DK, et al. Incidence and predictors of postdischarge nausea and vomiting in a 7-day population. J Clin Anesth 2013;25(7): 551–9.
3. Carroll NV, Miederhoff P, Cox FM, et al. Postoperative nausea and vomiting after discharge from outpatient surgery centers. Anesth Analg 1995;80:903–9.
4. Apfel CC, Philip BK, Cakmakkaya OS, et al. Who is at risk for postdischarge nausea and vomiting after ambulatory surgery? Anesthesiology 2012;117: 475–86.
5. Apfel CC, Korttila K, Abdalla M, et al. A factorial trial of six interventions for the prevention of postoperative nausea and vomiting. N Engl J Med 2004;350: 2441–51.
6. Macario A, Weinger M, Truong P, et al. Which clinical anesthesia outcomes are both common and important to avoid? The perspective of a panel of expert anesthesiologists. Anesth Analg 1999;88:1085–91.
7. Cohen MM, Duncan PG, DeBoer DP, et al. The postoperative interview: assessing risk factors for nausea and vomiting. Anesth Analg 1994;78:7–16.
8. Palazzo MG, Strunin L. Anaesthesia and emesis. I: etiology. Can Anaesth Soc J 1984;31:178–87.
9. Kovac AL. Prevention and treatment of postoperative nausea and vomiting. Drugs 2000;59:213–43.
10. Hill RP, Lubarsky DA, Phillips-Bute B, et al. Cost-effectiveness of prophylactic antiemetic therapy with ondansetron, droperidol, or placebo. Anesthesiology 2000;92:958–67.
11. Watcha MF. The cost-effective management of postoperative nausea and vomiting. Anesthesiology 2000;92:931–3.
12. Apfel CC, Läärä E, Koivuranta M, et al. A simplified risk score for predicting postoperative nausea and vomiting: conclusions from cross-validations between two centers. Anesthesiology 1999;91:693–700.
13. White PF, Sacan O, Nuangchamnong N, et al. The relationship between patient risk factors and early versus late postoperative emetic symptoms. Anesth Analg 2008;107:459–63.
14. Chinnappa V, Chung F. Post-discharge nausea and vomiting: an overlooked aspect of ambulatory anesthesia? Can J Anaesth 2008;55:565–71.
15. White PF, Tang J, Hamza MA, et al. The use of oral granisetron versus intravenous ondansetron for antiemetic prophylaxis in patients undergoing laparoscopic surgery: the effect on emetic symptoms and quality of recovery. Anesth Analg 2006; 102:1387–93.

16. Gan TJ, Candiotti KA, Klein SM, et al. Double-blind comparison of granisetron, promethazine, or a combination of both for the prevention of postoperative nausea and vomiting in females undergoing outpatient laparoscopies. Can J Anaesth 2009;56:829–36.

17. Gan TJ, Franiak R, Reeves J. Ondansetron orally disintegrating tablet versus placebo for the prevention of postdischarge nausea and vomiting after ambulatory surgery. Anesth Analg 2002;94:1199–200.

18. Pan PH, Lee SC, Harris LC. Antiemetic prophylaxis for postdischarge nausea and vomiting and impact on functional quality of living during recovery in patients with high emetic risks: a prospective, randomized, double-blind comparison of two prophylactic antiemetic regimens. Anesth Analg 2008;107:429–38.

19. Andrews PL. Physiology of nausea and vomiting. Br J Anaesth 1992;69(7 Suppl 1): 2S–19S.

20. Miller AD, Leslie RA. The area postrema and vomiting. Front Neuroendocrinol 1994;15:301–20.

21. Rueffert H, Thieme V, Wallenborn J, et al. Do variations in the 5-HT3A and 5-HT3B serotonin receptor genes (HTR3A and HTR3B) influence the occurrence of postoperative vomiting? Anesth Analg 2009;109:1442–7.

22. Wong EH, Clark R, Leung E, et al. The interaction of RS 25259-197, a potent and selective antagonist, with 5-HT3 receptors, in vitro. Br J Pharmacol 1995;114: 851–9.

23. Kovac AL, Eberhart L, Kotarski J, et al, Palonosetron 04-07 Study Group. A randomized, double-blind study to evaluate the efficacy and safety of three different doses of palonosetron versus placebo in preventing postoperative nausea and vomiting over a 72-hour period. Anesth Analg 2008;107:439–44.

24. Candiotti KA, Kovac AL, Melson TI, et al, Palonosetron 04-06 Study Group. A randomized, double-blind study to evaluate the efficacy and safety of three different doses of palonosetron versus placebo for preventing postoperative nausea and vomiting. Anesth Analg 2008;107:445–51.

25. Colin I, Blondeau C, Baude A. Neurokinin release in the rat nucleus of the solitary tract via NMDA and AMPA receptors. Neuroscience 2002;115:1023–33.

26. Minthorn E, Mencken T, King AG, et al. Pharmacokinetics and brain penetration of casopitant, a potent and selective neurokinin-1 receptor antagonist, in the ferret. Drug Metab Dispos 2008;36:1846–52.

27. Diemunsch P, Gan TJ, Philip BK, et al. Single-dose aprepitant vs ondansetron for the prevention of postoperative nausea and vomiting: a randomized, double-blind Phase III trial in patients undergoing open abdominal surgery. Br J Anaesth 2007;99:202–11.

28. Kim YY, Moon SY, Song DU, et al. Comparison of palonosetron with ondansetron in prevention of postoperative nausea and vomiting in patients receiving intravenous patient-controlled analgesia after gynecological laparoscopic surgery. Korean J Anesthesiol 2013;64:122–6.

29. Laha B, Hazra A, Mallick S. Evaluation of antiemetic effect of intravenous palonosetron versus intravenous ondansetron in laparoscopic cholecystectomy: a randomized controlled trial. Indian J Pharmacol 2013;45:24–9.

30. Moon YE, Joo J, Kim JE, et al. Anti-emetic effect of ondansetron and palonosetron in thyroidectomy: a prospective, randomized, double-blind study. Br J Anaesth 2012;108:417–22.

31. Park SK, Cho EJ. A randomized, double-blind trial of palonosetron compared with ondansetron in preventing postoperative nausea and vomiting after gynaecological laparoscopic surgery. J Int Med Res 2011;39:399–407.

32. Bajwa SS, Bajwa SK, Kaur J, et al. Palonosetron: a novel approach to control postoperative nausea and vomiting in day care surgery. Saudi J Anaesth 2011; 5:19–24.

33. Bhattacharjee DP, Dawn S, Nayak S, et al. A comparative study between palonosetron and granisetron to prevent postoperative nausea and vomiting after laparoscopic cholecystectomy. J Anaesthesiol Clin Pharmacol 2010;26:480–3.

34. Kim SH, Hong JY, Kim WO, et al. Palonosetron has superior prophylactic antiemetic efficacy compared with ondansetron or ramosetron in high-risk patients undergoing laparoscopic surgery: a prospective, randomized, double-blinded study. Korean J Anesthesiol 2013;64:517–23.

35. Park SK, Cho EJ, Kang SH, et al. A randomized, double-blind study to evaluate the efficacy of ramosetron and palonosetron for prevention of postoperative nausea and vomiting after gynecological laparoscopic surgery. Korean J Anesthesiol 2013;64:133–7.

36. Park JW, Jun JW, Lim YH, et al. The comparative study to evaluate the effect of palonosetron monotherapy versus palonosetron with dexamethasone combination therapy for prevention of postoperative nausea and vomiting. Korean J Anesthesiol 2012;63:334–9.

37. Blitz JD, Haile M, Kline R, et al. A randomized double blind study to evaluate efficacy of palonosetron with dexamethasone versus palonosetron alone for prevention of postoperative and postdischarge nausea and vomiting in subjects undergoing laparoscopic surgeries with high emetogenic risk. Am J Ther 2012; 19:324–9.

38. Gan TJ, Apfel CC, Kovac A, et al. A randomized, double-blind comparison of the NK1 antagonist, aprepitant, versus ondansetron for the prevention of postoperative nausea and vomiting. Anesth Analg 2007;104:1082–9.

39. Sinha AC, Singh PM, Williams NW, et al. Aprepitant's prophylactic efficacy in decreasing postoperative nausea and vomiting in morbidly obese patients undergoing bariatric surgery. Obes Surg 2014;24(2):225–31.

40. Vallejo MC, Phelps AL, Ibinson JW, et al. Aprepitant plus ondansetron compared with ondansetron alone in reducing postoperative nausea and vomiting in ambulatory patients undergoing plastic surgery. Plast Reconstr Surg 2012;129:519–26.

41. Hartrick CT, Tang YS, Hunstad D, et al. Aprepitant vs. multimodal prophylaxis in the prevention of nausea and vomiting following extended-release epidural morphine. Pain Pract 2010;10:245–8.

42. Habib AS, Keifer JC, Borel CO, et al. A comparison of the combination of aprepitant and dexamethasone versus the combination of ondansetron and dexamethasone for the prevention of postoperative nausea and vomiting In patients undergoing craniotomy. Anesth Analg 2011;112:813–8.

43. Lee SJ, Lee SM, Kim SI, et al. The effect of aprepitant for the prevention of postoperative nausea and vomiting in patients undergoing gynecologic surgery with intravenous patient controlled analgesia using fentanyl: aprepitant plus ramosetron vs ramosetron alone. Korean J Anesthesiol 2012;63:221–6.

44. Green MS, Green P, Malayaman SN, et al. Randomized, double-blind comparison of oral aprepitant alone compared with aprepitant and transdermal scopolamine for prevention of postoperative nausea and vomiting. Br J Anaesth 2012;109: 716–22.

45. Singla NK, Singla SK, Chung F, et al. Phase II study to evaluate the safety and efficacy of the oral neurokinin-1 receptor antagonist casopitant (GW679769) administered with ondansetron for the prevention of postoperative and postdischarge nausea and vomiting in high-risk patients. Anesthesiology 2010;113:74–82.

46. Altorjay A, Melson T, Chinachoit T, et al. Casopitant and ondansetron for postoperative nausea and vomiting prevention in women at high risk for emesis: a phase 3 study. Arch Surg 2011;146:201–6.

47. Gan TJ, Gu J, Singla N, et al. Rolapitant for the prevention of postoperative nausea and vomiting: a prospective, double-blinded, placebo-controlled randomized trial. Anesth Analg 2011;112:804–12.

48. Tang J, Wang B, White PF, et al. The effect of timing of ondansetron administration on its efficacy, cost-effectiveness, and cost-benefit as a prophylactic antiemetic in the ambulatory setting. Anesth Analg 1998;86:274–82.

49. Habib AS, Gan TJ. Postoperative nausea and vomiting. Anesth Analg 2012;115: 493–5.

Administrative Issues

Scheduling of Procedures and Staff in an Ambulatory Surgery Center

Joel Pash, DO, BCom, FRCPC[a,b,*], Bassam Kadry, MD[a],
Suhabe Bugrara, BSc[c], Alex Macario, MD, MBA[a]

KEYWORDS

- Operating room utilization • Surgical procedure scheduling
- Operating room allocation • Ambulatory surgical center • ASC • ASC management

KEY POINTS

- For ambulatory surgical centers (ASC) to succeed financially, it is critical for ASC managers to schedule surgical procedures in a manner that optimizes operating room (OR) efficiency.
- OR efficiency is maximized by using historical data to accurately predict future OR workload, thereby enabling OR time to be properly allocated to surgeons.
- Strategies to maintain a well-functioning ASC include recruiting and retaining the right staff and ensuring that patients and surgeons are satisfied with their experience.
- Understanding OR management terminology is essential to effective ASC management.
- OR scheduling is done according to 3 different systems: Fixed Hours, Reasonable Time, and Any Workday.
- OR delays can be categorized in order to pinpoint the relative contribution of a particular delay to a room's finish time.

INTRODUCTION

This article provides practitioners and residents with the current best practices for scheduling procedures and staff in ambulatory surgery centers (ASCs). Many anesthesiologists have leadership roles in ASCs because their participation in all perioperative periods provides the opportunity to develop a strong understanding of operating room

Financial support: None.

Conflicts of interest: B. Kadry and S. Bugrara have equity interest in WiseOR, a for-profit privately owned company.

[a] Department of Anesthesiology, Perioperative and Pain Medicine, Stanford University School of Medicine, 300 Pasteur Drive H3580, Stanford, CA 94305-5640, USA; [b] Department of Anesthesia, University of Calgary, Calgary, AB T2N 1N4, Canada; [c] Computer Science Department, Stanford University, Stanford, CA, USA

* Corresponding author. Department of Anesthesiology, Perioperative and Pain Medicine, Stanford University School of Medicine, 300 Pasteur Drive H3580, Stanford, CA 94305-5640.

E-mail address: joel.pash@gmail.com

http://dx.doi.org/10.1016/j.anclin.2014.02.020
1932-2275/14/$ – see front matter © 2014 Elsevier Inc. All rights reserved.
anesthesiology.theclinics.com

(OR) workflow. In addition, anesthesiologists are well placed to build relationships with nursing and other staff at all points of care. Furthermore, there are clinical, operational, and economic alignments between ASC management and anesthesiologists and anesthesiologists eventually work with all of an ASC's surgeons.

If veteran ASC medical directors were asked to give advice to a newly appointed ASC manager, several main points might be emphasized (**Box 1**) and objective criteria for measuring success may be suggested (**Box 2**). Although this article focuses on systematic approaches to scheduling, running an ASC is largely about personnel management. The top priority is to keep all customers, including the staff, patient, and surgeon, satisfied.[1]

BASIC DEFINITIONS

Basic definitions are required to properly execute a practical approach to ASC scheduling, allowing effective communication between team members (**Fig. 1, Table 1**).[2]

SYSTEMS FOR PROCEDURE SCHEDULING

One of the most important jobs in an ASC is scheduling procedures in the OR, which is the facility's scarcest and most expensive resource. The OR procedure scheduling function is usually overseen by 1 person such as the ASC director, or by a group of people that might include a triad of anesthesiologist, surgeon, and nurse. This entity examines OR times for each surgeon or group to predict future OR workload and compute the optimal allocated OR time to maximize OR efficiency. The goal is to maximize the number of surgical procedures that can be performed in each OR in the regularly defined workday while minimizing expenses. Because wages, salaries, and

---

Box 1
Strategies to maintain a well-functioning ASC

- Recruit and retain the right people

  Staff often choose to work at an ASC rather than a hospital for specific benefits (eg, more predictable hours, no call, less bureaucracy, faster decision making, no emergencies to disrupt the day, cordial team environment.) Therefore, keeping staff happy is a top priority. They are the most important resource. Move to remove the wrong people.

- Ensure that patients are satisfied with their experiences.

  Start procedures on time by ensuring appropriate preoperative consultation and laboratory work have been done, scheduling appropriately to avoid delays or cancellations, and minimizing postoperative pain, nausea, and vomiting.

- Manage the ASC to have happy surgeons

  Surgeons may have options to operate elsewhere. Starting on time, quick turnovers, knowledgeable staff, appropriate equipment and instruments, and providing easy access to OR time are surgeon satisfiers.

- Continuously work on the minor details to improve processes

- Make the case documentation and billing as clean as possible and have them work together

- Have the correct governance structure with properly defined responsibilities, authority, and policies and procedures.

Courtesy of Dr. Nanji M, President and CEO, Surgical Centers Incorporated, Calgary, Alberta, Canada. Personal interview. June 14, 2013.

Box 2
Characteristics of a well-functioning ASC

- Less than 45 minutes mean total delay of start times for elective procedures per OR per day
- Less than 5% procedure cancellation rate
- Less than 10% days with at least 1 delay greater than 10 minutes because the recovery room is full
- Less than 25 minutes average turnover times
- Less than 5% excess staffing costs
- Prolonged turnovers lasting greater than 60 minutes occur less than 10% of the time

From Macario A. Are your hospital operating rooms "efficient"? A scoring system with eight performance indicators. Anesthesiology 2006;105(2):237–40; with permission.

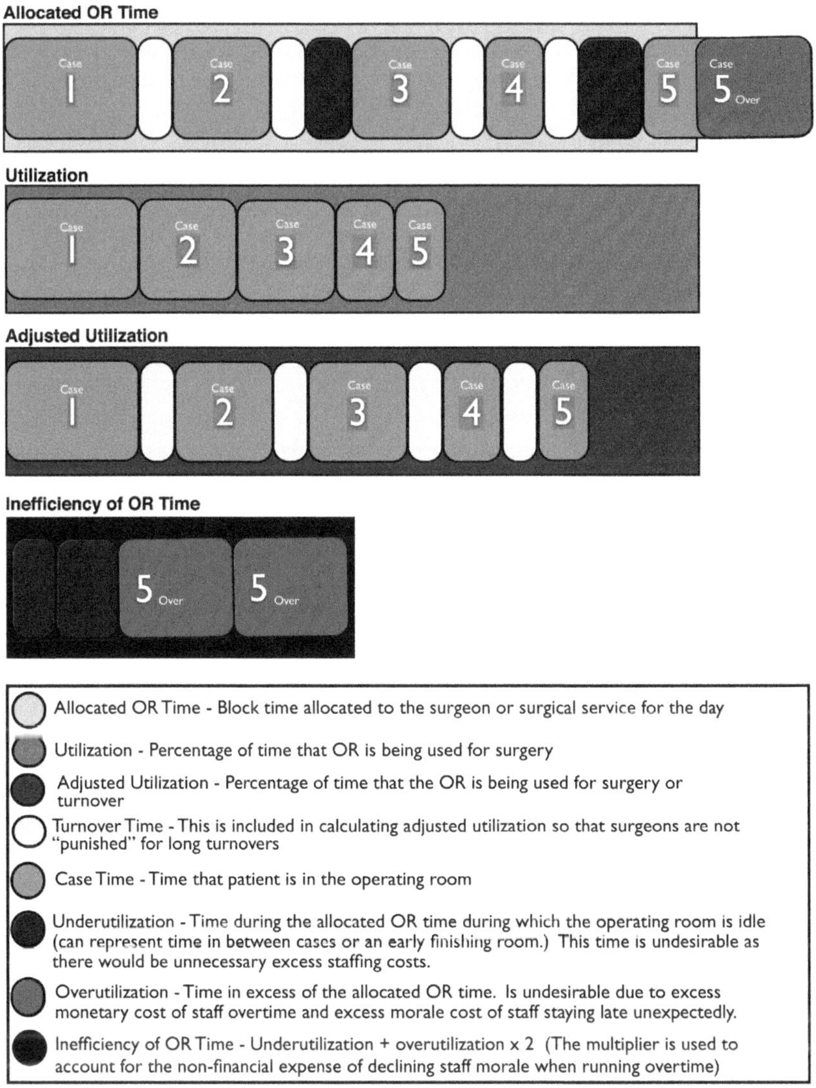
Allocated OR Time
Case 1
Case 2
Case 3
Case 4
Case 5
Case 5 Over
Utilization
Case 1
Case 2
Case 3
Case 4
Case 5
Adjusted Utilization
Case 1
Case 2
Case 3
Case 4
Case 5
Inefficiency of OR Time
5 Over
5 Over
Allocated OR Time - Block time allocated to the surgeon or surgical service for the day
Utilization - Percentage of time that OR is being used for surgery
Adjusted Utilization - Percentage of time that the OR is being used for surgery or turnover
Turnover Time - This is included in calculating adjusted utilization so that surgeons are not "punished" for long turnovers
Case Time - Time that patient is in the operating room
Underutilization - Time during the allocated OR time during which the operating room is idle (can represent time in between cases or an early finishing room.) This time is undesirable as there would be unnecessary excess staffing costs.
Overutilization - Time in excess of the allocated OR time. Is undesirable due to excess monetary cost of staff overtime and excess morale cost of staff staying late unexpectedly.
Inefficiency of OR Time - Underutilization + overutilization x 2 (The multiplier is used to account for the non-financial expense of declining staff morale when running overtime)

Fig. 1. Basic definitions of ASC scheduling.

Table 1	
ASC scheduling terminology and definitions	
Definition	**Explanation**
Staffing	The process of calculating the number of OR teams that must be available at each time during the week. For example, there may be staffing for 4 ORs Monday to Thursday between 7 AM and 3 PM, and 7 AM to noon on Fridays
Regular scheduled hours	The hours that an OR team member plans on working on the days when not on call (eg, 7 AM to 3 PM)
Master surgical schedule	A cyclic timetable that defines how many ORs are available, the hours that ORs are open, and the surgical groups given the OR time. Many ASCs use a schedule that repeats every 1 or 2 wk
Allocated OR time	Amount of OR time with a specified start and end time on a specified day of the week that is assigned by the ASC to a surgical group or surgeon. For example, the sports medicine surgeons may be allocated OR time from 7 AM to 3 PM every Tuesday. This allocation does not mean that additional cases would be turned away if the group could not finish them by 3 PM. Instead, OR time allocation indicates that the regularly scheduled hours planned for the surgeons are between 7 AM and 3 PM
Block time	A category of allocated OR time whereby an ASC does not schedule a procedure into block time unless it is predicted to finish within the block
Raw utilization	Equals the total hours of elective procedures performed by a surgeon or surgical group during allocated OR time, excluding turnover times, divided by the allocated OR time
Adjusted utilization	Equals the total hours of elective procedures, including the corresponding turnover times, performed within allocated OR time, divided by the allocated OR time. For example, if a surgeon is allocated 8 h of OR time and operates for an aggregate 7 h during the day with a 1-h aggregate turnover time, the adjusted utilization would be 100%
Underutilized OR time	Reflects how early a room finishes and becomes idle. If an anesthesiologist and OR nurse are scheduled to work from 8 AM to 5 PM and instead the room finishes early at 2 PM, then there would be 3 h of underutilized time. The excess staffing cost would be 33% (3 h/9 h). Excess staffing cost is one metric for assessing how well the ASC scheduling is being done
Overutilized hours	The hours that ORs run beyond scheduled time. For example, if 11 h of procedures (including turnovers) are performed with staff scheduled to work 9 h, there are 2 overutilized hours. Overutilized hours are at least twice as expensive because of the additional monetary and morale cost of staff staying late unexpectedly. The excess staffing cost is 44% (2 h/9 h = 22%, which is then multiplied by 2 to account for the incremental cost)

benefits of perioperative staff account for two-thirds of OR expenses, and overtime expenses are even higher, it is critical to minimize overtime.

There are 3 commonly used systems for managing procedure scheduling: Any Workday, Fixed Hours, or Reasonable Time (**Fig. 2**). Most ASCs in the United States

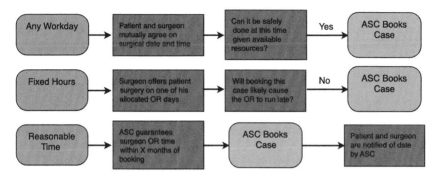

Fig. 2. The 3 commonly used systems for managing procedure scheduling.

handle cases using the Any Workday system, in which patients and surgeons determine the date on which they would like to have their surgery and the ASC complies with the requests provided the procedures can be done safely (ie, adequate resources are available.) Because surgeons can book procedures on almost any date at any time, the challenges inherent in the Any Workday system are to minimize the less obvious hidden, nonfinancial costs, such as staff dissatisfaction with working overtime. This scheduling is done months in advance through efficiency-based scheduling and on the day of surgery by creating incentives for the staff to work efficiently. One such example of a staff incentive is to allow nursing staff to go home early if their room is finished early.

The Fixed Hours system, which is less commonly used in the United States, is common in hospitals and ASCs in Canada.[3] In this system surgeons or surgical services are assigned block time during which they are expected to book their procedures. For example, a surgeon may be assigned OR time on every Tuesday from 7 AM until 4 PM. The surgeon is free to book any combination of procedures during this time with the expectation that they will not run late.

Some ASCs choose to schedule procedures in both the Any Workday and the Fixed Hours systems. For example, an ASC may prefer the Fixed Hours system because surgeons are given fixed blocks of OR time with clearly defined start and end times on specific days. As such, this may be more conducive to ensuring that rooms do not run late, thereby minimizing overtime expenses and staff dissatisfaction. Furthermore, insurance companies often reimburse the ASC with a fixed sum per procedure, regardless of the duration (ie, the ASC is not given extra compensation for a procedure that runs longer than expected.) Allowing a surgeon to operate at any time of day is not likely to increase revenue. In contrast, an exception may be made for procedures for which the patient pays cash (eg, elective plastic surgery), because reimbursement may be significantly higher and the surgeon and patient are free to use another ASC if their specific time preference cannot be accommodated. Furthermore, the reimbursement may be time based such that a procedure that runs longer than expected is reimbursed more. In this case, the Any Workday system may be used if it is tolerable to risk running overtime, given that reimbursement will adequately compensate for overtime expenses.

The Reasonable Time system is less commonly used in ASCs. In this system, the ASC makes an advance commitment to the surgeon that once a procedure is booked it will be scheduled within a predetermined time frame. For example, assuming that a surgeon has an agreement with the ASC that procedures be scheduled within 90 days of booking, the surgeon would be unable to guarantee the patient a specific date or time; they would only be able to guarantee the surgical date within a 90 day window. Having the ASC choose the surgical date, which may conflict with work or personal plans, could be unacceptable to many patients. For this reason, specifically in the United States, where many patients are not limited to a specific surgeon or ASC, this is the least desirable system.

USING UTILIZATION TO ASSIGN OR TIME

Some ASCs use prior utilization to assign OR time. For example, surgeons who show a pattern of failing to use their OR time may have it reduced, whereas surgeons who have high OR utilization may receive more time. This technique has several challenges (**Box 3**).[4]

PREDICTION OF PROCEDURE DURATION

If procedure times could be predicted accurately, it would be easy to schedule procedures in an ASC, but for several reasons the procedure duration may vary from predicted (**Box 4**).[7]

Box 3
Challenges to using OR utilization as criteria for changing the amount of OR time provided to an ASC surgeon

- Measuring OR utilization is tricky and may be done differently at different ASCs, and is therefore difficult to compare.

  Should add-on procedures be included? Does it matter whether the add-on was performed by the same surgeon who was in the room, or a different surgeon? What about a surgeon who does procedures out of the usual OR block time; should those be added to the OR utilization computation?

- Optimal OR utilization differs among surgical specialties

  Not all surgeons can achieve utilization greater than 90%. It is easier to achieve higher utilization in rooms with more predictable procedure durations. For example, cataract surgeons are more likely to know in advance which procedures they are doing and to fill up their OR time months in advance. Also, subspecialties with longer procedures may have lower utilization because long procedures cannot be fit neatly into block time as easily as several short procedures.

- Utilization is poorly related to contribution margin

  Contribution margin is the ASC revenue generated by a surgical procedure, less all the variable costs. For example, a slow surgeon decreases the contribution margin because the variable costs consume revenue.[5]

- Utilization measurements are not accurate for individual surgeons

  This inaccuracy arises because of random variations in the numbers of patients each week who request to be scheduled for surgery.[6]

- Utilization does not reflect strategic decisions by ASC to grow some subspecialties

  Providing more OR time for a specialty to build its activity may mean accepting a lower utilization initially

- Utilization can be artificially inflated

  For example, surgeons purposefully slow down at the end of the day to use their block fully, worrying that their block time will be reduced if their utilization is low.

Box 4
Accurate estimation of procedure duration is not straightforward for several reasons

- Procedure duration data are not normally distributed. They do not have a bell-shaped curve because long procedures skew the distribution to the right.

- The combination of a great variety of procedures and the large number of surgeons at many ASCs. As many as half of the procedures (defined by Current Procedural Terminology codes performed) scheduled may only have 5 or fewer previous procedures of the same type and the same surgeon during the preceding year.[8]

- An ASC may count multiple different procedure types and cases as the same when the patients are called into the scheduling office, because the required supplies, instruments, and surgical tray may be similar, even though the operation is different. Some hospitals use mnemonics to group such cases. Because of the variety of surgical procedures grouped together under one such mnemonic, procedure duration prediction based on the booking mnemonic is intrinsically flawed.

- Surgeons may try to underestimate the length of their procedures (so that the ASC allows them to book more procedures in their block) or overestimate their procedure duration (so no other surgeon can book procedures in that OR).[3]

- Some procedures may be particularly complex or easy compared with the typical so there is intrinsic variability that must be accepted and managed.

- Different information systems define procedure duration differently. Some from incision to close, others patient in to patient out, so the data may be flawed.

Furthermore, there are many different types of ASCs, including surgical ASCs, endoscopy ASCs, pain ASCs, or some combination thereof. For those ASCs that have a case mix with high variability of procedure times, it is more difficult to schedule times accurately and achieve maximum utilization without making patients wait, having the schedule extend past the end of the day, or idling staff.

Because most ASCs do not know until the day of surgery which procedures are scheduled in an OR, and it is difficult to accurately estimate the duration of any single procedure, the best way to optimize matching of staffing with workload is to allocate

---

Table 2
Categories of OR delays in ASC

Type of Delay	Example
First case delays	If a patient is scheduled to be in room at 7:30 AM and the patient is brought in at 7:40 AM then this delay is 10 min
Turnover takes longer than expected	If turnover is scheduled for 30 min but takes 40 min this is 10 min
Procedure duration went past scheduled duration	If the procedure is scheduled for 90 min but took 180 min this would be 90 min
Completing elective procedures on the wait list	Wait list cases are added to the OR schedule at the end of the day causing a late OR
Unused block time with an idle room	The room is sitting idle in between cases and it is not caused by first procedure delay or turnover
Overrun block time	The room runs unexpectedly late past the scheduled end of the OR time

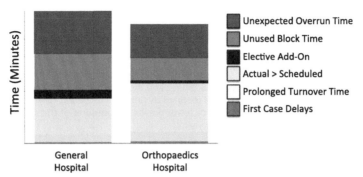

Fig. 3. The sum of all first-case delay minutes by month is in orange. In yellow is the sum of all prolonged turnover times. In red is the sum of all overutilized minutes from elective procedures in the same operating room suite that exceed block time. Instead of focusing on improving the scheduling accuracy of single cases, the ASC manager can analyze the historical data for how long each operation went each day and then compute the OR time allocation for each surgeon each day that minimizes OR inefficiency. (*Courtesy of* WiseOR, Inc. © 2013, Palo Alto, CA; with permission.)

appropriate time to each surgical service based on the history of how long each surgeon operated each day.[9]

CATEGORIES OF OR DELAYS

OR delays can be categorized into 6 types (**Table 2**). By comparing different types of OR delays it is possible to understand the magnitude of the contribution that each type of delay has on the OR's performance. This comparison can be broken down by specific ASCs (**Fig. 3**) or specific surgeons (**Fig. 4**). When the appropriate data are logged, information systems can be leveraged to produce reports that help ASC directors improve performance through meaningful predictions (**Table 3**).

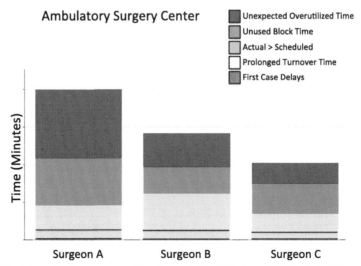

Fig. 4. OR delays for 3 surgeons. (*Courtesy of* WiseOR, Inc. © 2013, Palo Alto, CA; with permission.)

Table 3

Predicted ASC concurrency report that provides staff the ability to anticipate surges in workflow demand caused by concurrent turnovers or postanesthesia care unit (PACU) admissions by time of day

Type of Concurrency				Time of Day						
	7–8 AM	8–9 AM	9–10 AM	10–11 AM	11 AM–12 PM	12–1 PM	1–2 PM	2–3 PM	3–4 PM
4 or more concurrent turnovers	—	—	—	Rooms 1, 3, 5, 7	—	—	—	—	—
4 or more concurrent PACU arrivals	—	—	—	—	—	Rooms 2, 4, 6, 7, 9	—	Rooms 1, 2, 9, 11	—

Courtesy of WiseOR, Inc. © 2013, Palo Alto, CA; with permission.

First-case delays are often used as an OR performance indicator. When time is categorized in the manner shown in **Table 2**, it is clear that first-case delays tend to have only a minor effect on a late OR's finish time. Instead, other types of delays, such as longer-than-scheduled procedure durations and midday idle ORs are more responsible for later-than-scheduled finish times (see **Fig. 3**).[10] Although first-case delays cause dissatisfaction for patients and surgeons, they have a small effect on OR delays, although it may affect the providers' perception of a good day.[11]

SUMMARY

A successful ASC manager focuses attention on several tasks including the typical operational aspects of a business (ie, human resources, marketing, finance) and the scheduling of staff and surgical procedures.

This article presents basic definitions and several scheduling models to assist the ASC manager with scheduling surgical procedures including Any Workday, Fixed Hours, and Reasonable Time. Each model has its own merits, and the choice between these depends on the specifics of a particular facility. Although difficult to quantify and evaluate, utilization measurement is critical in order to maximize continuous optimization of OR utilization. The 6 categories of OR delays can simplify utilization analysis. Sources of dissatisfaction often include procedure delays, inability to schedule OR procedures, OR overutilization, and a priori knowledge of these. An understanding of each team member's needs and concerns helps the ASC manager to minimize dissatisfaction among patients and providers.

Using these tools, the ASC manager will be well prepared to best allocate resources and continuously evaluate performance, optimizing OR utilization and maximizing patient and provider satisfaction.

REFERENCES

1. Vitez TS, Macario A. Setting performance standards for an anesthesia department. J Clin Anesth 1998;10(2):166–75.
2. McIntosh C, Dexter F, Epstein RH. The impact of service-specific staffing, case scheduling, turnovers, and first-case starts on anesthesia group and operating room productivity: a tutorial using data from an Australian hospital. Anesth Analg 2006;103(6):1499–516.
3. Nanji M. Dr. President and CEO, Surgical Centers Incorporated, Calgary, Alberta, Canada. Personal interview. June 14, 2013.
4. Macario A. The limitations of using operating room utilisation to allocate surgeons more or less surgical block time in the USA. Anaesthesia 2010;65(6):548–52.
5. Dexter F, Blake JT, Penning DH, et al. Calculating a potential increase in hospital margin for elective surgery by changing operating room time allocations or increasing nursing staffing to permit completion of more cases: a case study. Anesth Analg 2002;94:138–42.
6. Dexter F, Macario A, Traub RD. Operating room utilization alone is not an accurate metric for the allocation of operating room block time to individual surgeons with low caseloads. Anesthesiology 2003;98:1243–9.
7. Macario A. Truth in scheduling: is it possible to accurately predict how long a surgical case will last? Anesth Analg 2009;108(3):681–5.
8. Zhou J, Dexter F, Macario A, et al. Relying solely on historical surgical times to estimate accurately future surgical times is unlikely to reduce the average length of time cases finish late. J Clin Anesth 1999;11:601–5.

9. Strum DP, Vargas LG, May JH. Surgical subspecialty block utilization and capacity planning. Anesthesiology 1999;90:1176–85.

10. Available at: www.wiseor.com.

11. Iverson TB, Anderson KA, Marolen KN, et al. Impact of determinants of a good day in the operating room (abstract). Anesthesiology 2012;117:A1183.

Practice Management/Role of the Medical Director

Douglas G. Merrill, MD, MBA

KEYWORDS

- Administration • Practice management • Medical director • Business
- Ambulatory surgery center • Anesthesiology • Outcomes • Quality

KEY POINTS

- The history of the ambulatory surgery center begins with Ralph Waters' inspiration to create a different kind of facility that catered to the needs of patients and the surgeon in a manner that the hospital could not.
- Today's medical director should actively manage the systems, policies, and providers using quantifiable outcomes of care and systems as well as planned process-improvement events.
- This work will ensure the medical director's ability to lead the center to excellence in care delivery, safety, and, by extension, the metrics of successful accreditation and finances.

INTRODUCTION

A medical director in an ambulatory surgery setting should be focused on the development and improvement of systems that support excellence in clinical and nonclinical outcomes. The effort requires individual patient's clinical and social assessment on a daily basis, personnel management, accreditation and compliance oversight, contracting, and strategic business planning. The role calls for the development of expertise in a wide variety of skills. Ideally, the medical director is on site most of the time to enforce policy but, more importantly, to provide coherence of attitude regarding service excellence and a full understanding of the challenges faced by the facility. Thus, an anesthesiologist, rather than a surgeon, is more often chosen for this role.

Anesthesiology, Center for Perioperative Services, Dartmouth-Hitchcock Medical Center, Geisel School of Medicine, Dartmouth, 1 Medical Center Drive, Lebanon, NH 03756, USA
E-mail address: douglas.g.merrill@hitchcock.org

Anesthesiology Clin 32 (2014) 529–540
http://dx.doi.org/10.1016/j.anclin.2014.02.021   **anesthesiology.theclinics.com**
1932-2275/14/$ – see front matter © 2014 Elsevier Inc. All rights reserved.

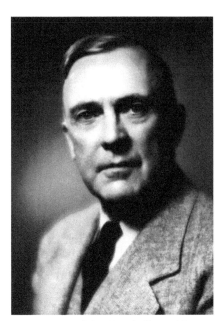

Fig. 1. Ralph Waters. (*Image courtesy* of the Wood Library-Museum of Anesthesiology, Park Ridge, IL.)

HISTORY AND DEVELOPMENT OF THE AMBULATORY SURGERY MEDICAL DIRECTOR

The first outpatient surgery center was developed by Dr Ralph Waters in Sioux City, Iowa in the years after World War I (**Figs. 1** and **2**). In creating the Downtown Anesthesia Clinic, Waters moved procedures out of the hospital with a primary aim:

> ...to give satisfaction to operator and patient and charge a fee that will pay expenses and a good profit...considerably less than for similar work in the hospital because less time and trouble is involved[1]...

He intended that this remarkable innovation target both patient and surgeon satisfaction. In his published account in an article in 1919, he noted the following wry customer service observations that remain accurate today:

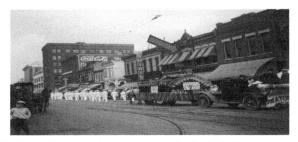

Fig. 2. Site of the Sioux City, Iowa downtown anesthesia clinic. *Arrow* shows the location of Dr Waters first "downtown anesthesia clinic". (*From* Waters RM. The down-town anesthesia clinic. Am J Surg 1919;33(7):71–73(S).)

We aim to keep an abundant supply of N2O-O2 and use it freely. Many patients and some doctors object to the fees, but they come back and their friends come back… Satisfactory anesthesia and too large fees work out better than bargain sale fees and unsatisfactory anesthesia…People forget the fee but they never forget the hurt, nor fail to tell their friends about it.[1]

In that short description, Waters distilled the essence of the modern ambulatory surgery industry and the role of the medical director in particular: provision of excellent customer service and outcomes and increased convenience for surgeons and patients, thereby ensuring a sustaining financial profit.

MANAGEMENT BY OUTCOMES AND PROCESS IMPROVEMENT

A modern, powerful means of maintaining the high quality and excellent service needed for an ambulatory surgery center is the ability to measure clinical and process outcomes. Outcome measurement may identify variation that is better than average, identifying practices that should be emulated, or worse than average, identifying opportunities for the guided revision of variable practice.

A long-term program of assessment of a few clinical and process outcomes in all patients can either validate or identify the needed revision of care pathways and/or systems that might benefit from the implementation of process-improvement projects.

Process improvement is best managed by the participation of all stakeholders so that the changes invoked are recognized as valid by all. Although relatively new to health care, the importance of providing outcome data to employees in an effort to support process improvement is well accepted in manufacturing[2]:

…(employees) experience a surprising mismatch between expected and actual results of action and respond to that mismatch through a process of thought and further action that leads them to modify their images of organization or their understandings of organizational phenomena and to restructure their activities so as to bring outcomes and expectations into line[1]…

The measurement and communication of outcomes to caregivers to direct process improvement has been shown to be of value in several health care settings.[3] One

RPIW - What is it?

- **3- 5 Day focused Improvement workshop:**
  - DMAIC based, leveraging the PDSA Cycle
  - Multiple employees from across the organization
  - Analyze and improve a complex, common process

- **Fundamental Operational Goals:**
  - Create a more reliable, efficient, patient driven process
  - Focus on higher quality with less time, energy and resources
  - Analyze and re-design with the patient as focal point

- **Educational Event:**
  - Training to understand a complex process in new ways
  - Draw upon upstream & downstream staff to strengthen performance
  - "See" the unit in new ways
  - Positioned to lead further change efforts

Fig. 3. RPIW basics. DMAIC, Define, Measure, Analyze, Improve, Control; PDSA, Plan, Do, Study, Act. (*Courtesy of* Daniel L. Herrick, BS, CPHQ, The Center for Perioperative Services and The Value Institute, Dartmouth-Hitchcock Medical Center, Lebanon, NH; with permission.)

RPIWs utilize the PDSA Cycle to test ideas

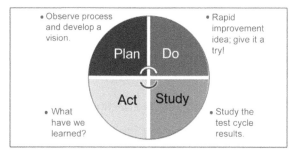

Fig. 4. The role of Plan, Do, Study, Act (PDSA) in an RPIW. (*Courtesy of* Daniel L. Herrick, BS, CPHQ, The Center for Perioperative Services and The Value Institute, Dartmouth-Hitchcock Medical Center, Lebanon, NH; with permission.)

approach, Lean Management, pioneered by the Toyota automobile company, was used to transform the Virginia Mason Medical Center and Clinics.[4] A short primer follows on the use of Rapid Process Improvement Workshop (RPIW), a helpful methodology drawn from Lean, in which a small group representing all interested parties meets in an intensive manner (2–5 days) to completely revise a process based on data analysis (**Figs. 3–6**).

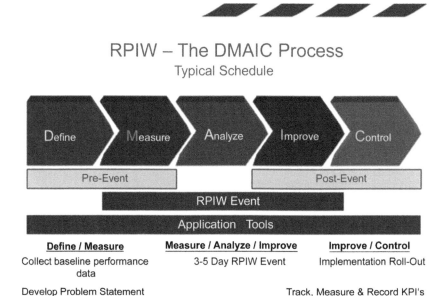

Fig. 5. The role of Define, Measure, Analyze, Improve, Control (DMAIC) in an RPIW process. KPI, key process improvements. (*Courtesy of* Daniel L. Herrick, BS, CPHQ, The Center for Perioperative Services and The Value Institute, Dartmouth-Hitchcock Medical Center, Lebanon, NH; with permission.)

Typical 5-Day RPIW
Event Agenda

Day 1	Day 2	Day 3	Day 4	Day 5
Event Kickoff	**Review Event Progress**	**Review Event Progress**	**Review Event Progress**	**Review Event Progress**
Team Introductions	Team "Check-In"	Team "Check-In"	Team "Check-In"	Update training Schedule
Event Charter Review				Continue training Affected
RPIW Event Overview	**Training / Review**	**Teamwork**	**Teamwork**	Workers
	Common Terminology	Design Improvements	Continue Design and Testing	
Training	DMAIC	Create Standard Work	of New Standard Work	Create Sustainability Plan
Common Terminology	Value Stream Analysis	Begin Testing Standard Work	Process Simulation	
DMAIC	Process mapping	Process Simulations	Obtain Workforce Input and	Finalize 30-Day List
Value Stream Analysis	5S	Obtain Stakeholder Input	Buy-In	
Process mapping	Root Cause	Update Future State process	Finalize Standard Work	Complete RPIW Report
5S	Cause and Effect Diagrams	Maps		Document Event Information
Root Cause	Charts and Plots		Prepare Training Materials	Prepare team Presentation
Cause and Effect Diagrams	Waste / Work / Re-Work		Set Training Schedule	
Charts and Plots	Styro Inc. Exercise		Begin Training Affected	**Hold Team Presentation**
Waste / Work / Re-Work			Workers	
Toast Video Exercise	**Teamwork**			
	Design Future State			
Teamwork	Brainstorm improvement			
Voice of Customer Review	Ideas			
Value Stream review	Select and Prioritize			
Current State	Crate Future State Process			
Future State	Maps			
Develop Process Maps				
Current State				
Wrap-Up Review / Briefing	**Wrap-Up Review / Briefing**	**Wrap-Up Review / Briefing**	**Wrap-Up Review / Briefing**	

Fig. 6. The typical RPIW cycle. KPI, key process improvements. (*Courtesy of* Daniel L. Herrick, BS, CPHQ, The Center for Perioperative Services and The Value Institute, Dartmouth-Hitchcock Medical Center, Lebanon, NH; with permission.)

Using this technique and targeted outcome measurements, any process or care pathway can be evaluated and revised, resulting in a standard process that will reduce variation-induced error or diminished patient care quality. An example of an action item list from an RPIW that successfully streamlined and reduced error in the author's institution's operating room setup process is shown in **Table 1**.

The use of outcome measurement to support process improvement can be used to improve quality one provider at a time or to transform the culture of an entire facility (**Table 2**).[5] For instance, when using one or a group of surgeons as risk adjustors, one can compare the outcomes for a set of anesthesia providers looking only at those cases that shared a similar surgeon or surgeons, thus, minimizing confounding variables.

Looking at those providers who have surgeons *F* and *G* in common, we see that anesthesia provider 4 tends toward longer turnovers than provider 8. If this trend were to hold over several quarters, it would provide an objective basis for a conversation with provider 4 to discuss differences in process between them. Number 8's lower

Table 1
Example of RPIW action item list

Action Items		Team	PDSAs			Rollout	
			First	Second	Third	Pilot	Final
1	End-of-day OR calling for final cleaning	Danni	Susan	—	—	5/3	6/3–6/14	6/17
2	End-of-day OR completion checklist	Danni	Susan	—	5/2	5/3	6/10–6/21	6/24
3	Standard room equipment templates, basic equipment counts and locations	Linda	Greg	—	5/2	5/3	6/10–6/21	6/24
4	Processing of anesthesia blades, dirty room to CSR to clean core	Greg	Glenda	5/1	5/2	5/3	6/10–6/21	6/24
5	Change in dinner break times for evening staff, new times from 16:15–16:45	Susan	—	5/1	5/2	5/3	6/3–6/14	6/17
6	Nonfolding of trash bags and linen, work order for improvements to shelving in OR core	Joyce	Merit	5/1	5/2	5/3	Work order entered 5/31	—
7	Housekeeping and PST staffing schedule adjustments, based on filling existing open positions	Matt	Glenda	Colleen	—	5/3	Pending staff hiring	—
8	Linen to be delivered, no longer retrieved by OR staff	Glenda	Matt	—	—	—	Future work	TBD
9	Standardize OR table and mattresses and identify surgeon preference options, specialty beds excluded	Mike	Michaela	—	—	—	Future work	TBD
10	Schedule all eye cases in same room (room 21 if possible or colocate with supplies)	Joyce	Merit	—	—	—	Future work	TBD
11	Dedicated cystoscopy room setup	Joyce	Merit	—	—	—	Future work	TBD
12	Check preference cards daily for accuracy and update, leverage current superusers	Danni	Linda	—	—	—	Future work	TBD

Abbreviations: CSR, central sterile reprocessing; OR, operating room; PDSA, Plan, Do, Study, Act; PST, patient support technician; TBD, to be determined.

Table 2

Outcome measurement

Surgeon	Anesthesiologist	Cases	Diaries	Average TO	N PACU (%)	V PACU (%)	N PD (%)	V PD (%)	Rated Excellent (%)	Recommend ASC (%)	Passport Defect (%)
A	1	39	32	11.12	0.00	0.00	16.67	8.00	85.19	95.65	43.75
AA	2	36	36	12.62	3.13	0.00	26.09	21.74	69.57	90.48	50.00
AA	3	43	42	12.66	5.41	2.70	25.71	14.29	82.86	100.00	28.57
B	4	25	25	18.81	0.00	0.00	6.67	0.00	93.75	100.00	68.00
C	5	25	22	11.17	0.00	0.00	0.00	0.00	88.89	100.00	54.55
D	5	26	24	17.37	0.00	0.00	5.00	5.00	85.00	100.00	25.00
EE	6	27	22	23.27	0.00	0.00	7.69	7.69	85.71	100.00	31.82
EE	7	25	21	21.29	0.00	0.00	8.33	8.33	78.57	87.50	38.10
F	4	106	95	15.85	6.02	3.61	6.06	5.88	84.06	100.00	33.68
F	8	45	43	12.83	0.00	0.00	8.70	8.70	66.67	100.00	27.91
G	4	62	51	17.83	2.00	4.00	21.43	17.86	85.71	100.00	50.98
G	6	25	25	20.11	0.00	0.00	0.00	10.53	72.22	91.67	44.00
G	8	79	79	14.14	0.00	0.00	3.92	3.92	87.76	100.00	46.84
H	3	27	26	33.25	0.00	0.00	22.73	18.18	68.18	100.00	46.15

Abbreviation: ASC, ambulatory surgery center; N, nausea; PACU, postanesthesia care unit; PD, post-discharge; TO, turnover; V, vomiting.

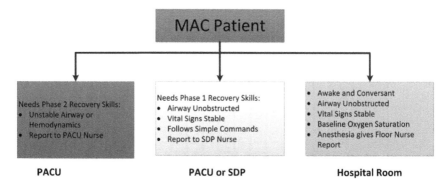

Fig. 7. Monitored Anesthesia Care (MAC) patient disposition and staffing algorithm. PACU, postanesthesia care unit; SDP, same day program.

postoperative nausea and vomiting (PONV) rate would also bear further observation, searching for emulative methods, particularly with regard to the kinds of cases performed by surgeon G.

CARE PATHWAY DEVELOPMENT: REDUCING ERROR AND IMPROVING QUALITY BY REDUCING VARIATION

The use of standard care pathways has been decried as cookbook medicine, which subverts the value of clinical autonomy and judgment. In reality, care pathways are the cornerstone of evidence-based medicine, drawing on the literature, expert opinion, and, most notably, the outcomes of local practice.[6] The use of standard algorithms allows the reduction of variation responsible for error.[7] Care pathway creation has reduced waste and cost, thereby improving margins in operating rooms.[8] In outpatient anesthesia, we take care of a narrow profile of procedures and patients and should take advantage of this because a narrow cohort of patients can be expected to respond relatively cohesively to similar therapies. Algorithms based on the literature and checked over time by local outcome assessment can be expected to produce improved outcomes and reduce error.

The use of safety events to drive algorithm creation can be an extremely successful means of improving safety for patients and a sense of teamwork for caregivers.[9] One example of a recovery room algorithm to manage patients who have had monitored anesthesia care is shown in **Fig. 7**, whereas an algorithm for adult PONV prevention appears in **Fig. 8**. An algorithm for anesthesia and surgical team interactions and procedures associated with breast reductions and liposuction that was created in response to a patient safety event (severe hypovolemia, unrecognized) is available in Appendix 1.

One value of sustained outcome measurement is to support the ongoing improvement of quality and safety required by facility accreditors, which is the responsibility of the medical director. A significant aspect of this work is the development of evidence-based policies.

SUMMARY

The history of the ambulatory surgery center begins with Ralph Waters' inspiration to create a different kind of facility that catered to the needs of patients and the surgeon in a manner that the hospital could not. His emphasis on quality of care and service excellence should be echoed in the modern medical director's role. Today's medical

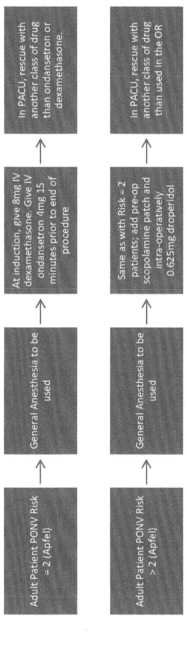

Fig. 8. Adult PONV prevention algorithm.

director should actively manage the systems, policies, and providers using quantifi-able outcomes of care and systems as well as planned process-improvement events. This work will ensure the medical director's ability to lead the center to excellence in care delivery, safety, and, by extension, the metrics of successful accreditation and finances.

REFERENCES

1. Waters RM. The down-town anesthesia clinic. Am J Surg 1919;33(7):71–73(S).
2. Argyris C, Schon D. Organisational learning: a theory of action perspective. New York: Addison-Wesley; 1978.
3. Available at: http://www.vnews.com/home/6122247-95/surgeons-take-critical-look-at-their-process. Accessed March 17, 2014.
4. Kenney C. Transforming health care: Virginia Mason Medical Center's pursuit of the perfect patient experience. New York: Productivity Press; 2011.
5. Gorenflo G. Achieving a culture of quality improvement. J Public Health Manag Pract 2010;16(1):83–4.
6. Sackett DL, Rosenberg WM, Gray JA, et al. Evidence based medicine: what it is and what it isn't. BMJ 1996;312:71–2.
7. Redberg RF. Getting to best care at lower cost. JAMA Intern Med 2013;173(2): 91–2.
8. Cima RR, Brown MJ, Hebl JR, et al. Use of lean and six sigma methodology to improve operating room efficiency in a high-volume tertiary-care academic med-ical center. J Am Coll Surg 2011;213:83–92.
9. McDonald TB, Helmchen LA, Smith KM, et al. Responding to patient safety inci-dents: the "seven pillars". Qual Saf Health Care 2010;19(6):e11.

APPENDIX 1: EXAMPLE OF A MULTIDISCIPLINARY ALGORITHM OF CARE RESULTING FROM A SAFETY EVENT
Surgical Team

Preoperative
- Surgeon orders preoperative hemoglobin (Hb)
  - On arrival in the preoperative area, a point-of-care Hb (outpatient surgery cen-ter) or blood draw Hb test (same day program) should be performed as a base-line. If anemia is present (Hb<10), the surgeon and anesthesia team should be alerted. Patients with anemia should not undergo large-volume liposuction.

Intraoperative
- The operating room should be kept at a relatively warm temperature.
- An underbody or other underbody warming device should be used for these procedures.
- Foley placement: The *surgeon* should determine the placement. (The recommen-dation is to place Foley for all liposuction cases and for large-volume breast reductions.)
- Time-out: The *surgical team* should announce what liposuction technique they will be using.

Estimated Blood Loss (EBL) estimation and fluid replacement during liposuction should follow this guideline:
  - Dry technique: The aspiration cannula is inserted directly into the space from which fat is to be removed, with no infiltration of the tissues. *The estimated blood loss is 20% to 45% of the aspirated volume.*

- Wet technique: Regardless of the amount aspirated, 200 to 300 mL of wetting solution is injected per area to be treated. Blood loss is difficult to assess, but *EBL may be as high as 30% of the aspirated volume.*
- Superwet technique: The amount of fluid injected (1 mL per estimated milliliter of expected aspirate) is equal to the amount of fat to be removed. *Blood loss is approximately 1% of the aspirated volume.*
- Tumescent technique: Large volume of fluid (3–4 mL per estimated milliliter of expected aspirate) is injected into the fat, raising the concerned areas to become turgid and firm. *Blood loss is approximately 1% of the aspirated volume.*

Fluid replacement guidelines

Liposuction fluid resuscitation guidelines

- *Small-volume aspirations* (less than 5 L): Replace routine maintenance fluid and anticipate that 70% of the subcutaneous infiltrate reaches the intravascular compartment when calculating the replacement of EBL (see earlier discussion).

Anesthesia Team

Preoperative
- Check the Hb value. (It should be ordered by the surgeon.)

Intraoperative
- Time-out: The time-out for these procedures should include an announcement by the *anesthesia team* that they are following this protocol.
- *A second intravenous (IV)* injection should be considered for any combination procedure.
- *IV fluid warmer* should be used for all of these procedures.
- EBL estimation and fluid replacement during liposuction should follow this guideline: (The anesthesiologist will announce which technique is being used during the time-out.)
  - Dry technique: The aspiration cannula is inserted directly into the space from which fat is to be removed, with no infiltration of the tissues. The *estimated blood loss is 20% to 45% of the aspirated volume.*
  - Wet technique: Regardless of the amount aspirated, 200 to 300 mL of wetting solution is injected per area to be treated. Blood loss is difficult to assess, but *EBL may be as high as 30% of the aspirated volume.*
  - Superwet technique: The amount of fluid injected (1 mL per estimated milliliter of expected aspirate) is equal to the amount of fat to be removed. *Blood loss is approximately 1% of the aspirated volume.*
  - Tumescent technique: A large volume of fluid (3–4 mL per estimated milliliter of expected aspirate) is injected into the fat, raising the concerned areas to become turgid and firm. *Blood loss is approximately 1% of the aspirated volume.*

Fluid replacement guidelines

Liposuction fluid resuscitation guidelines

  - *Small-volume aspirations* (less than 5 L): Replace routine maintenance fluid, and anticipate that 70% of the subcutaneous infiltrate reaches the intravascular compartment when calculating the replacement of EBL (see earlier discussion).
- Place and monitor an *esophageal or nasopharyngeal thermometer* for all of these cases.
- *Do NOT use ketorolac.*
- Do not manage hypotension without alerting the surgeon to its presence and the plan to remedy it.

- Use of vasoconstrictors should prompt an immediate discussion with the surgical team.
- IV volume should be used first to treat hypotension.
- Do not lighten anesthesia levels to remedy hypotension; use IV, normal saline, or lactated ringers boluses.
- As closure commences, hypotension should not be allowed to persist as it can also hide bleeding sites that later lead to hematoma formation.
- *Do not use hetastarch (Hespan).* If crystalloid is insufficient to maintain blood pressure (BP), obtain an Hb or hematocrit (Hct) to determine the potential need for transfusion.
- In all situations, active communication with the surgeon is of paramount importance.
- *Call the recovery nurse to obtain an Hb from the patient in the recovery room if*
  - Systolic BP remains 20% less than baseline despite IV fluid bolus therapy.
  - Heart Rate (HR) is greater than 100 despite IV fluid bolus therapy.
  - Breast swelling occurs (indicating hematoma formation).
  - The patient displays signs or symptoms of hypotension.
- *Call the surgeon if one of the aforementioned conditions exists and with the Hb result.*

Postoperative
- Call the surgeon if one of the aforementioned conditions exists, and report the Hb result if ordered.
  - Systolic BP remains 20% less than baseline despite IV fluid bolus therapy.
  - HR is greater than 100 despite IV fluid bolus therapy.
  - Breast swelling occurs (indicating hematoma formation).
  - The patient displays signs or symptoms of hypotension.

Pre-operative/Recovery Nurse

Preoperative
- If ordered on arrival in the preoperative area, a point-of-care/blood draw Hb test should be performed as a baseline. If anemia is present (Hb<10), the surgeon and anesthesia team should be alerted.

Postoperative
- Do NOT use ketorolac.
- Call the surgeon or anesthesia provider to provide an update on the patient's condition and obtain an order for a Hb from the patient in the recovery room if any of the following conditions exist:
  - Systolic BP remains 20% less than baseline despite IV fluid bolus therapy.
  - HR is greater than 100 despite IV fluid bolus therapy.
  - Breast swelling occurs (indicating hematoma formation).
  - The patient displays signs or symptoms of hypotension.
- Record the following on provided data sheet:
  - Hypotension in operating room or postanesthesia care unit
  - EBL
  - Placement of a Foley and urine volume for the case
  - Straight catheter and urine volume obtained
  - If patient had urinary incontinence on emergence

Legal Aspects of Ambulatory Anesthesia

Judith Jurin Semo, JD

KEYWORDS

- Legal issues • Anesthesiology • Ambulatory surgical center • Office practice

KEY POINTS

- This article informs anesthesiologists of some of the legal issues they may encounter in connection with ambulatory surgical center–based or office-based practice.
- The primary legal issues that anesthesiologists face in connection with practice in such settings can be broken down into practice-related issues and ownership-related issues.
- Given the complexity of legal issues relating to ambulatory anesthesia, anesthesiologists are advised to consult counsel at an early stage so as to understand the issues that may apply to their practice.

In the United States, medical practice is highly regulated and practice at ambulatory surgical centers (ASCs) and physicians' offices is no exception. The primary legal issues that anesthesiologists face in connection with practice in such settings can be broken down into 2 categories: (1) practice-related issues, and (2) ownership-related issues. This chapter provide an overview of these legal issues. Further resources are referenced in the endnotes.

PRACTICE-RELATED LEGAL ISSUES

Practice-related legal issues cover a wide range of aspects of practice. They include regulation of clinical practice, legal concerns related to clinical practice, and regulation of practice management, or business matters, including compliance with federal, state, and local regulatory requirements. This chapter provides anesthesiologists with summary information about how this category of legal issues affects their day-to-day practice.

Professional Liability

Professional liability, or medical malpractice, is often the first topic that physicians consider when they consider practice-related legal issues. Compliance with professional standards and the applicable standard of care is important in all settings. In

PLLC, 1800 M Street, Northwest, Suite 730 S, Washington, DC 20036, USA
E-mail address: jsemo@jsemo.com

Anesthesiology Clin 32 (2014) 541–549
http://dx.doi.org/10.1016/j.anclin.2014.02.009   **anesthesiology.theclinics.com**
1932-2275/14/$ – see front matter © 2014 Elsevier Inc. All rights reserved.

ambulatory settings, in which patients stay a shorter length of time than in inpatient facilities and in which there are fewer personnel and equipment resources, certain issues are even more important.

Patient selection

Patient section is important in any setting. In the ambulatory setting, patient selection is especially important for multiple reasons, including the shortened stay compared with inpatient facilities. The anesthesiologist needs to consider whether the patient is suited to the ambulatory setting, because surgeons and proceduralists may seek to perform a procedure in a facility they own, or in their office, rather than performing it in a hospital. The anesthesiologist serves as the gatekeeper, and may be held accountable for allowing the procedure to be performed in an ambulatory setting if there is an adverse outcome.

Issues can arise due to the patient's condition, such as unstable patients with multiple comorbidities, and there is the potential for problems to occur during the course of the procedure. In addition, patient selection concerns also relate to discharge of patients to a home environment in which there may be insufficient attention to the possible adverse reactions.

Patient selection is not only a professional liability concern; it is also is a matter of regulatory compliance for practice at an ASC. In the US Centers for Medicare & Medicaid Services (CMS) interpretive guidelines relating to the conditions for coverage (CfCs) for ASCs to participate in the Medicare program, CMS commented that even patients classified as ASA (American Society of Anesthesiologists) 3 may not be appropriate candidates for an ASC:

As the ASA PS level of a patient increases, the range of acceptable risk associated with a specific procedure or type of anesthesia in an ambulatory setting may narrow. An ASC that employed this classification system in its assessment of its patients might then consider, taking into account the nature of the procedures it performs and the anesthesia used, whether it will accept for admission patients who would have a classification of ASA PS IV or higher. For many patients classified as ASA PS level III, an ASC may also not be an appropriate setting, depending upon the procedure and anesthesia.[1]

State law also may bear on the patient selection process. For example, Alabama regulations require that "[p]atients must be individually evaluated for each procedure to determine if the office is an appropriate setting for the anesthesia required and for the surgical procedure to be performed."[2]

Informed consent

As in the case of patient selection, informed consent is a required element of anesthesia practice in all settings. In connection with ambulatory anesthesia, which covers both ASC and office settings, there may be additional legal requirements to consider in obtaining informed consent from a patient. In particular, the anesthesiologist needs to consider whether there are either (1) additional requirements for the patient's informed consent to having the procedure and the anesthesia performed in the ASC or office setting, or (2) additional substantive requirements relating to the nature of the informed consent provided.

Two examples illustrate the possible additional requirements. First, the CMS CfCs for ASCs to participate in the Medicare program require that patients be given information "needed to make an informed decision about whether to consent to a surgical procedure in the ASC."[3] CMS further requires that the informed consent process provide the patient with information on anesthesia risks and benefits. In describing a "well-designed" informed consent process, CMS explains that the informed consent process should cover the "material risks and benefits" related to anesthesia, which could include those risks with a high degree of likelihood but a low degree of severity, as well as those with a low degree of likelihood but a high degree of severity.[4]

Anesthesiologists also need to consider whether state law contains additional requirements relating to informed consent for anesthesia to be performed in the ambulatory setting. For example, Arizona law requires physicians who perform office-based surgery using sedation in an office, non-ASC, or nonhospital setting to obtain informed consent from the patient that "[a]uthorizes the office-based surgery to be performed in the physician's office."[5] Although this requirement may apply to the surgeon, it is important to consider how it may apply to anesthesiologists who perform office-based anesthesia.

Professional association standards

Anesthesiologists practicing in ambulatory and office-based settings should be familiar with professional association standards relating to ambulatory and office-based anesthesia. Compliance with such standards assists in demonstrating compliance with the standard of care. Applicable standards include those of the Society for Ambulatory Anesthesia (such as the *Consensus Statement on Preoperative Selection of Adult Patients with Obstructive Sleep Apnea Scheduled for Ambulatory Surgery*, and the *Guidelines for the Management of Postoperative Nausea and Vomiting*) and the ASA (such as the *Guidelines for Ambulatory Anesthesia and Surgery* and the *Guidelines for Office-Based Anesthesia*).

Regulatory Considerations

Anesthesiologists practicing in ambulatory settings also need to consider legal requirements that apply to their practice.

CMS conditions for coverage

The CMS CfCs are requirements for ASCs to participate in the Medicare program. The CMS regulations require that a physician "examine the patient immediately before surgery to evaluate the risk of anesthesia and of the procedure to be performed,"[6] and that a physician or anesthetist evaluate the patient before discharge for "proper anesthesia recovery,"[7] and they limit the individuals who may administer anesthetics to an anesthesiologist, a certified registered nurse anesthetist (CRNA) or anesthesiologist's assistant (AA), or a "supervised trainee in an approved educational program."[8] Except in opt-out states (states that have opted out of the physician supervision requirement for CRNAs), the nonphysician anesthetist must be under "the supervision of the operating physician"; an AA must be "under the supervision of an anesthesiologist."[9]

The CMS Interpretive Guidelines provide further guidance regarding the regulatory requirements. Several sections of the Interpretive Guidelines relate to anesthesia. The requirements related to anesthetic risk and evaluation are discussed earlier. Other sections of the Interpretive Guidelines outline requirements relating to the requirement of a predischarge evaluation by a physician or anesthetist. The guidelines reference ASA recommendations for routine postanesthesia assessment and monitoring, and reference assessment of the following factors:

1. Respiratory function, including respiratory rate, airway patency, and oxygen saturation
2. Cardiovascular function, including pulse rate and blood pressure
3. Mental status
4. Temperature

5. Pain
6. Nausea and vomiting
7. Postoperative hydration[10]

Because the evaluation must be done by a physician or anesthetist, it is not sufficient for the postanesthesia care unit nurse to monitor and document these indicators.

The Interpretive Guidelines also provide additional information on who may administer anesthesia and the supervision requirements.[11]

State law requirements

Specific requirements relating to administration of anesthesia in ASCs frequently are based on state law. Many states regulate ASCs and, as part of the regulations, outline requirements relating to such matters as who may perform anesthesia; who must perform the preanesthetic assessment; and, in some states, the supervision requirements for nonphysician anesthetists.[12]

Some states regulate office-based surgery and office-based anesthesia. As noted earlier, Alabama and Arizona both have regulations governing office-based surgery. The Federation of State Medical Boards has assembled information regarding states that regulate office-based surgery[13]; those rules often contain specific requirements relating to the administration of anesthesia in offices.

Kickbacks

The federal antikickback statute[14] makes it a criminal offense knowingly and willfully to offer, pay, solicit, or receive any remuneration to induce referrals of items or services that are reimbursable by federal health care programs. "Remuneration" includes the transfer of anything of value, no matter what form the value takes (whether cash, services, or other items of value), and regardless whether it is paid directly or indirectly. Courts have interpreted the statute to cover an arrangement if even 1 purpose of the remuneration is to obtain money (or other value) for the referral of services or to induce further referrals.[15] Thus, a transaction can be illegal even if funds are paid for legitimate services, if any purpose of the remuneration is to induce referrals or to pay for referrals.

A persistent issue related to anesthesia practice at ASCs and in office-based settings has been the efforts of referring physicians to obtain money or other items of value in order to allow the anesthesiologists to provide services at the ASC or office. These efforts have taken many different forms, including having the anesthesiologists absorb some of the ASC's or physician's costs by paying for or providing drugs, equipment, or personnel, or paying for space at the ASC or office. Other efforts have involved so-called "company models" or other structures in which the referring physician's bill for the anesthesia services that either the anesthesiologists or CRNAs provide, pay the anesthesia personnel some amount for their services, and then retain the balance of the anesthesia professional fee.

The legality of many of these arrangements has been the topic of active debate in the legal and medical communities. On June 1, 2012, the Office of Inspector General (OIG) within the Department of Health and Human Services issued an advisory opinion on 2 different proposed arrangements relating to the provision of anesthesia services at ASCs owned by referring physicians or their professional corporations or limited liability companies. The OIG expressed concern that both arrangements might violate the antikickback statute.

In the first arrangement, the anesthesiologists were to pay the ASC owners for management services, which were to include preoperative nursing assessments; adequate space for all of the anesthesiologists, including their personal effects; adequate space for the anesthesiologists' materials, including documentation and records; and assistance with transferring billing documentation to the anesthesiologists' billing office. The management services fee was to be payable only on non–federal health care program patients. In the second arrangement, the ASC owners would set up a separate company that would provide anesthesia services to the ASC's patients. The anesthesiologists would work for the anesthesia company, the referring physicians would bill for their services and pay the anesthesiologists a negotiated rate, and the referring physicians would retain the balance of the professional fees paid for anesthesia services.

The OIG first determined that separating the federal health care program patients from payment of the fee did not avoid implicating the antikickback statute, because there was a risk that the anesthesiologists would be paying the management services fees for non–federal health care program patients to induce the referring physicians to refer of all of their patients, including federal health care program patients. It is significant that the ASCs owned by the referring physicians planned to continue to charge a facility fee, which pays for some of the same services that the management services fee was to cover.

The OIG expressed concern about the company model arrangement, noting that it "appears that [the arrangement] is designed to permit the Centers' physician-owners [the referring physicians] to do indirectly what they cannot do directly; that is, to receive compensation, in the form of a portion of the Requestor's [the anesthesiologists'] anesthesia services revenues, in return for their referrals to the Requestor."[16] Even if the payments to the anesthesiologists could be protected under a so-called safe harbor, a business arrangement that meets regulatory requirements and is not subject to prosecution (discussed later), the retained profit was not subject to such protection. The legality of an arrangement depends on the intent of the parties, so the absence of safe harbor protection does not mean that the arrangement is illegal. The OIG was concerned that the anesthesia company was set up just to provide services to the referring physicians' own patients, and that the referring physicians would not actually participate in the operation of the anesthesia company, which reflected long-standing concerns of the OIG with "suspect contractual joint ventures."

Advisory opinions apply only to the specific facts outlined in the request for the advisory opinion. Nonetheless, they are viewed as helpful guidance to the industry. The referring physician community is trying to restructure arrangements to conform to the OIG guidance, and the anesthesia community is continuing to seek guidance from federal and state agencies on the legality of these arrangements.

Anesthesiologists need to consider whether state law may render arrangements such as the 2 outlined in the OIG advisory opinion and variations on those arrangements unlawful. In particular, state laws barring kickbacks and physician self-referrals and state laws prohibiting fee-splitting may make such arrangements unlawful.

Stark and physician self-referrals

The federal law that limits physician self-referrals, known as Stark II,[17] is a civil federal statute, in contrast with the antikickback statute, which is a criminal law. Stark II prohibits physicians from making referrals for designated health services (DHS) to an entity in which they or their immediate family members have a financial interest, either by way of ownership or compensation, unless an exception applies. The law prohibits the entity from billing Medicare, the patient, or a third party payor for the services or goods provided as a result of such a referral.

The term DHS includes the following services: (1) clinical laboratory services; (2) physical therapy, occupational therapy, and speech-language pathology services; (3) radiology services, including magnetic resonance imaging, computed axial tomography scans, and ultrasound services; (4) radiation therapy services and supplies; (5) durable medical equipment and supplies; (6) parenteral and enteral nutrients, equipment, and supplies; (7) prosthetics, orthotics, and prosthetic devices and supplies; (8) home health services; (9) outpatient prescription drugs; and (10) inpatient and outpatient hospital services.[18]

Neither ASC services nor anesthesia services are DHS, so anesthesiologists performing surgical anesthesia services in an ASC or office typically do not refer for DHS. (In contrast, in a hospital setting, anesthesiologists may refer for inpatient or outpatient hospital services in connection with ordering testing of patients.) Pain physicians may refer for certain categories of DHS and may need to consider how Stark affects their practice.[19]

There is further discussion of how Stark applies to ambulatory anesthesia practice and the exceptions of interest to anesthesiologists in the American Society of Anesthesiologists publication, *Ambulatory Surgical Centers: A Manual for Anesthesiologists* (chapter VII).

Contracts

Contracts and contract interpretation are part of the business of ambulatory anesthesia practice, because anesthesiologists often enter into professional services agreements with ASCs and physician offices. The contracts typically reflect the business terms agreed to by the parties. There is a detailed discussion of contract issues that arise in ASC agreements in the American Society of Anesthesiologists publication, *Ambulatory Surgical Centers: A Manual for Anesthesiologists* (chapter III).

If the ASC or office owners ask the anesthesiologists to provide items or services of value, or require the anesthesiologists to allow the referring physicians or a company they own to bill for the anesthesia services (with the anesthesiologists receiving less than their full professional fees), in exchange for the right to provide services at the ASC or office, the anesthesiologists should consult counsel regarding the legality of the arrangement (discussed earlier).

OWNERSHIP-RELATED LEGAL ISSUES

The other category of legal issues relates to who may own an ASC and the regulatory requirements relating to such ownership. Ownership of an office is not regulated for purposes of Medicare and federal health care programs, in large part because Medicare does not pay a facility fee for procedures performed in offices.

Federal Antikickback Statute Restrictions on Ownership

The concern with investment interests in ASCs is that the ownership interests might be given to physicians as an inducement for them to refer business to the investment ASC. As noted earlier, the antikickback statute is broad in its prohibition. It prohibits offering or paying, or soliciting or receiving any remuneration that is intended to induce referrals of items or services payable under federal health care programs. That prohibition is broad, so Congress directed the OIG to issue so-called safe harbors; practices that, although potentially capable of inducing referrals of business under federal and state health care programs, are not treated as criminal offenses under the antikickback statute. Because the antikickback statute is intent based, the failure to fit within a safe harbor does not mean that the arrangement is illegal. It does mean that it is necessary to review the transaction to assess whether it violates the antikickback statute.

Given the high degree of interest in physician ownership of ASCs, the OIG promulgated a safe harbor relating to investment interests in ASCs.[20] The purpose of the ASC safe harbor is to protect investment interests held by physicians who use the ASC as an extension of their practices. It is focused on surgeons and other physicians who agree to perform no less than one-third of their outpatient procedures at the investment ASC. The safe harbor does not extend to ownership by primary care physicians, because of the concern that ASC ownership by such physicians may be a way to reward them for referrals to surgeons and other investors.

In issuing the safe harbor, the OIG stated that it would look for indicia that the ASC investment represents the extension of a physician's office space, and not a means to profit from referrals.[21] Some of the requirements listed later (in particular the requirements related to [1] performance of one-third of the procedures at the investment ASC, and [2] deriving at least one-third of each physician investor's medical practice income from all sources for the prior fiscal year or prior 12-month period from performance of Medicare-covered procedures [the so-called one-third/one-third test]) are designed to ensure that the investment ASC is an extension of the investing physician's practice.

The safe harbor for ASC investments covers 4 types of ASCs: (1) surgeon-owned ASCs, (2) single-specialty ASCs, (3) multispecialty ASCs, and (4) hospital/physician ASCs. There are detailed requirements pertaining to each type of ASC.[22] Investments in multispecialty ASCs are typically the type in which anesthesiologists wish to invest. The requirements for the safe harbor applicable to multispecialty ASCs include the one-third/one-third test noted earlier. (The safe harbors for the 3 other types of ASCs similarly require that all eligible investors derive at least one-third of their individual medical practice incomes from all sources for the prior fiscal year or prior 12-month period from performance of Medicare-covered procedures.) Because anesthesia services are not on the list of procedures,[23] anesthesiologists do not meet the requirements of the safe harbor for ASC investments. In contrast, pain medicine physicians may be able to satisfy the one-third/one-third test.

As noted earlier, it is not necessary for a transaction to satisfy a safe harbor to be legal. The question is the intent of the parties. Because anesthesiologists do not refer procedures to the investment ASC, an ownership interest is unlikely to be intended as an inducement for the anesthesiologists to refer items or services to the investment ASC. (Pain medicine physicians are in a position to refer cases to an investment ASC, so their situation needs to be assessed separately. As noted earlier, pain medicine physicians may be able to satisfy the one-third/one-third test.) Moreover, to the extent that the one-third/one-third test is intended to ensure that the investment ASC is an extension of the investing physician's practice, that goal is met in the case of anesthesiologists. Their practice at ASC is an extension of their practice. Anesthesiologists often are given opportunities to invest in ASCs to reward them for their efforts in working hard to make the ASC successful, not for any illegal purpose.

In summary, it is not illegal for anesthesiologists to invest in ASCs, but they typically do not satisfy the requirements of the safe harbor for ASC investments.

Stark Law Considerations

The Stark law is unlikely to be implicated in connection with an anesthesiologist's ownership of an ASC. It would be necessary to consider the Stark law issues if the anesthesiologist were to refer to the investment ASC for DHS. In such an unlikely event, it would be necessary to consider what exceptions might apply to cover the ownership interest. Stark law analysis is complex, so anesthesiologists who are concerned with potential Stark issues in connection with ASC practice should consult experienced health law counsel.

State Law Requirements

State law may apply to an anesthesiologist's ownership interest in an ASC. States have passed many types of laws relating to ASC ownership, including the following:

Requirements that referring physicians perform the services themselves

Some state laws require physicians investing in health care facilities to perform clinical services at those facilities in order to refer patients to those facilities. Such laws essentially bar self-referrals, although the term "referral" generally does not include a service provided by the referring physician or a member of the referring physician's group practice. North Carolina is an example of a state with such a self-referral statute.[24]

Disclosure or sunshine requirements

Some states do not prohibit investments in ASCs. Instead, they require disclosure to the patient of the referring physician's ownership interest. For example, in Washington State, if a physician owns an interest in an ASC, the physician must provide the following disclosure before referring a patient to that ASC[25]:

1. Disclose to the patient in writing that the physician has a financial interest in the ASC
2. Provide the patient with a list of effective alternative facilities
3. Inform patients that they have the option to use one of the alternative facilities
4. Assure patients that they will not be treated differently by the referring physician if the patient chooses one of the alternative facilities

Anesthesiologists considering an ASC investment should understand the extent to which state law may regulate their practices, based on such ownership interest. Additional information regarding state law governing ASC investments is available in the American Society of Anesthesiologists publication, *Ambulatory Surgical Centers: A Manual for Anesthesiologists* (chapter VIII). Given the changing nature of state law, anesthesiologists should check for any updates to the laws in the state(s) in which they practice.

SUMMARY

This article is intended to sensitize anesthesiologists to some of the legal issues they may encounter in connection with ASC or office-based practice. Given the complexity of legal issues relating to ambulatory anesthesia, anesthesiologists are advised to consult counsel at an early stage so as to understand the issues that may apply to their practices.

REFERENCES

1. *State operations manual*, appendix L, guidance for surveyors: ambulatory surgical centers, section Q-0061, at page 59. Available at: http://www.cms.gov/Regulations-and-Guidance/Guidance/Manuals/downloads/som107ap_l_ambulatory.pdf. Accessed September 2, 2013.
2. ALA. ADMIN. CODE r. 540-X-10-.01(2)(b) (2013).
3. *State operations manual*, appendix L, guidance for surveyors: ambulatory surgical centers, section Q-0229, at page 133.
4. *State operations manual*, appendix L, guidance for surveyors: ambulatory surgical centers, section Q-0229, at page 134.

5. ARIZ. ADMIN. CODE § R4-16-702.A.5.
6. 42 C.F.R. § 416.42(a)(1).
7. 42 C.F.R. § 416.42(a)(2).
8. 42 C.F.R. § 416.42(b)(1) and (2).
9. 42 C.F.R. § 416.42(b)(2).
10. *State operations manual*, appendix L, guidance for surveyors: ambulatory surgical centers, section Q-0062, at pages 60–1. Available at: http://www.cms.gov/Regulations-and-Guidance/Guidance/Manuals/downloads/som107ap_l_ambulatory.pdf. Accessed September 2, 2013.
11. *Id.* at section Q-0063, at pages 62–4.
12. A detailed listing of state law requirements regarding administration of anesthesia in ASCs as of 2007 is available in *Ambulatory Surgical Centers: A Manual for Anesthesiologists*, published by the American Society of Anesthesiologists, at pages 49–55.
13. Available at: http://www.fsmb.org/pdf/grpol_regulation_office_based_surgery.pdf and http://www.fsmb.org/pdf/GRPOL_Office_Based_Surgery_N-Z.pdf. Accessed March 20, 2014.
14. 42 U.S.C. § 1320a-7b(b).
15. *United States v. Kats*, 871 F.2d 105 (9th Cir. 1989); United States v. Greber, 760 F.2d 68 (3d Cir.), *cert. denied*, 474 U.S. 988 (1985).
16. OIG, advisory opinion 12-06 (2012), at page 10. Available at: http://oig.hhs.gov/fraud/docs/advisoryopinions/2012/AdvOpn12-06.pdf. Accessed September 2, 2013.
17. 42 U.S.C. § 1395nn (section 1877 of the Social Security Act).
18. 42 U.S.C. § 1395nn (h)(6); 42 C.F.R. § 411.351.
19. Further discussion of the Stark law appears in *Ambulatory Surgical Centers: A Manual for Anesthesiologists*, published by the American Society of Anesthesiologists, Chapter VII, at pages 91–115.
20. 64 *Fed. Reg.* 63, 517 (1999). The ASC safe harbor appears in 42 C.F.R. § 1001.952(r).
21. 64 *Fed. Reg.* at 63,535–36.
22. Further detail on the specifics of the requirements appears in *Ambulatory Surgical Centers: A Manual for Anesthesiologists*, published by the American Society of Anesthesiologists, Chapter VI, pages 67–75.
23. The term "procedures" means any procedure(s) on the list of Medicare-covered procedures for ASCs. See 42 C.F.R. § 1001.952(r)(5).
24. N.C. GEN. STAT. §; 90–406.
25. WASH. REV. CODE § 19.68.010(2).

Accreditation of Ambulatory Facilities

Richard D. Urman, MD, MBA*, Beverly K. Philip, MD

KEYWORDS

- Ambulatory surgery center • Accreditation • Ambulatory anesthesia
- Quality improvement • Patient safety

KEY POINTS

- There are significant benefits to accreditation, in addition to fulfilling federal and individual state requirements.
- Accreditation provides external validation of safe practices, benchmarking performance against other accredited facilities, and demonstrates to patients and payers the facility's commitment to continuous quality improvement.
- There are several options for accreditation of ambulatory facilities, and each accrediting organization has its own unique philosophy, standards, process measures, and pricing structures.
- Accreditation organizations are increasingly emphasizing continuous quality improvement and outcomes measurement.

INTRODUCTION

With the continued growth of ambulatory surgical centers (ASC), the regulation of facilities has evolved to include new standards and requirements on both state and federal levels. Accreditation allows for the assessment of nursing and medical practice, improves accountability, and better ensures quality of care.[1–3]

ASCs are heavily regulated in most states, where specific licensure and other local regulatory prerequisites must be satisfied. It is important to differentiate the concepts of licensure, certification, and accreditation. *Licensure* allows the facility to operate and provide services and is granted by and required in the most states. *Certification* is granted by the Centers for Medicare and Medicaid Services (CMS) and is a regulatory requirement for all ASCs that intend to provide care to Medicare or Medicaid beneficiaries.[4] The number of Medicare-certified ASCs increased more than 18% from 4441 in 2005 to 5260 in 2009, and total Medicare payments also increased from $2.7 to $3.2 billion.[5] The facility must meet CMS Conditions of Participation in the

Departments of Anesthesiology, Perioperative and Pain Medicine, Brigham and Women's Hospital, Harvard Medical School, 75 Francis Street, Boston, MA 02115, USA
* Corresponding author.
E-mail address: rurman@partners.org

Anesthesiology Clin 32 (2014) 551–557
http://dx.doi.org/10.1016/j.anclin.2014.02.016 **anesthesiology.theclinics.com**
1932-2275/14/$ – see front matter © 2014 Elsevier Inc. All rights reserved.

Medicare program before it is allowed to bill for medical services it provides.[6] *Accreditation* is granted by various private organizations and indicates that a facility has met certain standards. For example, the Healthcare Facilities Accreditation Program is authorized by CMS to survey hospitals, laboratories, and other facilities to ascertain compliance with CMS standards.

ACCREDITING ORGANIZATIONS

In some states, ambulatory surgery centers may choose to voluntarily apply for accreditation from a recognized organization, but in others it is mandated. The facility must show compliance with standards regarding the environment of care, the provision of care, and the quality of care. Regular surveys of the organization's performance by the accrediting agency are intended to ensure the quality of care provided to the patients. The accreditation process provides evidence to all stakeholders such as patients, payers, and regulators that the facility meets nationally accepted standards.[7] Accreditation from one of the nationally recognized accrediting organizations is achieved via an onsite visit from surveyors with significant clinical experience. The survey determines if the facility can be accredited based on meeting a specific set of criteria. Currently, ASC accrediting organizations include The American Association for Accreditation of Ambulatory Surgery Facilities (AAAASF), The Accreditation Association for Ambulatory Health Care (AAAHC), and The Joint Commission (TJC). Although the goal of each organization is to ensure quality by providing an external source for evaluating provision of care, each agency has its own unique mission, scope, oversight, and organizational histories, and each develops their own accreditation processes and programs and sets their own accreditation standards.[3]

Up-to-date information about the accreditation process can be found on each organization's Web site. The AAAASF Regular Standards and Checklist for Accreditation of Ambulatory Surgery Facilities Manual[8] contains the most recent surgical program standards and is summarized in **Table 1**. These standards emphasize the need for an effective operating room policy, addressing such things as facility maintenance and safety, safe administration of fluids and medications, record keeping, anesthesia services and post-anesthesia care, and quality assessment and improvement programs.

The AAAHC evaluation process is based on a facility's own unique set of criteria. Although the actual content of their standards is proprietary, it is found in the 2013

Table 1	
AAAASF surgical program standards	
Manual Section #	**Section Title**
100	Basic mandates
200	Operating room policy, environment and procedures
300	Post-anesthetic care unit (PACU)
400	General safety in the facility
500	Intravenous fluids and medications
600	Medical records
700	Quality assessment/quality improvement
800	Personnel
900	Anesthesia

Data from Refs.[7,8,9,15,16,18]

Accreditation Handbook Including Medicare Requirements for Ambulatory Surgery Centers. **Box 1** shows a general outline of AAAHC standards.

The third nationally recognized accrediting organization is TJC, which accredits and certifies more than 19,000 health care organizations and programs in the United States.

During the last decade, TJC revised its survey process by offering a new format using tracer methodology.[9] The emphasis is on greater standardization in the quality management process with the currently used approach called "Shared Visions-New Pathways", which also emphasizes periodic self-assessment.[10] Standards and other requirements are outlined in the Comprehensive Accreditation Manual for Ambulatory Care and Comprehensive Accreditation Manual for Office-Based Surgery. Both manuals contain patient-focused standards organized around health care functions and processes. **Box 2** outlines key areas of assessment emphasized by TJC.[11]

DEEMED STATUS

An accrediting organization may apply and qualify for so-called *deemed status* with CMS, which is an effort by the federal government to find cost-effective and efficient ways to ensure quality of care in ASCs by allowing another organization to serve as its proxy. Nationally recognized accrediting organizations such as TJC, AAAHC, and AAAASF have secured such an agreement with CMS whereby they provide CMS with evidence that the accredited facility meets the required federal regulations, including the "Conditions for Coverage." After the verification process is complete, the facility can receive CMS accreditation without undergoing a separate survey.[4] CMS Conditions for Coverage include several elements, such as compliance with state licensure laws; governing body and management; surgical and nursing services; and evaluation of quality, environment, medical staff, medical records, pharmaceutical, laboratory, and radiologic services.[6]

Box 1
AAAHC standards for ASCs

1. Patient rights
2. Governance
3. Administration
4. Quality of care provided
5. Quality management and improvement
6. Clinical records and health information
7. Infection prevention and control and safety
8. Facilities and environment
9. Anesthesia services
10. Surgical and related services
11. Pharmaceutical services
12. Diagnostic and other imaging services

Adapted from Mercier DW, Philip B. Is your ambulatory surgery center licensed, accredited or certified? ASA Newsl 2008;72(10):10–2; and Accreditation Association for Ambulatory Health Care (AAAHC). Medicare deemed status surveys for ASCs. Available at: http://www.aaahc.org/en/accreditation/ascs/test-medicare-deemed-status-surveys-for-ascs/. Accessed September 14, 2013, with permission.

Box 2
Summary of TJC standards and other requirements for ambulatory health care

Environment of Care: How safe, functional and effective the environment for patients, staff, and other individuals is in the organization.

Emergency Management: Ensures the provider has a disaster plan in place.

Human Resources: Processes for staff and physician management.

Infection Prevention and Control: How the provider identifies and reduces the risk of acquiring and transmitting infections.

Information Management: How well the ambulatory care provider obtains, manages, and uses information to provide, coordinate, and integrate services.

Leadership: Reviews structure and relationships of leadership, the maintenance of a culture of safety, quality, and operational performance.

Life Safety: Only applicable to organizations designated as "ambulatory health care occupancy." Covers requirements for ongoing maintenance of building safety requirements during and after construction.

Medication Management: Addresses the stages of medication use, including selection, storage and safe management of medications, ordering, preparing and dispensing, administration, and monitoring of effect and evaluation of the processes.

National Patient Safety Goals: Specific actions ambulatory care organizations are expected to take to prevent medical errors, such as miscommunication and medication errors.

Provision of Care: Covers 4 basic areas: planning care, implementing care, special conditions, and discharge or transfer.

Performance Improvement: Focuses on using data to monitor performance, compiling and analyzing data to identify improvement opportunities, and taking action on improvement priorities.

Record of Care: Covers the planning function (components of clinical records, authentication, timeliness, and record retention) as well as documentation of items in the patient record.

Rights of the Individual: Informed consent, receiving information, participating in decision making, and services provided to respect patient rights.

Transplant Safety: Applies only to ambulatory organizations using tissues as part of the provision of care.

Waived Testing: Covers policies identifying staff responsible for performing and supervising waived testing, competency requirements, quality control, and record keeping.

Required Written Documentation: Identifies elements of performance in the *Comprehensive Accreditation Manual for Ambulatory Care* and *Comprehensive Accreditation Manual for Office-Based Surgery* requiring written documentation. See the Required Written Documents article in the manual for complete details.

From The Joint Commission. Ambulatory care accreditation overview: a snapshot of the accreditation process. 2013. Available at: http://www.jointcommission.org/ambulatory_care_accr_overview/. Accessed September 14, 2013; with permission.

AMBULATORY FACILITY REGULATION BY STATES

Each state has a specific set of regulations governing ASC and office-based practice. Unlike ASCs, only a handful of states require accreditation of office-based facilities, although an increasing number of states are tightening their control over office-based practices[12] and a growing number of states now require accrediting entities to evaluate office practices instead of using state inspections.[5] Roughly 30 states have specific regulations, statues, or guidelines regarding anesthetic practice in an office setting.[13] For example, New York ASCs must obtain accreditation from AAAHC or another named accrediting organizations within 2 full years of operation. After an initial licensing inspection, the state accepts accreditation surveys in lieu of its own relicensing inspections. In the case of office-based surgery (OBS), 2009 legislation (S.6052) requires that OBSs may only be performed by physicians in accredited settings and performing surgery in an unaccredited setting would constitute professional medical misconduct. The new law also requires physicians in these practices to report adverse events to the state Health Department's Patient Safety Center within 24 hours. This includes patients who die within 30 days of a procedure, unplanned transfers to hospitals, or other "serious or life-threatening" events. Data from these reports are protected under the new legislation and are not subject to public disclosure under state "freedom of information" act requests, but can be included in reports that aggregate such outcome data.[14]

Florida accepts the survey report of an accrediting organization as substantial compliance, but those ASCs not accredited by AAAHC or another approved accrediting organization are subject to an annual licensure inspection survey. Regarding OBS, Florida law requires Department of Health inspections for physician office facilities where certain levels of surgery are performed, unless a nationally recognized accrediting agency or another accrediting organization approved by the Board of Medicine accredits the offices. Physicians performing certain levels of surgery in an office are required to register with the board and indicate whether their office is accredited or subject to a state inspection. Although the rules recognize AAAHC as an approved accrediting agency, the rules also require compliance with several state standards for OBS.[14]

In California, Senate Bill 100 became effective on January 1, 2012 and amended the existing law requiring the accreditation of outpatient settings. Accreditation agencies are now required to query the Medical Board of California concerning any adverse accreditation decisions rendered against physician owners of an organization applying for accreditation. For outpatient settings that failed accreditation by another accrediting agency, the subsequent accreditation agency must determine that prior deficiencies were corrected. The law also requires the Medical Board to post certain survey reports of accreditation agencies on its Web site.[14]

QUALITY REPORTING AND OUTCOMES

CMS recently announced details of its new quality reporting program for ASCs. Under this program, ASCs that fail to report required information face a 2% reduction in their Medicare payments. As of October 1, 2012, ASCs are required to report data on the following 5 quality measures: patient burn, patient fall, wrong site/side/patient/procedure/implant, hospital admission/transfer, and prophylactic intravenous antibiotic timing. Additional measures introduced for 2013 include using the Safe Surgery Checklist[15] and reporting the volume of certain procedures.[16]

Regulatory and accreditation processes have traditionally concentrated on processes of care and looked at structural and process measures rather than actual outcomes.[7,17,18] There is now a trend toward outcomes research and accreditation. It is increasingly being viewed as a desirable process to establish standards and provide quality care, although there is limited evidence that accredited organizations actually provide higher-quality health care.[3] A recent study compared quality outcomes from accredited ASCs with those from nonaccredited facilities located in Florida,[17] analyzing patient discharge data and rates of unexpected hospitalizations between nationally accredited and nonaccredited ASCs. The only significant finding was that patients at TJC-accredited facilities were 10.9% less likely to be hospitalized after colonoscopy within 7 days of the procedure. No other differences in unexpected hospitalization rates were detected in the other procedures analyzed in this study. It is possible that the lack of differences in patient outcomes may be due to the already tight state regulation of ASC facilities in Florida.

In summary, there are significant benefits to accreditation, in addition to fulfilling state and federal CMS requirements. It provides external validation of safe practices, benchmarking performance against other accredited facilities, and demonstrates to patients and payers the facility's commitment to continuous quality improvement.[4] There are several options for accreditation of ambulatory facilities, and each accrediting organization has its own unique philosophy, standards, process measures, and pricing structures. Accreditation organizations are increasingly emphasizing continuous quality improvement and outcomes measurement.

REFERENCES

1. Lapetina EM, Armstrong EM. Preventing errors in the outpatient setting: a tale of three states. Health Aff (Millwood) 2002;21(4):26–39.
2. Vallejo BC, Flies LA, Fine DJ. A comparison of hospital accreditation programs. J Clin Eng 2011;32–8.
3. Viswanathan HN, Salmon JW. Accrediting organizations and quality improvement. Am J Manag Care 2000;6(10):1117–30.
4. Mercier DW, Philip B. Is your ambulatory surgery center licensed, accredited or certified? ASA Newsl 2008;72(10):10–2.
5. Becker's ASC review: 25 Statistics on Medicare reimbursements in ambulatory surgery centers. Available at: http://www.beckersasc.com/asc-coding-billing-and-collections/25-statistics-on-medicare-reimbursements-in-ambulatory-surgery-centers.html. Accessed September 14, 2013.
6. Centers for Medicare and Medicaid Services: Ambulatory Surgery Centers. Available at: http://www.cms.gov/Medicare/Provider-Enrollment-and-Certification/GuidanceforLawsAndRegulations/ASCs.html. Accessed September 14, 2013.
7. Saufl NM, Fieldus MH. Accreditation: a "voluntary" regulatory requirement. J Perianesth Nurs 2003;18(3):152–9.
8. American Association for the Accreditation of Ambulatory Surgical Facilities (AAAASF). Regular standards and checklist for accreditation of ambulatory surgery facilities version 13. 2011. Available at: http://www.aaaasf.org/aboutus.html. Accessed September 14, 2013.
9. DeLorenzo M. Shared visions-new pathways: what to expect at your next JCAHO survey. Nurs Manage 2005;36(3):26–30 [quiz: 1].
10. Cohen JA, Brull SJ, Maurer WG. Quality management, regulation, and accreditation. In: Twersky RS, Philip BK, editors. Handbook of ambulatory anesthesia. 2nd edition. New York: Springer Press; 2008. p. 372–93.
11. The Joint Commission. Ambulatory care accreditation overview: a snapshot of the accreditation process. 2013. Available at: http://www.jointcommission.org/ambulatory_care_accr_overview/. Accessed September 14, 2013.
12. Urman RD, Punwani N, Shapiro FE. Patient safety and office-based anesthesia. Curr Opin Anaesthesiol 2012;25(6):648–53.
13. Federation of State Medical Boards. Office-based surgery states A-M: board-by-board statutes, regulations and policies. Available at: http://www.fsmb.org/pdf/GRPOL_Regulation_Office_Based_Surgery.pdf. Accessed September 14, 2013.

14. Accreditation Association for Ambulatory Health Care (AAAHC). State requirements for accreditation. Available at: http://www.aaahc.org/en/news/State-Laws-and-Regulations/. Accessed September 14, 2013.
15. World Alliance for Patient Safety. WHO surgical safety checklist and implementation manual. 2008. Available at: http://www.who.int/patientsafety/safesurgery/ss_checklist/en/. Accessed December 30, 2013.
16. Ambulatory Surgery Center Association. Quality reporting FAQs. Available at: http://www.ascassociation.org/ASCA/FederalRegulations/Medicare/QualityReporting/QualityReportingFAQs. Accessed September 14, 2013.
17. Menachemi N, Chukmaitov A, Brown LS, et al. Quality of care in accredited and nonaccredited ambulatory surgical centers. Jt Comm J Qual Patient Saf 2008; 34(9):546–51.
18. Pawlson LG, Torda P, Roski J, et al. The role of accreditation in an era of market-driven accountability. Am J Manag Care 2005;11(5):290–3.

Anesthesia Information Management Systems in the Ambulatory Setting

Benefits and Challenges

Ori Gottlieb, MD

KEYWORDS

- Anesthesia information management system • AIMS • EHR • EMR
- Electronic medical record • Electronic health record • Anesthesia • Informatics

KEY POINTS

- The salient benefits of using an anesthesia information management system include medical record review, support links, organization of information, automatic transfer of vitals, legibility, integration with the electronic health record, decision support, menus, compliance, icons that communicate patient status, and registries.
- The challenges of implementing an anesthesia information management system include report management, the so-called forest-for-the-trees dilemma, garbage in/garbage out, the requirement of experience for short cases, device integration, support and downtimes, alerts after the fact, workstation reliability/availability, cost, and medicolegal concerns.
- Once implemented, the benefits of an anesthesia information management system outweigh the challenges, but understanding where the potential obstacles lie is critical to removing them efficiently and effectively.
- As different anesthesia information management systems continue to spread throughout the medical world, so will their benefits.

The anesthesia record is the most detailed general physiologic and pharmacologic account in routine clinical practice.[1] Its two main uses are for support of patient care during the delivery of an anesthetic and for review.[2] An anesthesia information management system (AIMS) captures and produces this record electronically during the periprocedural period. The AIMS is often the last component of the electronic health record (EHR) installed at institutions because of the challenges associated

Disclosure: The author has no relationships with any commercial companies that have a direct financial interest in the subject matter discussed in this article.
Department of Anesthesia and Critical Care, University of Chicago, 5841 South Maryland Avenue, MC 4028, Chicago, IL 60637, USA
E-mail address: ori@uchicago.edu

Anesthesiology Clin 32 (2014) 559–576
http://dx.doi.org/10.1016/j.anclin.2014.02.019
1932-2275/14/$ – see front matter © 2014 Elsevier Inc. All rights reserved.

with capturing the enormous quantity of data and presenting it in a useful and coherent manner.

BENEFITS
Medical Record Review

Because the anesthesiologist has limited time in which to review a patient's record before a procedure, scrutinizing a paper chart for relevant information can be frustrating and can leave the clinician with incomplete information. With the introduction of an AIMS, much of the preanesthesia evaluation is transformed into a report, largely compiled from the EHR. The anesthesiologist completes the preanesthesia evaluation by reviewing the report with the patient, asking time-sensitive questions (eg, nil-by-mouth status), and formulating an assessment and plan. If the patient's medical status was evaluated before the day of the procedure, much of the data may already have been entered into the electronic chart. The provider may even prepare for the anesthetic several days before the procedure by reviewing the chart from another room, another hospital, or even from home. Already having much of the patient's information previously reviewed may be more reassuring to the patient than asking for information at the bedside.[3]

All anesthesiologists are familiar with having to ask: 'who has the chart?' (**Fig. 1**). With an AIMS, the paper chart contains only those documents that have yet to be scanned into the EHR (eg, consent form). Questions that arise during treatment, like details of a previous surgery, can be answered with a few clicks (**Fig. 2**). The anesthesiologist can review not only the preanesthesia evaluation, but how the case is proceeding, as well as every other part of the patient's record. A supervising anesthesiologist can follow along from a postanesthesia care unit (PACU) terminal or another room.

Perhaps the greatest benefit is the ability to review a patient's previous anesthetic records for airway management and other medical concerns. Surgeons can prescribe antibiotics in advance, and anesthesiologists can ensure that a pregnancy test or

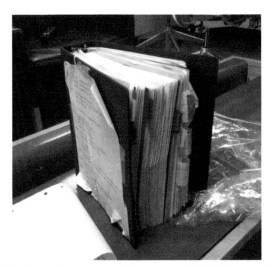

Fig. 1. It does not take long after go-live to forget how difficult it was to find information in a paper chart. The benefit of having the data so readily available to the anesthesiologist is soon taken for granted.

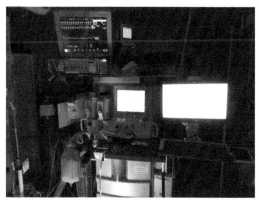

Fig. 2. With the computer equipped for access to the AIMS mounted on either the right side of the anesthesia machine (as seen above), on the left, or both, patient data are only a few clicks away. After using the system for only a short period of time, the method of documenting events, medications, and procedures becomes second nature.

glucose reading was performed. Workflow is standardized and communication is enhanced to increase efficiency.

Support Links (Information Buttons)

As an anesthesiologist reviews the chart, some items in the lists of medical diagnoses, surgeries, and medications may be unfamiliar. The EHR links terms to databases for additional information, which enables point-of-care referencing. Eponyms that once required a pocket reference booklet can now be defined with a mouse click. Some institutions award continuing medical education credits when clinicians review articles they access from within the EHR.

Organization of Information

Anesthesiologists can navigate from one section to another, finding a potassium level in Labs, a chest radiograph in Images, or a surgeon's entry filed by name and date of the encounter in Notes. Filters help to find a specific document, such as a previous anesthesia record. The provider locates the relevant data in the place they should reside with confidence that, if a radiograph or test is not found, it likely was not performed.

Automatic Transfer of Vital Signs

The anesthesiologist is responsible for creating a document that provides a clinically accurate portrayal of what occurred during delivery of an anesthetic. An intraoperative AIMS is superior to handwritten records in the categories of completeness and efficiency in recording vital signs.[4] On paper, blood pressure carets may be placed in the wrong spot or medications may be charted in the wrong row or with incorrect/missing units. With an AIMS, the anesthesiologist does not have to allocate attention and time to transcribing data onto paper during a procedure. Vital signs are transmitted and documented throughout the procedure, even during unstable periods. Although the vital signs may not reflect as smooth a delivery of an anesthetic as they would on paper, it can be argued that paper records never contain all the irregularities they should. A pulse oximeter reading of 65% because of electrocautery interference does not reflect reality, nor does an arterial line reading from a transducer that is set 20 cm too high (**Fig. 3**). Once these artifacts are identified and corrected and/or

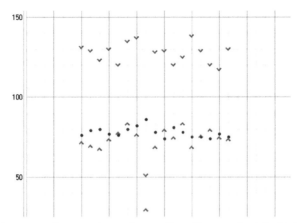

Fig. 3. A blood pressure that was deemed an artifact. The anesthesiologist is left with a decision of whether to leave the grid or to delete it. Regardless, a note is appropriate explaining that the patient's blood pressure likely did not decrease to 50/30 mm Hg.

explained, the accuracy of the AIMS is increased. However, it has been argued that without manually charted vital signs an automated record can be created without ever passing through the consciousness of the anesthesiologist.[5]

Automatic transfer of vital signs requires the occasional attention of an anesthesiologist but is far less than that required by continual documentation on a paper record. Because an anesthesiologist is responsible for producing a record that accurately reflects the procedure's events, data should be edited when appropriate.[6] The nearly ubiquitous concern regarding automatic transfer of vital signs disappears once the anesthesiologist becomes accustomed to using the system and can appreciate its benefits (see **Fig. 3**).

Legibility

There are many benefits of being able to read a medical chart, especially for anesthesiologists who have to review previous records, consult notes, and consent forms (**Fig. 4**). Anesthesiologists caring for the patient on a future date, professionals reviewing charts for quality of care, auditors, researchers, lawyers, and others can determine what was done during delivery of an anesthetic. From the medicolegal perspective, defending decisions made during a procedure is easier with a legible chart that describes events clearly than with an illegible chart that can be misinterpreted to reflect malpractice.

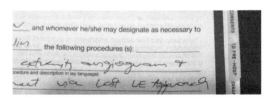

Fig. 4. Checking a consent form before performing a regional block is a key element of the preblock time-out. However, in this case it is not clear whether the operative site is an arm or leg. When consents become digital with electronic signatures, illegible entries such as this will be eliminated.

AIMS is Integrated with the EHR

Just as a diagnosis of asthma entered by an internist can be seen by an anesthesiologist, when an anesthesiologist documents a procedure such as an axillary block, it becomes part of the patient's EHR. Another example is the documentation of medications. If a β-blocker is given (a compliance issue), the documented dose in the AIMS is displayed in the medication administration record. Safety may be affected by the timing of antibiotic and heparin administration, which may become clearer with an AIMS.

As fluid administration is documented during a procedure, the system tabulates totals and merges them with the comparable section in the EHR. Total surgery time is reported easily, as well as other relevant metrics (eg, tourniquet time). These data can be pulled into notes or reports, further increasing consistency among the different teams. For instance, the total volume of crystalloid infused can be updated throughout the procedure and then fed into the handoff note, brief operative note, and nursing notes. The surgeon no longer needs to ask how much fluid was given.

Decision Support

With the goal of reducing errors, federal initiatives exist under the term meaningful use to incentivize institutions to incorporate EHRs. One example is decision support for computerized physician order entry. When a medication such as an antibiotic is ordered in the preprocedure area, the EHR can cross-check it against an allergy list as well as other medications and alert the physician of any conflicts (**Fig. 5**). The system may even suggest an antibiotic and dose based on the patient's planned procedure and body mass index. When blood is treated as a medication, antibodies listed in the problem list or allergy list can be cross-checked with blood transfusion orders (see **Fig. 5**).

Other examples of preprocedure decision support include reminders to order and document the result of a pregnancy test, consider stress-dose steroids, check a potassium level for patients on dialysis, prepare for a difficult airway for a patient with such a history, and send a sample of blood for a patient who may have blood antibodies (**Fig. 6**).

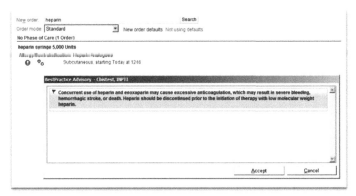

Fig. 5. An allergy alert for a patient with an intolerance to heparin and a best-practice advisory alert notifying the clinician that administering heparin while the patient is already taking enoxaparin may be dangerous. Both are forms of clinical decision support and a key benefit to using an EHR.

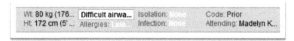

Fig. 6. The anesthesia information management system can be programmed to display alerts. In this case, "difficult airway" is highlighted in the header.

Parameters such as a low temperature can be set during the procedure period that alert the clinician to a change in patient status and may suggest placing a warming device. Algorithms and protocols may be programmed into the AIMS to help the clinician decide which antibiotic to administer. An antibiotic pop-up reminder can appear before incision, assisting with a surgical care improvement project metric that tracks preoperative antibiotic administration.[6] Prompts for airway documentation may appear after the anesthesiologist documents administration of a muscle relaxant. Although clinical judgment cannot be replaced, computerized decision-support systems with practice guidelines should help improve patient care and safety.[7]

Menus

Drop-down menus assist with documentation before, during, and after a procedure. Templates built into preanesthesia evaluations, with the required elements highlighted, help an anesthesiologist fill out a complete and compliant evaluation (**Fig. 7**). Identifying the most commonly observed review of system items and including them in easy-to-select Yes/No menus saves the clinician time. During the procedure,

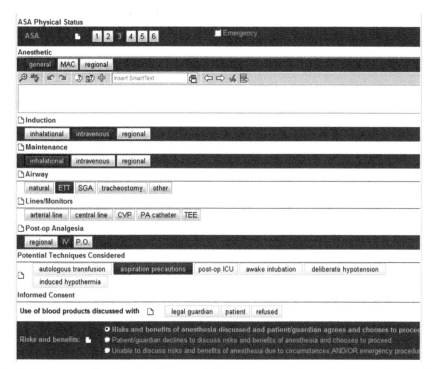

Fig. 7. This preanesthesia evaluation template includes several required elements, as listed by the interpretive guidelines published by the Centers for Medicare and Medicaid Services. A purple background has been added to the required elements.

reminders alert the anesthesiologist to tasks yet to be completed and, when clicked, lead directly to a series of menus for documentation of airway management, staffing, positioning, and monitoring (**Fig. 8**).

Once the most commonly used medications are identified by the department, menus can be built that list them by category, removing the need to search for a medication and select the appropriate concentration, dose, and route.[8] The same concept is applied to airway maneuvers, regional nerve blocks, and other interventions. After the procedure, the handoff note can remind the clinician to include certain fields (eg, vital signs, pain score, absence of nausea).

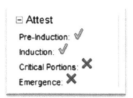

Fig. 8. One of the many ways icons and reminders can help the anesthesiologist complete required tasks and stay compliant.

Compliance

Documenting on a standard template for both the preanesthesia and postanesthesia evaluation may improve compliance and chart completion. Clinicians not only know where to enter every required data element but they can scan to see whether an item was missed. Checks can be used in real time, alerting the anesthesiologist to incomplete sections (eg, discussion of risks and benefits for informed consent). Hard stops may be programmed to require completion of certain elements, such as attestations.[6,9] Audits of charts are straightforward because the elements on these forms can be created directly from guidelines set forth by regulatory agencies. Even naming conventions can assist with inspections and reviews (eg, postanesthesia evaluation) (**Fig. 9**).

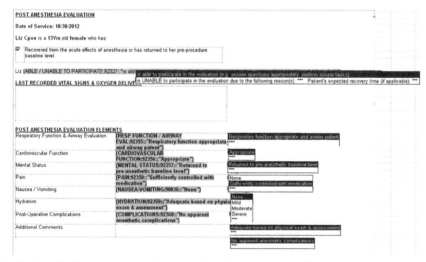

Fig. 9. As with the preanesthesia evaluation, the postanesthesia evaluation template can force the anesthesiologist to answer a set list of queries to comply with the requirements of the Centers for Medicare and Medicaid Services.

Icons Communicate Patient Status

As the patient progresses from one location to another and certain elements are completed, icons can be triggered by nurses and physicians to appear on status boards. These status boards can be viewed from a computer, tablet, or cell phone, as well as locations in the procedural suite (**Fig. 10**) A simplified status board without patient identifiers can be placed in the waiting room for families (**Fig. 11**).

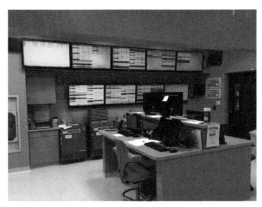

Fig. 10. Status boards have revolutionized communication among team members. As the patient's status changes, colors and icons communicate those changes to others. Here the charge nurse is sitting at the central command center. The boards on the wall reflect the status of each patient having a procedure that day.

Status Board - Full Screen - CD7 Sky Lobby CD5 GI & CERT SB (fs) [500631] for 9/13/2013

GI PROCEDURES		GI PROCEDURES		GI PROCEDURES	
AB.3208	OUT OF ROOM	FF.2840	IN PRE	MK.3403	IN ROOM
AG.3857	IN POST	GH.1943	IN ROOM	MS.9088	Scheduled
AG.5808	Scheduled	GL.3932	Scheduled	PK.6585	Scheduled
AG.9049	IN PRE	GM.5507	IN PRE	PP.8881	Scheduled
AK.2077	SENT FOR	GR.3092	IN PRE	RB.3055	IN WAITING
AM.5770	IN POST	HK.0822	SENT FOR	RD.5644	Scheduled
BB.6132	Scheduled	HS.0653	Scheduled	RE.7640	IN WAITING
BF.0391	Scheduled	JL.7418	IN PRE	RL.6933	IN PRE
CG.3646	Scheduled	JM.7869	Scheduled	SG.4428	Scheduled
CH.8751	Scheduled	JP.0425	Scheduled	SG.7087	IN ROOM
CL.9049	IN POST	JW.1756	IN POST	SP.4741	IN ROOM
CS.9834	IN POST	KC.7624	Scheduled	TD.0133	DISCHARGED
DK.6517	Scheduled	KJ.2667	Scheduled	TJ.7727	Scheduled
DN.2152	DISCHARGED	LJ.4028	Scheduled	VB.9511	SENT FOR
DP.0044	SENT FOR	MC.5079	Scheduled	VW.8088	Scheduled
EG.0163	Scheduled	MH.4938	IN PRE		

Fig. 11. The patient's status is updated during perioperative progression. This information helps clinicians and the patient's family. The status board can be displayed in the family waiting room. Patient privacy is protected with initials and code numbers. Families waiting for news can track the family member's progress.

Icons can reflect task completion, proceduralist availability, consent status, isolation status, delay codes, American Society of Anesthesiologists physical status, and the activities that have been completed in the preanesthesia evaluation. During a procedure, icons can help the anesthesiologist keep track of whether key elements have been performed (eg, airway documentation), orders have been entered, and attestations signed. After the procedure, clinicians can determine whether a patient needs to be or has been discharged from the PACU simply by reviewing a status board. The anesthesiologist can be confident that, if certain icons are displayed on the status board, certain activities have taken place.

Registries

There are several databases (eg, Anesthesia Quality Institute, the Society of Ambulatory Anesthesia Clinical Outcome Registry, the Multicenter Perioperative Outcomes Group) that collect data for the purpose of quality, outcomes, research, and education. Once an institution agrees to submit data to these registries, it is granted access to data submitted by other institutions. As a common dictionary of terms is standardized, merging data and compiling information becomes possible. Because anesthesiologists practice in greater solitude than most other clinicians, information about what colleagues are doing is helpful. This information can include length of procedures (**Fig. 12**), type of anesthetic (**Fig. 13**), and American Society of Anesthesiologists physical status by age (**Fig. 14**).

Feedback about variance from what is commonly done potentially improves care and reduces cost.[10] Using these registries, individuals and groups can benchmark their performance against larger aggregates of practitioners.[6,11] How often are certain anesthesia techniques being used? How many patients get certain complications? How long do certain procedures take? What staffing do other institutions devote to certain procedures?

Do academic centers take longer to do hips?				
Facility type	Case #	% Redo	Mean duration (min)	StDev (min)
Outpt SC	75	11%	158	54
Freestanding	162	1.8%	157	31
Specialty	239	2.5%	106	24
Unknown	865	16%	152	56
Academic	1,004	20%	228	77
Small	2,026	7.4%	155	41
Large	9,364	14%	148	53
Medium	25,929	12%	155	93

Fig. 12. The Anesthesia Quality Institute registry indicates that total hip arthroplasties take longer at academic institutions than in large private hospitals. Time at free-standing surgicenters is between the two. (*From* Anesthesia Quality Institute. Available at: http://www.aqihq.org/index.aspx. Accessed February 12, 2014; with permission.)

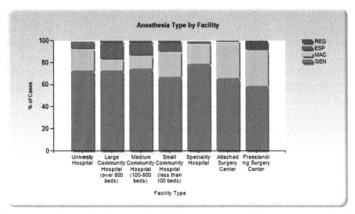

Fig. 13. The types of anesthetics used at different types of facilities. ESP, epidural/spinal anesthesia; GEN, general anesthesia; MAC, monitored anesthesia care; REG, regional anesthesia. (*From* Anesthesia Quality Institute. Available at: http://www.aqihq.org/index.aspx. Accessed February 12, 2014; with permission.)

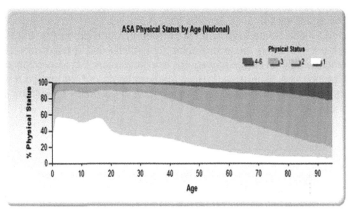

Fig. 14. The Anesthesia Quality Institute provides a perspective beyond each clinician's institution. American Society of Anesthesiologists (ASA) physical status graphed against age. (*From* Anesthesia Quality Institute. Available at http://www.aqihq.org/index.aspx. Accessed February 12, 2014; with permission.)

Summary of benefits

The benefits of using an AIMS go beyond those that have been discussed here. Residents who have never charted on paper find it difficult to understand how it was ever done and clinicians who have made the transition may miss certain aspects of old days, but few would abandon the AIMS to revert to paper. Going digital has brought the rest of the chart into the anesthesia record and, perhaps more importantly, has introduced the anesthesia record to other clinicians. The end result is an intraprocedural anesthesia record that is complete, easy to read, and does not fade with copying or time.[7]

CHALLENGES
Report Management

With an EHR, a chronologic or linear chart is replaced by events that result in the generation of reports. There must be strict rules for how each event report is constructed and where it resides, and the institution should define parameters and conduct education sessions on a regular basis to ensure uniformity and conformity. The anesthesiologist must know whether the results from a nuclear stress test are found under Procedures, Radiology, Cardiology, or Results. Clear protocols that are integrated into training courses and subsequently enforced help to keep clinicians on the same (correct) page.

Forest-for-the-trees Dilemma

Largely because of the prevalence of templates, copy forwarding, and the pulling in of data, EHR notes are often longer than comparable paper notes. Identifying significant and relevant clinical points within documents can be challenging because clinicians include any data they think might be important. Comprehensive laboratory values or results from a complex procedure may yield a note that is excessively long. Limiting results to the most recent tests may not be helpful if it is weeks, months, or years old.

There are 2 ways to view this problem: (1) the important points may be lost among the abundance of noisy data, or (2) abundant data points provide so much detail that they obscure the bigger picture. A solution may be for the clinician to enter a deliberate note with the relevant points focused in a well-crafted assessment and plan, just as was done on paper. The reader then reviews the rest of the note as necessary.

Garbage In, Garbage Out

Worse than excessively long notes are notes containing errors. The EHR makes it easier to propagate an error (eg, an allergy, contact status, or diagnosis) from visit to visit. Clinicians are often reluctant to remove or even change patient data for fear of making a mistake. To minimize this problem, the institution must clearly designate which team is responsible for cleaning up the chart. The obvious choice is the admitting and discharging primary care teams rather than the anesthesiologist.

Short Cases Require an Experienced AIMS User

Short cases are likely to require proportionately more time for record keeping[4] and an AIMS may delay throughput.[7] Time-saving case-specific templates for a wide variety of cases may be helpful. This problem is most significant immediately after implementation (known as go-live) and diminishes as proficiency improves. Shadow charting with the AIMS while using paper before go-live greatly reduces anxiety and reduces inefficiency with short procedures.

Device Integration

Device integration is defined as processing patient data from devices (eg, monitors, pumps, ventilators) and transferring them into the AIMS. More and more devices will be connected to the EHR, including medication dispensers, cardiac pacemakers, so-called smart pumps, endoscopic capsules, and intrathecal pumps. A medical device integration solution is needed to package the output, translate each variable, and assign it to a destination cell within the EHR (**Fig. 15**). Integration is critically important when patients move from one area to another because vital signs and other data have to reflect the correct patient as information is acquired from different devices in different locations. Device integration is often underappreciated before go-live and

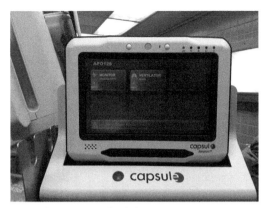

Fig. 15. Choosing among the many medical device integration companies can be difficult. The most widely used products, made by Cerner, iSirona, and Capsule, all have advantages and disadvantages. For instance, Capsule's Neuron is a solid performer when working correctly but struggles with buffering problems and user interface.

continues to affect systems well beyond. Charting on the wrong patient in the EHR is an example of what may happen when device integration is applied incorrectly.

Support and Downtimes

It is challenging to determine the correct level of support during the AIMS go-live period and beyond. Although at-the-elbow support is critical during the first few days after go-live, it must be scaled back at a rate that is appropriate for each institution. Tweaks to the system will continue and a mechanism for a quick response is critical. Immediately addressing changes to the system after go-live is paramount for 2 reasons: (1) the habits of clinicians have yet to be formed, and (2) information technology support and resources are still focused on the AIMS. As time passes, users become resistant to changes in workflow, and information technology staff will be assigned to other projects.

Downtime occurs, whether upgrades and adjustments are planned or unplanned because of a system failure. During these times, the anesthesiologist must be prepared to enter vital signs manually into the AIMS or return to paper documentation. Paper options for preanesthesia evaluations, intraoperative records, order sets, requests for or results from laboratory tests, and image viewers must be available and familiar to clinicians. Although system failures during the before and after periods may only cause inefficiencies, those during the intraoperative phase distract the anesthesiologist in the midst of a procedure and may potentially create an unacceptable clinical situation.

Alerts After the Fact

Although the EHR offers decision support and acts as a safety mechanism before and after a procedure, it is less helpful during a procedure. Anesthesiologists typically administer a medication first and document it second, eliminating the benefit of a cross-check; for example, with Allergies. It is still unclear how radio frequency identification or barcode scanning of medications will be integrated into the workflow of the anesthesiologist, but the technologies have such promise that they are likely to be incorporated.

Workstation Reliability and Availability

To benefit from the AIMS, clinicians must be able to easily access a reliable workstation. There must be enough workstations equipped with rapid log-on functionality to support the needs of anesthesiologists, surgeons, and nurses. When they fail, support must be available immediately.[12] Because of the urgent nature of the anesthesiologist's work, a rapid-access bypass of the hospital's general help line should be created.

Many AIMS let sessions roam from one workstation to another. For instance, an anesthesiologist leaving an operating room with a patient may secure the computer, enter the recovery room, and log into another terminal that loads where the record was left. The advantage is quick access to the patient's chart. However, such a system may have problems, particularly with multiple open sessions trying to migrate across different platforms. The result is a confusing array of error messages and unfamiliar screen images, leaving the clinician wondering why all of the workstations cannot be programmed to behave in similar ways (**Fig. 16**). The solution is to use a standardized rapid log-on program that is installed on identical workstations throughout the work area.

Cost

The initial investment can be large and varies from vendor to vendor. The 5 main components are hardware, software, implementation assistance (workflow redesign), training, and ongoing maintenance.[13] Although the incentives from federal agencies help, they do not cover the costs and, as the incentives are converted to withholding of reimbursement, they may even add to the cost rather than defray it.

In 2012 and 2013, Athena Health conducted a survey of 507 and 1199 physicians, respectively. The overall opinion of an EHR's impact on patient care remained favorable at 70% each year. The perception of cost/benefit was mixed, with only 50% stating that the financial benefits outweighed the costs (**Figs. 17** and **18**).[14] Long-term benefits may offset some of the costs (eg, reduced testing, increased efficiency) (**Fig. 19**), but a perspective that goes beyond short-term financial considerations is required. For the AIMS, cost recovery may be found in reducing anesthetic-related drug costs, improving staff scheduling, increasing anesthesia billing by capture of anesthesia-related charges, and improving hospital reimbursement through accurate coding.[15]

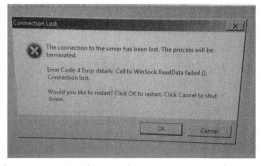

Fig. 16. Anesthesiologists accessing the EHR do not want to see obscure error messages. The help-desk experts they call may not understand or appreciate the time-sensitive context within which the anesthesiologist often works.

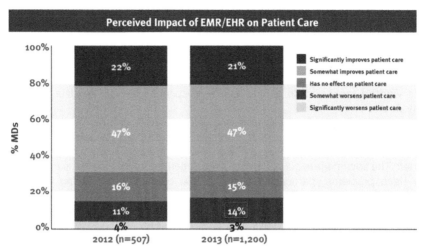

Fig. 17. From surveys in 2013, most physicians (MDs) think that the EHR has at least some positive impact on patient care; in 2013, 68% had that opinion. EMR, electronic medical record. (*From* Athena Health. 2013 Physician sentiment index. Available at: http://www.athenahealth.com/physician-sentiment-index/_doc/2013_Physician_Sentiment_Index.pdf. Accessed February 12, 2014; with permission.)

However, an AIMS that stands alone without integration into institution-wide EHRs is of limited value.[7,11] Until an institution implements system-wide EHRs, adding an AIMS is marginally helpful. Even with an installed EHR, the anesthesiologist is only slightly better off than with paper charts if the EHR does not integrate with the AIMS.

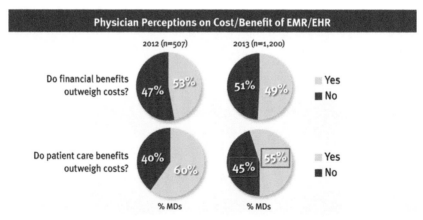

Fig. 18. The Athena Health Survey found that, by a slight margin, most physicians thought that patient care was worth the cost of the EHR. Opinion was divided on whether the program was cost-effective. (*From* Athena Health. 2013 Physician sentiment index. Available at: http://www.athenahealth.com/physician-sentiment-index/_doc/2013_Physician_Sentiment_Index.pdf. Accessed February 12, 2014; with permission.)

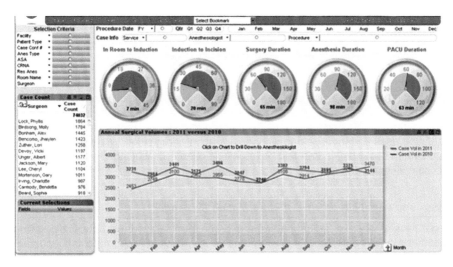

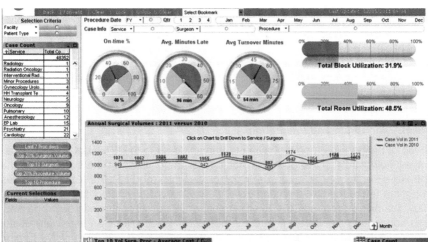

Fig. 19. Two examples from Surgical Information Systems show dashboards that reflect metrics of efficiency. They can be run automatically on a schedule and highlight areas of efficiency and areas that need improvement. (*Image courtesy* of Surgical Information Systems, LLC, Alpharetta, GA. Copyright © 2013 Surgical Information Systems LLC. All rights reserved.)

Medicolegal Concerns

The anesthesia record is critical to the determination of the standard of care given to any patient. Expert witnesses use the anesthesia record as the most objective rendition of events during a procedure. When the standard of care is met, the ideal record is accurate, legible, and supports an effective defense. When it is not met, it is better to explain a problem that did occur and was properly charted than to have to defend against charges of cover-up and fraud.[16] A well-maintained AIMS record is superior to a handwritten record in malpractice cases. It is unclear whether all data captured by the AIMS are discoverable, including those points that do not ultimately make it to the official anesthesia record.[17,18] Until federal standards are secure, the database of all AIMS should either be erased after an official anesthesia record is signed or be kept in a separate repository.

THE FUTURE
Standardization

There are already some standards with which EHR data must comply, such as the International Classification of Disease (ICD), Current Procedural Terminology (CPT), Systematic Nomenclature of Medicine, and Health Level Seven. The next step will be to standardize the language with which anesthesiologists communicate. For instance, within the AIMS, the term pulse may have to yield to the more accurate term heart rate. CPT and ICD codes define procedure and diagnosis terms that every institution uses and these, along with the adoption of registries, will likely force standardization. Data entry in free-text boxes will be reduced, resulting in easy and reliable record review.

Access and Portability in a Health Information Exchange

Regardless of where a patient receives care, the medical record is accessible, giving anesthesiologists potentially lifesaving data as they develop and implement an anesthesia plan. There may be a central depository of medical charts that health care institutions can access, with little personal patient information stored at the health care facility. Privacy concerns will continue, and the conflict of keeping health records private while ensuring their availability must be resolved. A patient chart will be divided into public and private sections, and passwords and other security measures will limit access. At some point, patients will carry their health records on a chip embedded in a bracelet, necklace, or watch. It is likely that in the future patients will have these chips implanted inside them.

Wireless Monitoring and Integration

Instead of the bedside monitor having to transmit data to the EHR, data from the patient will flow wirelessly to both the monitor (for the clinician at the scene) and to a centralized server where it can be incorporated into the EHR. As a patient moves throughout the procedure area and beyond, wirelessly transmitted data will continue to flow seamlessly into the EHR. Even in transport, data will continue to be processed. Wires connecting monitors will become obsolete, which will be an especially useful evolution during procedures on prone patients and procedures that involve turning an operating room table.

Standard pump technology will aid in the integration of data from devices into the AIMS, freeing the clinician from documenting adjustments for each pump. Because of standardization through a central server, pump medication libraries will be updated regularly, reducing programming errors. With the pump integrated into the AIMS, checks within the program will prevent miscalculations and other errors.[7]

Mobile Technology

Clinicians are rapidly incorporating technology into everyday workflow. Carrying a display device wirelessly linked to a patient's EHR, anesthesiologists can better monitor their patients. Such a device will be customizable and trigger alerts preset by the anesthesiologist. In addition to being notified when the patient enters the room, the system will be able to communicate information such as when vitals migrate beyond a percentage of baseline or when laboratory values are abnormal. These devices will replace phones and pagers and improve efficiency and communication among the team members.

SUMMARY

Moving to an AIMS is a challenge for an anesthesia department. The transition requires a physician champion and the support of members in every section. This change can be facilitated by visiting similar institutions that are already using AIMS, shadow charting for a sufficient period of time, and understanding that optimization continues after the go-live date. Once implemented, the benefits outweigh the challenges, but understanding where the potential obstacles lie is critical to removing them efficiently and effectively. As different AIMS continue to spread throughout the medical world, so will their benefits. Patients will endure fewer repeat tests, hospitals will address care concerns with comprehensive information, and anesthesiologists will appreciate having patient data a mouse click away.

REFERENCES

1. Cook RI, McDonald JS, Nunziata E. Differences between handwritten and automatic blood pressure records. Anesthesiology 1989;71:385–90.
2. Ream AK. Automating the recording and improving the presentation of the anesthesia record. J Clin Monit 1989;5:270–83.
3. Klafta JM, Roizen MF. Current understanding of patients' attitudes toward and preparation for anesthesia: a review. Anesth Analg 1996;83:1314–21.
4. Edsall DW, Deshane P, Giles C, et al. Computerized patient anesthesia records: less time and better quality than manually produced anesthesia records. J Clin Anesth 1993;4:275–83.
5. Noel TA II. Computerized anesthesia records may be dangerous [letter]. Anesthesiology 1986;64:300.
6. Douglas JR Jr, Ritter MJ. Implementation of an anesthesia information management system (AIMS). Ochsner J 2011;11:102–14.
7. Balust J, Macario A. Can anesthesia information management systems improve quality in the surgical suite? Curr Opin Anaesthesiol 2009;22:215–22.
8. Marian AA, Dexter F, Tucker P, et al. Comparison of alphabetical versus categorical display format for medication order entry in a simulated touch screen anesthesia information management system: an experiment in clinician-computer interaction in anesthesia. BMC Med Inform Decis Mak 2012;12:46.
9. Driscoll WD, Columbia MA, Peterfreund RA. An observational study of anesthesia record completeness using an anesthesia information management system. Anesth Analg 2007;104:1454–61.
10. Frank SM, Savage WJ, Rothschild JA, ot al. Variability in blood and blood component utilization as assessed by an anesthesia information management system. Anesthesiology 2012;117:99–106.
11. Kadry B, Feaster WW, Macario A, et al. Anesthesia information management systems: past, present, and future of anesthesia records. Mt Sinai J Med 2012;79:154–65.
12. Muravchick S, Caldwell JE, Epstein RH, et al. Anesthesia information management system implementation: a practical guide. Anesth Analg 2008;107:1598–608.
13. Available at: www.healthit.gov. Accessed October 7, 2013.
14. Athena Health Survey. Available at: http://www.athenahealth.com/physician-sentiment-index/future-of-medicine.php?intcmp=PSI/MEANINGFUL-USE-INCENTIVES.PHP&intcmp=l000859. Accessed October 7, 2013.
15. O'Sullivan CT, Dexter F, Lubarsky DA, et al. Evidence-based management assessment of return on investment from anesthesia information management systems. AANA J 2007;75:43–8.

16. Lane P, Feldman JM. Legal aspects of AIMS. In: Stonemetz J, Ruskin K, editors. Anesthesia informatics. London: Springer-Verlag; 2008. p. 227–46.
17. Epstein RH, Vigoda MM, Feinstein DM. Anesthesia information management systems: a survey of current implementation policies and practices. Anesth Analg 2007;105:405–11.
18. Feldman JM. Do anesthesia information systems increase malpractice exposure? Results of a survey. Anesth Analg 2004;99:840–3.

Quality Management and Registries

Richard P. Dutton, MD, MBA

KEYWORDS

- Ambulatory anesthesia • Quality management • Registries
- Anesthesia Quality Institute • National Anesthesia Clinical Outcomes Registry

KEY POINTS

- Continuous improvement in outcomes is a professional obligation of all anesthesiologists.
- What is not measured cannot be improved; data collection is critical to quality management in anesthesia.
- Participation in national registry efforts allows an ambulatory anesthesia practice to benchmark its performance against other practices and providers.
- Reporting outcome data is a sensitive topic, and must be customized for each practice and each piece of information.

WHY QUALITY MANAGEMENT IS IMPORTANT AND HOW TO DO IT

Striving to improve patient outcomes is a professional obligation of every anesthesiologist. This obligation applies no less in ambulatory practice than in office-based practice. Most patients in the outpatient setting are in good health and most procedures are routine, but there is always opportunity for improvement. Major adverse events are rare, but operational metrics are as important as in any practice, and patient-centered outcomes even more so. This article describes basic principles of quality management (QM) in ambulatory anesthesiology, provides resources for external benchmarking and education, lists the indicators and outcome measures that should be pursued, and concludes with some ideas for reporting QM data and reacting to unusual events.

In addition to professional obligation, QM reporting will soon be needed for practice viability. The notion of pay for performance is strongly influencing government and private-payor activities.[1] Although efforts such as the Physician Quality Reporting

Dr R.P. Dutton is Executive Director of the Anesthesia Quality Institute, a nonprofit public charity devoted to creation and maintenance of the National Anesthesia Clinical Outcomes Registry.
Anesthesia Quality Institute, 520 North Northwest Highway, Park Ridge, IL 60068, USA
E-mail address: r.dutton@asahq.org

Anesthesiology Clin 32 (2014) 577–586
http://dx.doi.org/10.1016/j.anclin.2014.02.014
1932-2275/14/$ – see front matter © 2014 Elsevier Inc. All rights reserved.

System (PQRS) began as incentive programs designed to encourage public reporting of clinical outcomes, they are transitioning now to penalty programs that will rapidly escalate into mandatory requirements for provider payment. Both public and private quality reporting are strongly emphasized under the Affordable Care Act. Under new payment models incorporating bundled and capitated payments, quality measures are a necessary public safeguard to protect against skimping on indicated care. Participation in a national benchmarking registry is an emerging standard for anesthesia practices, and is likely to become the most expedient way to meet multiple regulatory requirements. In the specific realm of ambulatory surgical care, institutional requirements for quality data reporting are just as important. Organizations such as the Accreditation Association for Ambulatory Health Care (AAAHC) are developing performance metrics for public reporting that will necessitate the participation of anesthesiologists.[2]

W. Edwards Deming, the father of QM in American business, is famously paraphrased as saying that those things that cannot be measured cannot be improved.[3] The essence of QM is the ability to measure and to understand a practice in a way that encourages continual improvement. This process requires the collection and reporting of objective data. In a perfect world, anesthesiologists would learn something from every patient for whom they provide care. **Box 1** summarizes the basic steps in creating a QM program, including the collection and reporting of patient-based data. A few of these points are worthy of comment.

First, anesthesia practice culture and human dynamics are such that best results are achieved with a single person in charge. Designating a QM officer for the practice and making it this person's responsibility to do the job creates a level of accountability that leads to tangible results. Other opinions are welcome and should be included, especially when considering outcomes in different subspecialty areas, but the project works better with a single individual in charge.

Once the administrative structure is created, the QM officer and assistants should begin a search for data. In the so-called Information Age, there is a lot of data already in existence and a good QM program begins by harvesting all available material before creating anything new. In our present fee-for-service health care system, every anesthetic is remunerated from a digital record, meaning that somewhere in every practice (or its billing company) is a record of every case performed. This file includes patient specifics (age, sex, American Society of Anesthesiologists [ASA] physical status,

---

Box 1
Essential steps in creation of an anesthesia QM program

- Designate a single individual to lead the effort
- Recruit interested participants from the practice
- Collect and investigate sentinel cases
- Collect structured data for every case from billing and medical record systems
- Collect relevant clinical outcomes (may require creating new data capture tools)
- Benchmark practice performance to internal trends and external peers
- Identify outliers in the data, and determine why
- Create reports for the public, for facility leadership, for the practice, and for individuals
- Make changes to improve care
- Repeat continuously

medical record number), the time and location of the case, the specific surgical and anesthetic procedures performed (typically represented by Current Procedural Terminology [CPT] codes), and the identity of all providers involved.[4] This information provides a critical overview of the practice, reveals demographic changes over time, and provides denominator data for interpretation of events and outcomes.

A minority of anesthesia practices today have a system in place for capturing patient outcomes from every case, but this will soon be a requirement. One role of the QM committee is to define outcomes of interest and develop the infrastructure needed to collect these data. The guiding principle in this effort should be to steal, collaborate, and create. Because physicians have little desire to fill out additional forms, no matter how valuable the resulting data might be, the effective QM officer must build a system that operates as much as possible through passive data collection. Inquiry might reveal that someone in the facility is already collecting much of the relevant data. For example, measurement of patient satisfaction is a requirement for hospital systems, whereas identification of unexpected admission after outpatient surgery is a required activity for accredited ambulatory surgery centers (ASCs).[2] Rather than creating a new form to gather these data, the QM officer should find out who already has it and request a copy. If the data do not exist, the next step should be a collaboration with facility QM personnel. It is often the case that these individuals are happy to gather data on the part of the anesthesia department when provided with some input on what measures to collect (discussed later) and some reassurance that the data will be put to good use. As a last resort, the QM officer should consider asking practitioners to generate new data. This step is most likely to be necessary for outcomes that are specific to anesthesia practice, such as the occurrence of a difficult airway or an inadvertent dural puncture. This data collection should be built into existing documentation tools (such as the Anesthesia Information Management System [AIMS]), and should be as simple and structured as possible. Examples of anesthesia department quality capture forms, and technical suggestions for how to implement them, are available on the Anesthesia Quality Institute (AQI) Web site at www.aqihq.org.

As a final piece of data collection infrastructure, the QM officer should build a pipeline for identifying unusual cases and sentinel events. Although the collection of aggregate and structured case data represents top-down QM, there is just as much to be learned from a bottom-up approach that begins with review of individual cases in which something went wrong. This kind of peer review is familiar to most providers, and in many groups leads to the traditional morbidity and mortality conference. Single case review is complementary to data-driven QM, and the ideal QM program includes both elements working in a synergistic fashion.[5]

With data in hand, the QM committee should turn its attention to analysis and response. Often, simple awareness of results provides the necessary impetus for change. A single provider who can see that the practice is out of step with peers is already highly motivated to improve; methods for QM data reporting that are intended to enhance this effect are discussed later. Some problems require either a more proactive approach on the part of the committee or a more global perspective. Participation in a national data registry provides access to performance benchmarks that can indicate areas in need of improvement for the group. Options for this are presented later. The QM committee should be unafraid to tinker with department and facility policy, especially when the data suggest that improvement is possible. Examples include changes to preoperative patient assessment, new rules for operating room (OR) use, or revised postanesthesia care unit (PACU) order sets to improve pain management. Identifying an area for improvement, making a change in practice, and then using QM data to document the benefit creates a story that shows the value of the QM program to internal participants and external stakeholders.

In addition, all parties concerned should recognize that QM is an infinite activity conducted with finite resources. Improvement in patient care is always possible. The job of the QM officer is to apply the resources available in the institution to resolve the issue of greatest importance at that moment, recognizing that, as soon as one problem is addressed, another will present itself. Although this kind of never-ending cycle can seem frustrating at first, it becomes highly rewarding when looking back on the improvement in patient outcomes that occurs over time. This kind of iterative progress, leading from small steps to big improvements, has distinguished anesthesiology in the house of medicine and is something of which to be justly proud.

EXTERNAL RESOURCES AND REGISTRIES

The initial benefit of a QM program arises from internal use of the data collected. At first, this is no more than a snapshot of what the practice does: numbers and types of cases and patients. As time passes, accumulating data reveal trends over time that can be used to make changes in practice. One of the most obvious might be the gradually increasing number of cases done on an outpatient basis; **Fig. 1** shows this rate on the national level with data abstracted from the National Anesthesia Clinical Outcomes Registry (NACOR). Even over the 4 years of this registry's scope, a significant change can be seen; other sources confirm that this change in practice demographics has been underway for decades.[6]

When a practice has a good understanding of its own data, the next step is to seek external comparators. Human curiosity and innate competitive spirit make anesthesiologists and their groups eager to compare performance with their peers. The emerging federal regulations described earlier provide a powerful incentive to understand how one clinician's outcomes compare with other anesthesiologists and groups. Even before financial rewards for good performance become meaningful, an internal understanding of the benchmarked performance of the group is critical

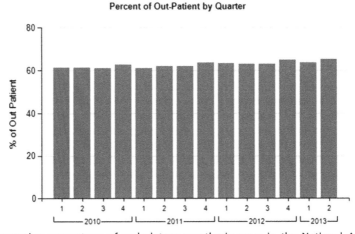

Fig. 1. Increasing percentage of ambulatory anesthesia cases in the National Anesthesia Clinical Outcomes Registry: 2010 to 2013. There has been a 5% increase nationally since the inception of the registry.

for internal operations and for acquiring and defending hospital and facility contracts. Where can these external benchmarks be obtained?

The most granular and specific registry of ambulatory anesthesia care is the Clinical Outcomes Registry (SCOR), created by the Society for Ambulatory Anesthesia (SAMBA).[7] Practices participating in SCOR complete an electronic data form for every case, which includes patient demographics, procedure specifics, technical details of the anesthetic, and short-term patient outcomes (OR and PACU complications). These forms are periodically uploaded to the national registry, and the participating practices receive regular reports on their performance, benchmarked across all participating groups. SCOR was designed by practicing anesthesiologists with interest and experience in ambulatory care, and has been refined over several iterations to be as user friendly as possible. Participation in SCOR is strongly recommended for any group with a large portfolio of ambulatory anesthetics, although strong leadership is needed to achieve buy-in for data collection, or to build in the SCOR metrics to an existing electronic record.

Participation in SCOR requires commitment by the members of the practice; both in paying the modest membership fees charged by SAMBA and in investing the individual time and effort required to complete the data forms for every case. Another option, more in keeping with the principle of minimizing the need for the provider or group to input data, is participation in the NACOR, operated by the AQI.[8] NACOR participation is open to any anesthesia practice in America, and costs are waived for ASA members. NACOR accumulates data by direct monthly collection from existing digital sources, including billing systems, QM and patient satisfaction programs, and AIMS. No additional effort is required of individual practitioners, beyond the documentation already routine in their practice, which has led NACOR to grow rapidly, with more than 20% of all anesthesiologists nationwide now participating. The downside is the heterogeneity of the data collected. Although analysis of SCOR data and benchmarking across groups is easy because every group is gathering the same data using the same technology, analysis of data in NACOR requires careful interpretation and sorting, to ensure apples-with-apples comparisons. The depth of data in NACOR is also less than in SCOR, because most practices do not yet capture clinical outcomes in an accessible digital format.

Several private groups also collect QM data from anesthesia practices. These groups may be organized across large commercial entities (eg, Kaiser Permanente or the Hospital Corporation of America), be based in university or academic networks (eg, the Multicenter Perioperative Outcomes Group or the University Healthcare Consortium), be run by billing and practice management companies, or be the result of loose coalitions of independent practices (eg, the Anesthesia Business Group). These collaboratives are good for generating peer-group benchmarks from the participating practices, and many of them can also serve as conduits to send data to the AQI.

In the long term, ambulatory anesthesia practices that take QM seriously should participate in both SCOR and NACOR. A memorandum of understanding is in place between SAMBA and the AQI that allows free exchange of data between the two. The goal for the practice is to collect granular information using the SCOR template from ambulatory cases, while also sending the bulk of practice data (including a duplicate of the SCOR information) to NACOR. Reporting from SAMBA provides detailed and subject-specific benchmarks for ambulatory cases, benefitting from the intellectual capital of this group of experts. Reporting from NACOR puts the ambulatory subset into context within the total operations of the practice and the experience of a national peer group.

WHAT DATA TO COLLECT

Box 2 shows AQI recommendations for data collection in ambulatory anesthesia cases. This list should be viewed as aspirational; no practice yet collects all of this information for every case, although every item suggested here is collected by at least one group. The QM officer should begin at the top of the list, and seek every possible method to steal, collaborate on, and (if necessary) create these data.

Clinical outcomes are the core of this list and are of the greatest interest to providers. It is appropriate to begin with the outcomes that can be easily observed in the OR and PACU, such as intraoperative cardiac arrest, difficult airway management or reintubation, anaphylaxis, and serious neurologic injury. In the future,

---

Box 2
Suggested data to support ambulatory anesthesia QM. Data elements are organized from most to least accessible in current practice

Demographics (for each case)
- Case type (CPT code)
- Surgical or procedural service
- Surgeon or proceduralist
- Anesthesia providers
- Anesthesia type
- Case duration (start and stop times)

Patient information
- Age
- Sex
- ASA Physical Status
- Height and weight (or body mass index)
- Comorbidities, by present-on-admission ICD-9 (International Classification of Diseases, Edition 9) code

Outcomes
- Administrative issues
  - Case canceled
  - Case delayed (list reasons)
  - Delayed PACU discharge (list reasons)
- Safety issues
  - Major complications (list)
  - Unplanned admission or emergency room transfer
  - Minor adverse events (corneal abrasion, dental injury, and so forth)
- Patient experience
  - Overall satisfaction
  - Satisfaction with anesthesia providers
  - Occurrence of postoperative nausea or vomiting
  - Adequacy of pain management

more robust information technology connectivity will enable collection of longer-term outcomes: return to preoperative health, 30-day and 1-year survival, myocardial infarction, late pulmonary complications, and so forth, which are examples of shared accountability measures that reflect the performance of the entire team (facility, surgeon, and anesthesiologist), and thereby avoid the biases that result from attempts to attribute outcomes to a particular service or provider. Although adverse outcomes are sometimes the result of one provider (eg, dural puncture headache), it is more likely that an adverse outcome is multifactorial (eg, perioperative myocardial ischemia). All-cause, shared accountability measures are the easiest to interpret and will be of greatest significance to payors, regulators, and patients in the future.

The final section of recommended measures discussed here relates to patient experience. The idea of patient-centered outcome measures is becoming established in federal regulatory efforts, and is embedded in the Affordable Care Act's creation of a Patient-Centered Outcomes Research Institute (PCORI) to fund and coordinate work in this area.[9] Efforts to measure global patient satisfaction with ambulatory surgery have been underway for years, especially on the facility side of the team. Few anesthesia departments see these results and there is a universal opportunity for anesthesiologists to collaborate with facility QM personnel to collect, analyze, and report these data. Key components of patient satisfaction with anesthesia are safety, communication skills, postoperative nausea and vomiting, and the adequacy of pain management.[10] Few ASCs collect structured information on these topics and report it back to providers, but this is likely to change in the near future. The easy availability of software to support text, email, online, and voice-response data collection systems is reducing the traditional burden of nurses making postoperative phone calls to outpatients. Recommendations for how to collect patient experience data and links to information technology vendors that support these efforts are available at www.aqihq.org.

HOW TO USE QM DATA

In order to motivate change in practice, QM data must be turned into information for clinicians, which is accomplished through analysis and reporting. As was indicated earlier, the QM officer and committee should reflect on the best way to report their data. This information can range from purely private information, shared with no one but the individual provider, to metrics shared within the department and reports prepared specifically for public consumption. Each approach has its own merits and shortcomings, and QM reporting should be customized to the specifics of the practice, the patients, and the public climate.

Reporting at the individual level that shows variation across providers within the group can be useful for metrics that are within a provider's control. Because public disclosure might be embarrassing (eg, patient satisfaction data), private reporting could be considered first. The practices that best manage this are currently those that arrange for individual physician data to go straight to the physician, without being seen by anyone else, including the QM officer. Anesthesiologists in the group see their own results compared with the group average and are free to improve their own practices. Educational materials can be provided and accessed anonymously, often through the satisfaction-reporting software. Although definitive studies have yet to be performed, anecdotal experience suggests that such a reporting system will lead to improvements in patient satisfaction overall, yielding a group result that can and should be reported publicly.[11]

Private reporting at the group level is appropriate for unadjusted data, serious outcomes, and individual contributions to group metrics. One example might be the rate of occurrence of rare events, such as intraoperative cardiac arrest. With an average rate of about 1 per 1800 cases (current NACOR data) the statistical power to identify differences at the level of an individual provider is limited. Differences are just as likely to occur from bad luck as from bad practice and, because this is a serious occurrence, there will be substantial resistance to any kind of public reporting without extensive risk adjustment and highly accurate data.[12] This type of metric should be gathered at the group level, benchmarked to other similar practices (through a registry such as NACOR), and addressed only when the data show significant deviation from the norm.

Public reporting can occur at the group, facility, or national level. Within the group, it is reasonable to share most data about business operations, overall financial returns, and those process indicators (such as completion of required documentation) that are deemed critical to group success. Sometimes public embarrassment within the group can create the peer pressure needed to turn performance around. Another area in which public discussion is valuable is in the discussion of sentinel events. The QM officer should strive to create a climate in which open dialogue about difficult situations and bad outcomes is accepted. Creation of this kind of culture depends both on laws protecting peer-review activities from legal discovery and on the faith of those present that the discussions will go no further than their circle of colleagues. Most states have laws protecting this kind of internal discussion, but Florida and Kentucky are notable exceptions. Facilitating these conversations is an important activity of the QM officer.

Reporting from the QM program to external stakeholders, such as the hospital or ASC, should be carefully considered. Current Joint Commission standards require that physician credentialing be based on individual performance metrics (the Ongoing Professional Practice Evaluation),[13] but this thinking is increasingly incompatible with team-based care. Most practices have chosen only innocuous metrics to report in this way, such as compliance with antibiotic administration or attendance at department meetings. Of more value are data that show improvement by the group in processes that are important to the hospital. Patient satisfaction has already been mentioned; other examples include on-time first case starts, adequacy of postoperative pain management, and reintubation rate in the PACU. Data showing steady and sustained performance by the group are valuable in internal discussions, contract negotiations, and as exemplars to share with external auditors.

An exception to the general preference for group rather than individual metrics is the use of QM data for maintenance of certification and licensure. These activities are necessarily individual, but can be facilitated by a QM program that can share practitioner-level data when needed.[14] On the national level, both SAMBA and the AQI are working to provide practice reports that can be used in this way.

At the highest level of reporting are data intended for submission to government programs such as PQRS. By design, the provider-level data submitted to these programs, incentivized by financial rewards (or future penalties), are intended for transparent sharing with the public. This requirement has led to predictable evolution of bureaucratic detail in defining and risk adjusting the measures, and to a paradoxic unwillingness to report data that show substantial variation across providers or practices. Anesthesiology currently has the highest rate of PQRS participation of any specialty,[15] but the measures reported (**Box 3**) are not what might be considered critical to anesthesia quality. Future modifications to PQRS are expected to expand the available measures for anesthesiologists and emphasize participation in external registries, but it will take many years of building confidence in the reporting mechanisms

> **Box 3**
> **Measures available to anesthesiologists under the PQRS**
>
> - Timely administration of indicated perioperative antibiotics
> - Observation of a bundle of sterile precautions during central line placement
> - Normothermia on PACU arrival for cases lasting more than 60 minutes, or evidence of active warming efforts in the OR

and the risk-adjustment methodology before the results are widely accepted as accurate.

SUMMARY

QM is an important part of any anesthesia practice and is just as important for ambulatory surgery as for any other specialty. Although the overall principles are similar, QM in outpatient surgery practices should focus on patient satisfaction and operational efficiency. Adverse events will be rare, but should be collected and discussed within the group on a case-by-case basis. The group should contribute their data to a national registry such as SCOR or NACOR, and should take advantage of the benchmarking information that will then be available.

REFERENCES

1. Curfman GD, Morrissey S, Drazen JM. High-value health care — a sustainable proposition. N Engl J Med 2013. [Epub ahead of print].
2. Available at: http://www.aaahc.org/en/institute/clinical-performances/. Accessed September 18, 2013.
3. Gabor A. The man who discovered quality: how W. Edwards Deming brought the quality revolution to America. New York: Penguin; 1992. ISBN: 0-14-016528-2.
4. Dutton RP, Dukatz A. Quality improvement using automated data sources: The Anesthesia Quality Institute. Anesthesiol Clin 2011;29(3):439–54.
5. Macario A. Managing quality in an anesthesia department. Curr Opin Anaesthesiol 2009;22:223–31.
6. Horton B, Doyle B. Day case surgery: a modern view. Br J Hosp Med (Lond) 2005;66:631–3.
7. Available at: http://www.sambahq.org/professional/scor-clinical-outcomes-registry/. Accessed September 18, 2013.
8. Grissom TE, DuKatz A, Kordylewski H, et al. Bring out your data: the evolution of the National Anesthesia Clinical Outcomes Registry. Int J Comput Models Algorithms Med 2011;2:51–69.
9. Available at: http://pcori.org/. Accessed September 18, 2013.
10. Chanthong P, Abrishami A, Wong J, et al. Systematic review of questionnaires measuring patient satisfaction in ambulatory anesthesia. Anesthesiology 2009;110:1061–7.
11. Frenzel JC, Kee SS, Ensor JE, et al. Ongoing provision of individual clinician performance data improves practice behavior. Anesth Analg 2010;111(2):515–9.
12. Glance LG, Neuman M, Martinez EA, et al. Performance measurement at a "tipping point". Anesth Analg 2011;112:958–66.
13. Available at: http://www.jointcommission.org/mobile/standards_information/jcfaqdetails.aspx?StandardsFAQId=213&StandardsFAQChapterId=74. Accessed September 18, 2013.

14. Culley DJ, Sun H, Harman AE, et al. Perceived value of board certification and the Maintenance of Certification in Anesthesiology Program (MOCA®). J Clin Anesth 2013;25:12–9.

15. Available at: http://www.cms.gov/Medicare/Quality-Initiatives-Patient-Assessment-Instruments/PQRS/index.html?redirect=/PQRS/. Accessed September 18, 2013.

Index

Note: Page numbers of article titles are in **boldface** type.

A

Accreditation, of ambulatory facilities, **551–557**
    accrediting organizations, 552–553
    deemed status, 553–554
    quality reporting and outcomes, 555–556
    regulation by states, 554–555
Acetaminophen, rectal dosing for pediatric ambulatory surgical patients, 420–422
Acute pain management. *See* Pain Management, acute.
Administrative issues, in office-based surgery, 432–437
Airway management, **445–461**
   anesthetic emergence and extubation, 456–458
    Bailey maneuver, 456–458
   assessment of airway, 453–456
    developing a strategy for, 454–455
    supraglottic airway tips for success, 455–456
    videolaryngoscopy tips for success, 456
   emergency equipment, 458–460
   lessons learned from recent studies, 446–453
    ASA Difficult Airway Algorithm, 2013 update, 448–449, 450
    Fourth National Audit Project of United Kingdom, 446–448
    on failure of supraglottic airway, 449
    on videolaryngoscope, glottic view *vs.* successful intubation, 449–452
Ambulatory anesthesia, 309–586
   accreditation of ambulatory facilities, **551–557**
   acute pain management, **495–504**
   airway management, **445–461**
   anesthesia information management systems, **559–576**
   for cardiac catheterization and electrophysiology laboratories, **381–386**
   for chronic pain-relieving procedures, **395–409**
   for diagnostic and therapeutic radiology procedures, **371–380**
   for gastrointestinal endoscopy suite, **387–394**
   Initial results from National Anesthesia Outcomes Registry on, **431–444**
   legal aspects of, **541–549**
   neuraxial anesthesia for, **357–369**
   new medications and techniques in, **463–485**
   pediatric, **411–429**
   perioperative evaluation and management, 309–339
    of cardiac disease, **309–320**
    of diabetes medications, **329–339**
    of obstructive sleep apnea, **321–328**
   peripheral nerve blocks for, **341–355**
   postoperative issues, **487–493**

Anesthesiology Clin 32 (2014) 587–598
http://dx.doi.org/10.1016/S1932-2275(14)00046-9
1932-2275/14/$ – see front matter © 2014 Elsevier Inc. All rights reserved.

Ambulatory (*continued*)
    practice management and role of medical director, **529–540**
    quality management and registries, **577–586**
        data to collect, 581–583
        external resources, 580–581
        how to use the data, 583–585
        importance of, 577–580
    scheduling of procedures and staff, **517–527**
    serotonin antagonist and NK-1 receptor antagonists, **505–516**
Ambulatory surgery centers, accreditation of, **551–557**
    accrediting organizations, 552–553
    deemed status, 553–554
    quality reporting and outcomes, 555–556
    regulation by states, 554–555
Ambulatory surgery centers. *See also* Ambulatory anesthesia.
    role of the medical director, **529–540**
        care pathway development, 536
        history and development of role, 530–531
        management by outcomes and process improvement, 531–536
    scheduling of procedures and staff, **517–527**
        categories of OR delays, 524–526
        prediction of procedure duration, 522–524
        systems for, 518–522
        using utilization to assign OR time, 522
American Society of Anesthesiologists (ASA), Difficult Airway Algorithm, 2013 revision, 448–449, 450
    practice guidelines for acute perioperative pain management, 496
Analgesia. *See* Pain management.
Anesthesia information management systems (AIMS), in ambulatory settings, **559–576**
        benefits of, 560–569
            automatic transfer of vital signs, 561–562
            compliance, 565
            decision support, 563–564
            icons communicate patient status, 566–567
            integration with electronic health record, 563
            legibility, 562
            medical record review, 560–561
            menus, 564–565
            organization of information, 561
            registries, 567–568
            support links, 561
        challenges of, 569–574
            alerts after the fact, 570
            cost, 571–573
            device integration, 569–570
            medicolegal concerns, 573
            report management, 569
            support and downtimes, 570
            workstation reliability and availability, 571
        future of, 574
            access and portability in health information exchange, 574

mobile technology, 574

standardization, 574

wireless monitoring and integration, 574

Anesthesia Quality Institute, data analysis on NACOR from, 437–441

recommendations for data to support ambulatory anesthesia quality management, 582–583

Anesthetics, local, neuraxial anesthesia for ambulatory surgery with, **357–369**

Anxiolysis, nonpharmacological preoperative, in pediatric ambulatory surgery, 416, 418

audiovisual material and games, 418

clowns and magicians, 416, 418

humor and verbal methods, 418

Aortic stenosis, evaluation of in ambulatory surgery setting, 313–314

Aortic valve replacement, transcatheter, in ambulatory setting, 384

Apnea risk, in infants presenting for ambulatory surgery, 413–414

Apnea. *See* Obstructive sleep apnea.

Aprepitant, efficacy of NK-1 receptor antagonists for PDNV, 508–509, 511–512

Axillary block, for ambulatory surgery, 348

B

Benzodiazepine receptor agonists, new, for ambulatory anesthesia, 469–470

Bupivacaine, new formulation for ambulatory anesthesia, 476–477

C

Cardiac catheterization laboratory, ambulatory anesthesia for, **381–386**

general strategies for, 382

higher risk procedures in, 382–384

complex catheter ablation, 382–383

lead extractions for cardiovascular implantable electronic devices, 383–384

transcatheter aortic valve replacement, 384

multidisciplinary approach to consultation, 381–382

radiation safety, 384–385

Cardiac disease, perioperative evaluation and management in ambulatory surgery setting, **309–320**

aortic stenosis, 313–314

cardiovascular implantable electronic devices, 312–313

coronary artery disease, 310–311

coronary stents, 312

functional capacity, 310

heart failure, 311–312

hypertension, 310

in the near future, 318

medical management, 315

preoperative testing, 315

prophylaxis for infective endocarditis, 315–316

prosthetic heart valves, 314–315

stepwise practical approach for, 316–318

Cardiac risk, in children presenting for ambulatory surgery, 414

Cardiovascular implantable electronic devices, evaluation of in ambulatory surgery setting, 312–313

lead extraction for, in the ambulatory setting, 383–384

Casopitant, efficacy of NK-1 receptor antagonists for PDNV, 508–509, 511–512
Catheter ablation, complex, in the ambulatory setting, 382–383
Children. *See* Pediatric ambulatory anesthesia.
Chronic pain. *See* Pain management.
Circumcision, pain management for outpatients, 420
Colonoscopy. *See* Gastrointestinal endoscopy.
Compliance, improvement of, with AIMS, 565
Contracts, in management of ambulatory surgery centers, 546
Contrast media, for ambulatory diagnostic and therapeutic radiology procedures, 372–373
Coronary artery disease, evaluation of in ambulatory surgery setting, 310–311
Coronary stents, evaluation of in ambulatory surgery setting, 312

D

Decision support, with AIMS, 563–564
Diabetic patients, management of medications for ambulatory surgery, **329–339**
    anesthesia care, 336–337
        abnormal blood glucose values, 337
        glucose measurement, 337
        postoperative care, 337
    hypoglycemia, 330–332
    preoperative, 332–336
        insulin dosing, 332–335
        oral medications, 335–336
    preoperative inquiries, 329–330
        insulin, 330
        insulin pumps, 330
        medications for type 2, 329–330
    significance of diabetes in, 332
        evidence for glycemic control, 332
        glycemic disturbances, 332
Difficult Airway Algorithm, 2013 revision, from ASA, 448–449, 450
Discharge criteria, after ambulatory surgery, **487–493**
    after regional anesthesia, 489–491
    fast tracking, 488–489
    postanesthetic recovery, 487–488
    postdischarge instructions, 491–493
    scoring system, 488

E

Electronic health records (EHR). *See* Anesthesia information management systems (AIMS).
Electrophysiology laboratory, ambulatory anesthesia for, **381–386**
    general strategies for, 382
    higher risk procedures in, 382–384
        complex catheter ablation, 382–383
        lead extractions for cardiovascular implantable electronic devices, 383–384
        transcatheter aortic valve replacement, 384
    multidisciplinary approach to consultation, 381–382
    radiation safety, 384–385
Endocarditis, infective, prophylaxis for in ambulatory surgery setting, 315–316

Endoscopy
    gastrointestinal, anesthesia in the ambulatory setting for, **387–394**
        anesthesia techniques for, 389–392
        increasing role for anesthesia in GI endoscopy suite, 392–393
        patients, 388
        postanesthesia care, 392
        preanesthesia preparation for, 390
        procedures, 388–389
Epidural anesthesia, for ambulatory surgery, 360–364
Esophagogastroduodenoscopy. See Gastrointestinal endoscopy.
Etomidate derivatives, new, for ambulatory anesthesia, 470–472
EXPAREL, new, for ambulatory anesthesia, 476–477

F

Fast tracking, for discharge after ambulatory surgery, 488–489
Femoral nerve block, for ambulatory surgery, 349
Functional capacity, evaluation of in ambulatory surgery setting, 310

G

Gantacurium, in ambulatory anesthesia, 473
Gastrointestinal endoscopy
    anesthesia in the ambulatory setting for, **387–394**
        anesthesia techniques for, 389–392
        increasing role for anesthesia in GI endoscopy suite, 392–393
        patients, 388
        postanesthesia care, 392
        preanesthesia preparation for, 390
        procedures, 388–389
Glucose measurement, in diabetic patients during ambulatory surgery, 337

H

Heart failure, evaluation of in ambulatory surgery setting, 311–312
Heart valves, prosthetic, evaluation of in ambulatory surgery setting, 314–315
Hyperkalemic cardiac arrest, in pediatric ambulatory surgery, 415–416
Hypertension, evaluation of in ambulatory surgery setting, 310
Hypoglycemia, in diabetics, 330
        during ambulatory surgery, 332, 337
Hypotonia, undiagnosed, in children presenting for ambulatory surgery, 415–416, 417
        hyperkalemic cardiac arrest, 415–416
        malignant hyperthermia, 415
        propofol infusion syndrome, 416

I

Implantable cardioverter defibrillators, evaluation of in ambulatory surgery setting, 312–313
Infective endocarditis, prophylaxis for in ambulatory surgery setting, 315–316
Informatics. See Anesthesia information management systems (AIMS).
Information management systems. See Anesthesia information management systems (AIMS).

Informed consent, professional liability issues with ambulatory anesthesia, 542–543
Infraclavicular block, for ambulatory surgery, 346–348
Insulin, management of in diabetic patients undergoing ambulatory surgery, **329–339**
    dosing before and during, 332–335
    preoperative inquiries, 330
Interscalene block, for ambulatory surgery, 344–346
Interventional pain-relieving procedures, 396–402
  complications related to anesthetic techniques in, 402–407
  history of, 395–396
Interventional radiology, for ambulatory procedures, 375–379
    anesthetic considerations, 376–377
    monitoring and equipment, 377
    postprocedure care, 379
    procedures, 377–378
    radiation safety, 375–376

K

Kappa-opioid agonists, new, in ambulatory anesthesia, 474–475

L

Legal aspects, of ambulatory anesthesia, **541–549**
    ownership-related issues, 546–548
      Federal anti-kickback statute restrictions, 546–547
      Stark law considerations, 547–548
      state law requirements, 548
    practice-related issues, 541–546
      contracts, 546
      informed consent, 542–543
      patient selection, 542
      professional liability, 541–543
      regulatory considerations, 543–546
Liability, professional, with ambulatory anesthesia, 541–542
Local anesthetics, neuraxial anesthesia for ambulatory surgery with, **357–369**
  new, for ambulatory anesthesia, 476–477
Lower extremity peripheral nerve blocks, for ambulatory surgery, 348–350
    femoral, 349
    sciatic, 349–350

M

Magnetic resonance imaging (MRI), ambulatory procedures using, 372–375
    anesthetic considerations, 372–375
    magnet safety, 372
Malignant hyperthermia, in pediatric ambulatory surgery, 415
Management. See Practice management.
Medical director, role in ambulatory surgery centers, **529–540**
    care pathway development, 536
    history and development of role, 530–531
    management by outcomes and process improvement, 531–536

Medical records, electronic. *See* Anesthesia information management systems (AIMS).

Medications, for diabetes, management in patients undergoing ambulatory surgery, **329–339**

for PDNV, **505–516**

long-acting serotonin antagonist (palonosteron), 508, 509–511

NK-1 receptor antagonists, 508–509, 511–512

new, in ambulatory anesthesia, **463–485**

novel analgesics and analgesic delivery systems, 473–479

kappa-opioid agonists, 474–475

local anesthetics, 475–479

novel neuromuscular blocking/reversal agents, 472–473

gantacurium, 473

sugammadex, 473

novel sedative-hypnotics and delivery systems, 464–472

alternate propofol emulsion formulations, 464–466

benzodiazepine receptor agonists, 469–470

etomidate derivatives, 470–472

melatonin, 472

nonemulsion propofol formulations, 466–467

propofol formulations, 464

propofol prodrugs, 467–469

remifentanil, intubation with, in pediatric ambulatory surgery patients, 416, 417

Melatonin, in ambulatory anesthesia, 472

Multimodal analgesia, perioperative, in ambulatory surgery setting, **495–504**

ASA practice guidelines for management of, 496

implementation of, 497–500

nonpharmacologic techniques, 500

pharmacotherapy and, 499–500

recovery room rescue, 500

regional anesthesia and, 497–499

risk stratification and preprocedural planning, 497

N

National Anesthesia Clinical Outcomes Registry (NACOR), and quality management for ambulatory anesthesia, 580–581

initial results from, **431–444**

administrative and safety issues, 432–437

accreditation, 434–435

facility, patient, and procedure selection, 435–437

literature review, 432–434

data analysis from Anesthesia Quality Institute, 437–441

future directions for office-based anesthesia, 442

Nausea, postoperative. *See* Postdischarge nausea and vomiting (PDNV).

Nerve blocks, peripheral, for ambulatory surgery, **341–355**

lower extremity, 348–350

femoral, 349

sciatic, 349–350

upper extremity, 344–348

axillary, 348

infraclavicular, 346–348

Nerve (*continued*)
        interscalene, 344–346
        supraclavicular, 346
Neuraxial anesthesia, for ambulatory surgery, **357–369**
      epidural anesthesia, 360–364
      selection of agents, 357–360, 364
      side effects, 365–367
Neuromuscular blockade, intubation without, in pediatric ambulatory surgery patients,
    416, 417
Neuromuscular blocking/reversal agents, new, in ambulatory anesthesia, 472–473
      gantacurium, 473
      sugammadex, 473
NK-1 receptor antagonists, long-acting, for PDNV, **505–516**

    O

Obstructive sleep apnea, in children presenting for ambulatory tonsillectomy for, 414
    perioperative consideration of, in ambulatory surgery, **321–328**
      diagnostic criteria, 322
      outcome of patients with, 324
      perioperative care of patients with, 324–325
      perioperative screening methods for, 322
      postoperative disposition and unplanned admission after, 325–326
      preoperative evaluation of patient with suspected or diagnosed, 322–324
      risk factors and pathophysiology, 322
Office-based surgery. *See* Ambulatory surgery.
Operating room (OR) allocation, scheduling staff and procedures in ambulatory surgery
    centers, **517–527**
Opioid agonists, new kappa-, in ambulatory anesthesia, 474–475
Outcomes, initial results from National Anesthesia Clinical Outcomes Registry, **431–444**
    management of ambulatory surgery center by process improvement and, 531–536
Outpatient surgery. *See* Ambulatory surgery.
Ownership, of ambulatory surgery center, legal issue related to, 546–548
      Federal anti-kickback statute restrictions, 546–547
      Stark law considerations, 547–548
      state law requirements, 548

    P

Pacemakers, evaluation of in ambulatory surgery setting, 312–313
Pain management, acetaminophen rectal dosing for pediatric ambulatory surgical patients,
    420–422
    acute postoperative, in ambulatory surgery setting, **495–504**
      ASA practice guidelines for management of, 496
      implementation of multimodal analgesia, 497–500
        nonpharmacologic techniques, 500
        pharmacotherapy and, 499–500
        recovery room rescue, 500
        regional anesthesia and, 497–499
      risk stratification and preprocedural planning, 497
    chronic pain, anesthesia for in ambulatory settings, **395–409**

interventional pain-relieving procedures, 396–402
    complications related to anesthetic techniques in, 402–407
    history of, 395–396
for circumcision in ambulatory setting, 420
Palonosetron, efficacy for PDNV, **505–516**
Pediatric ambulatory anesthesia, **411–429**
    intraoperative management, 418–422
        acetaminophen, rectal dosing, 420–422
        intubation with remifentanil, 418–419
        pain management for circumcision, 420
    patient selection, 412–416
        apnea risk in infants, 413–414
        cardiac risk, 414
        preoperative pregnancy testing, 416, 417
        sleep apnea and tonsillectomy, 414
        undiagnosed weakness or hypotonia, 415–416, 417
            hyperkalemic cardiac arrest, 415–416
            malignant hyperthermia, 415
            propofol infusion syndrome, 416
        upper respiratory infection, 412–413
    preoperative management, 416–418
        nonpharmacological anxiolysis, 416, 418
            audiovisual material and games, 418
            clowns and magicians, 416, 418
            humor and verbal methods, 418
Peripheral nerve blocks, for ambulatory surgery, **341–355**
    lower extremity, 348–350
        femoral, 349
        sciatic, 349–350
    upper extremity, 344–348
        axillary, 348
        infraclavicular, 346–348
        interscalene, 344–346
        supraclavicular, 346
Pharmacotherapy, and multimodal analgesia for perioperative pain, 499–500
Postdischarge nausea and vomiting (PDNV), after ambulatory surgery, **505–516**
    pharmacologic intervention, 506–512
        aprepitant, casopitant, rolapitant, 508–509, 511–512
        palonesetron, 508, 509–511
    risk factor identification, 506
Postoperative issues, in ambulatory anesthesia, **487–493**
    discharge after regional anesthesia, 489–491
    discharge scoring system, 488
    fast tracking, 488–489
    postanesthetic recovery, 487–488
    postdischarge instructions, 491–493
Practice management, accreditation of ambulatory facilities, **551–557**
    accrediting organizations, 552–553
    deemed status, 553–554
    quality reporting and outcomes, 555–556
    regulation by states, 554–555

Practice (*continued*)
  in ambulatory surgery centers, **517–527, 529–540**
    role of the medical director, **529–540**
      care pathway development, 536
      history and development of role, 530–531
      management by outcomes and process improvement, 531–536
    scheduling of procedures and staff, **517–527**
      categories of OR delays, 524–526
      prediction of procedure duration, 522–524
      systems for, 518–522
      using utilization to assign OR time, 522
  legal aspects of ambulatory anesthesia, **541–549**
    ownership-related issues, 546–548
      Federal anti-kickback statute restrictions, 546–547
      Stark law considerations, 547–548
      state law requirements, 548
    practice-related issues, 541–546
      contracts, 546
      informed consent, 542–543
      patient selection, 542
      professional liability, 541–543
      regulatory considerations, 543–546
Pregnancy testing, preoperative, in adolescent ambulatory surgery patients, 416, 417
Preoperative evaluation, of cardiac disease in ambulatory surgery setting, **309–320**
  of diabetes medications, **329–339**
Prophylaxis, for infective endocarditis in ambulatory surgery setting, 315–316
Propofol, novel formulations for ambulatory anesthesia, 464–469
      alternate emulsion formulation, 464–466
      nonemulsion formulation, 466–467
      prodrugs, 467–469
Propofol infusion syndrome, in pediatric ambulatory surgery, 416
Prosthetic heart valves, evaluation of in ambulatory surgery setting, 314–315

Q

Quality improvement, reporting for accreditation of ambulatory facilities, 555–556
Quality management, and registries in ambulatory anesthesia, **577–586**
      data to collect, 581–583
      external resources, 580–581
      how to use the data, 583–585
      importance of, 577–580
  care pathway development in ambulatory surgery centers, 536

R

Radiation safety, in the cardiac catheterization and electrophysiology laboratories, 384–385
Radiology, anesthesia for ambulatory diagnostic and therapeutic procedures, **371–380**
      chemotoxic effects of intravascular contrast media, 372–373
      interventional, 375–379
        anesthetic considerations, 376–377

monitoring and equipment, 377
postprocedure care, 379
procedures, 377–378
radiation safety, 375–376
magnetic resonance imaging (MRI), 372–375
anesthetic considerations, 372–375
magnet safety, 372
other contrast media, 372
Regional anesthesia, and multimodal analgesia for perioperative pain, 497–499
discharge after ambulatory surgery with, 489–491
Registries, and anesthesia information management systems, 567
and quality management in ambulatory anesthesia, **577–586**
data to collect, 581–583
external resources, 580–581
how to use the data, 583–585
importance of, 577–580
Regulatory considerations, in ambulatory surgery settings, 543–546
for accreditation, **551–557**
Remifentanil
intubation with, in pediatric ambulatory surgery patients, 416, 417
Respiratory infection, upper, in children presenting for ambulatory surgery, 412–413
Rolapitant, efficacy of NK-1 receptor antagonists for PDNV, 508–509, 511–512

S

Safety issues, in office-based surgery, 432–437
Scheduling, of procedures and staff in ambulatory surgery center, **517–527**
categories of OR delays, 524–526
prediction of procedure duration, 522–524
systems for, 518–522
using utilization to assign OR time, 522
Sciatic nerve block, for ambulatory surgery, 349–350
SEDASYS system, for propofol anesthesia, 468–469
Sedative-hypnotics, novel medications and delivery systems, 464–472
alternate propofol emulsion formulations, 464–466
benzodiazepine receptor agonists, 469–470
etomidate derivatives, 470–472
melatonin, 472
nonemulsion propofol formulations, 466–467
propofol formulations, 464
propofol prodrugs, 467–469
Serotonin antagonist, long-acting, for PDNV, **505–516**
Sleep apnea. *See* Obstructive sleep apnea.
Society for Ambulatory Anesthesia, Clinical Outcomes Registry created by, 581–582
Spinal anesthesia, for ambulatory surgery, **357–369**
epidural anesthesia, 360–364
selection of agents, 357–360, 364
side effects, 365–367
Staffing issues, scheduling staff in ambulatory surgery centers, **517–527**
Sugammadex, new, in ambulatory anesthesia, 473
Supraclavicular block, for ambulatory surgery, 346

Supraglottic airway, in airway management, **445–461**
    failure of, 449
    tips for success, 455–456

T

Tonsillectomy, obstructive sleep apnea in children presenting for ambulatory, 414

U

Upper extremity peripheral nerve blocks, for ambulatory surgery, 344–348
    axillary, 348
    infraclavicular, 346–348
    interscalene, 344–346
    supraclavicular, 346
Upper respiratory infection, in children presenting for ambulatory surgery, 412–413

V

Videolaryngoscopes, in airway management, **445–461**
    glottic view *versus* successful intubation, 449–452
    tips for success, 456
Vomiting, postoperative. *See* Postdischarge nausea and vomiting (PDNV).

Moving?

Make sure your subscription moves with you!

To notify us of your new address, find your **Clinics Account Number** (located on your mailing label above your name), and contact customer service at:

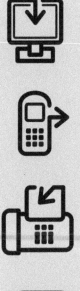

Email: journalscustomerservice-usa@elsevier.com

800-654-2452 (subscribers in the U.S. & Canada)
314-447-8871 (subscribers outside of the U.S. & Canada)

Fax number: 314-447-8029

Elsevier Health Sciences Division
Subscription Customer Service
3251 Riverport Lane
Maryland Heights, MO 63043

*To ensure uninterrupted delivery of your subscription, please notify us at least 4 weeks in advance of move.

Printed and bound by CPI Group (UK) Ltd, Croydon, CR0 4YY

03/10/2024

01040486-0013